With compliments of
Merck Serono, a division of
Merck KGaA, Darmstadt, Germany

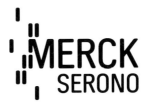

The Thyroid and Reproduction

Merck
European Thyroid Symposium

Riga 2008, May 22–25

Chairpersons

John Lazarus
Valdis Pirags

Edited by

John Lazarus
Valdis Pirags
Sigrid Butz

28 figures
26 tables

Georg Thieme Verlag
Stuttgart · New York

John H. Lazarus
Centre for Endocrine and Diabetes Sciences
Cardiff University, University Hospital of Wales
Heath Park, Cardiff CF14 4XN
United Kingdom

Valdis Pirags
Pauls Stradins Clinical University Hospital
Pilsonu iela 13
Riga LV1002
Latvia

Sigrid Butz
Merck Serono, a divison of Merck KGaA
Frankfurter Straße 250
64293 Darmstadt
Germany

Bibliographic Information published by
Die Deutsche Nationalbibliothek

Die Deutsche Nationalbibliothek lists this
publication in the Deutsche Nationalbibliografie;
detailled bibliographic data are available on
the internet at http://dnb.d-nb.de.

This publication has been sponsored by Merck KGaA.

© 2009 Georg Thieme Verlag KG
Rüdigerstraße 14
70469 Stuttgart, Germany
http://www.thieme.de
Thieme New York, 333 Seventh Avenue
New York, NY 10001, USA
http://www.thieme.com

Printed in Germany

Cover design by Thieme Verlagsgruppe
Figures by Ziegler + Müller, Kirchentellinsfurt
Typesetting by Ziegler + Müller, Kirchentellinsfurt
Printing and Bookbinding by Grafisches Centrum
Cuno, Calbe

ISBN 978-3-13-146721-8 (TPS)

1 2 3 4 5 6

Important Note: Medicine is an ever-changing science undergoing continual development. Research and clinical experience are continually expanding our knowledge, in particular our knowledge of proper treatment and drug therapy. Insofar as this book mentions any dosage or application, readers may rest assured that the authors, editors, and publishers have made every effort to ensure that such references are in accordance with **the state of knowledge at the time of production of the book.**

Nevertheless, this does not involve, imply, or express any guarantee or responsibility on the part of the publishers in respect to any dosage instructions and forms of applications stated in the book. **Every user is requested to examine carefully** the manufacturers' leaflets accompanying each drug and to check, if necessary in consultation with a physician or specialist, whether the dosage schedules mentioned therein or the contraindications stated by the manufacturers differ from the statements made in the present book. Such examination is particularly important with drugs that are either rarely used or have been newly released on the market. Every dosage schedule or every form of application used is entirely at the user's own risk and responsibility. The authors and publishers request every user to report to the publishers any discrepancies or inaccuracies noticed.

Preface

Abnormalities of thyroid function in pregnancy are now known to be quite frequent with potential adverse effects on the foetus and neonate. This volume reports the proceedings of a meeting devoted to thyroid and pregnancy sponsored by Merck Serono. The conference is one of a series of Merck European Thyroid Symposia (METS), which take place every 2 years. We have been fortunate on this occasion to have the input of experts in the field of infertility and assisted reproduction to introduce the meeting.

We were all impressed with the advances in these fields and the optimism for future developments. The rest of the programme explored the current status of aspects of thyroid function and disease in pregnancy and postpartum. There is a wealth of new data, which have appeared during the last decade and we are extremely grateful to our speakers for sharing these findings with us in Riga.

We would like to thank Dr. Sigrid Butz and her colleagues at Merck Serono for organising such an excellent educational event and hope that this volume will serve as an important publication in the field.

John Lazarus, Cardiff, UK
Valdis Pirags, Riga, Latvia

Corresponding Contributors

Marcos Abalovich
Sarmiento 2012, 2° A (CP 1044), Buenos Aires, Argentina
e-mail: mabalovich@intramed.net

Fereidoun Azizi
Endocrine Research Centre, Research Institute
for Endocrine Sciences, Shaheed Beheshti University
of Medical Sciences, P.O. Box 19395-4763, Tehran, I.R.
Iran
e-mail: azizi@endocrine.ac.ir

Jacky Boivin
School of Psychology, Cardiff University, Psychology
Building, Cardiff CF10 3 AT, Wales, U.K.
e-mail: Boivin@cardiff.ac.uk

Ulla Feldt-Rasmussen
Department of Medical Endocrinology, Rigshospitalet,
National University Hospital, Blegdamsvej 9,
DK-2100 Copenhagen, Denmark
e-mail: ufeldt@rh.dk

Natalie Fokina
Endocrinology Department, Pauls Stradiņš Clinical
University Hospital, Pilsoņu iela 13, LV-1002 Riga, Latvia
e-mail: nfokina@inbox.lv

Simona Gaberscek
University Medical Centre Ljubljana, Department of
Nuclear Medicine, Zaloska 7, 1525 Ljubljana, Slovenia
e-mail: simona.gaberscek@kclj.si

Una Gailisa
Paula Stradina Clinical University Hospital
Children's University Hospital, Pilsoņu iela 13,
LV-1002 Riga, Latvia
e-mail: unagailisa@inbox.lv

Daniel Glinoer
University Hospital Saint Pierre, Division of Endocrinology, 322 rue Haute, B-1000 Brussels, Belgium
e-mail: dglinoer@ulb.ac.be

Peter Laurberg
Department of Endocrinology and Medicine, Aalborg
Hospital, Aarhus University Hospital, DK-9000 Aalborg,
Denmark
e-mail: peter.laurberg@rn.dk

Stefan Karger
Department of Internal Medicine III, University of
Leipzig, Ph.-Rosenthal-Str. 27, D-04103 Leipzig,
Germany
e-mail: Stefan.Karger@medizin.uni-leipzig.de

Mark D. Kilby
Division of Reproduction and Child Health, Birmingham
Women's Foundation Trust, University of Birmingham,
Edgbaston, Birmingham B15 2TG, U.K.
e-mail: m.d.kilby@bham.ac.uk

Gerasimos E. Krassas
Department of Endocrinology, Diabetes and Metabolism, Panagia General Hospital, N. Plastira 22,
551 32 Thessaloniki, Greece
e-mail: krassas@the.forthnet.gr

Ieva Lase
Department of Endocrinology, Pauls Stradiņš Clinical
University Hospital, Pilsoņu iela 13, LV-1002 Riga, Latvia
e-mail: ievalase@gmail.com

John H. Lazarus
Centre for Endocrine and Diabetes Sciences,
Cardiff University, University Hospital of Wales,
Heath Park, Cardiff CF14 4XN, U.K.
e-mail Lazarus@cf.ac.uk

Edward Limbert
Portuguese Cancer Institute, R. Professor Lima Basto,
1099-023 Lisboa, Portugal
e-mail: elimbert@ipolisboa.min-saude.pt

Paolo Emidio Macchia
Dipartimento di Endocrinologia ed Oncologia Molecolare e Clinica, Università degli Studi di Napoli Federico II,
Via S. Pansini 5, 80131, Napoli Italy
e-mail: pmacchia@unina.it

Nick S. Macklon
Department of Reproductive Medicine and Gynaecology, University Medical Center Utrecht, Heidelberglaan
100, 3584 CX Utrecht, The Netherlands
e-mail: N.S.Macklon@umcutrecht.nl

Mara Marga
Institute of Experimental and Clinical Medicine, University of Latvia, 4 Ojara Vaciesa str., Riga, LV-1004, Latvia
e-mail: mara_marga@dr.lv

Bryan McIver
Mayo Clinic and Foundation, Rochester, Minnesota
55905, U.S.A.
e-mail: mciver.bryan@mayo.edu

Svetlana Miceva Ristevska
Institute of Pathophysiology & Nuclear Medicine,
Vodnjanska 17, Skopje, Republic of Macedonia
e-mail: svetlana.miceva.ristevska@gmail.com

Roberto Negro
Department of Endocrinology, "V. Fazzi" Hospital,
Piazza F. Muratore, 73 100 Lecce, Italy
e-mail: robnegro@tiscali.it

Valdis Pirags
Pauls Stradiņš Clinical University Hospital,
Pilsoņu iela 13, LV-1002 Riga, Latvia
e-mail: pirags@latnet.lv

Kris Poppe
Department of Endocrinology, Universitair Ziekenhuis
Brussel, Free University Brussels (VUB), Laarbeeklaan
101, B-1090 Brussels, Belgium
e-mail: kris.poppe@uzbrussel.be

Ludvik Puklavec
University Hospital Maribor, Department for Nuclear
Medicine, Ljubljanska 5, 2000 Maribor, Slovenia
e-mail: ludvik.puklavec@sb-mb.si

Peter Smyth, UCD Conway Institute of Biomolecular and
Biomedical Research, School of Medicine and Medical
Science, University College Dublin, Ireland
e-mail:peter.smyth@ucd.ie

André Van Steirteghem
Centre for Reproductive Medicine, UZ Brussel,
Laarbeeklaan 101, B-1090 Brussels, Belgium
e-mail: Andre.VanSteirteghem@uzbrussel.be

Mark Vanderpump
Department of Endocrinology, Royal Free Hampstead
NHS Trust, London NW3 2QG, U.K.
e-mail: mark.vanderpump@royalfree.nhs.uk

Contents

Special Lecture

The History of Assisted Reproduction

30 Years of IVF: The Legacy of Patrick Steptoe and Robert Edwards

P. R. Brinsden

Bourn Hall Clinic, Cambridge, United Kingdom

In this chapter the early history of in vitro fertilisation (IVF) will be reviewed from the perspective of Patrick Steptoe and Robert Edwards, who together "created" the World's first "test tube" baby, Louise Brown. In 2008, we are celebrating the 30th anniversary of this momentous event and also the 20th anniversary of the death of Patrick Steptoe. An understanding and knowledge of the early history of IVF is important to our understanding of the practice of IVF in the present day. Although others had been involved in the early development of animal and, later, human IVF, it was through the determination and dedication of Steptoe and Edwards, together with their colleague Jean Purdy, to achieve the birth of the first baby. This was some two years before other specialists in Australia, and later still the United States, achieved their first births. The story of the Steptoe and Edwards collaboration, their early years of disappointment and failure, culminating in their eventual success with the birth of Louise Brown is a fascinating story. Their influence on today's practice of the assisted reproductive technologies (ART) and even on our future practice is still relevant.

Patrick Steptoe was born in 1913, the seventh of a family of ten children. He qualified as a doctor from St George's Hospital in London and served in the Royal Navy in the Second World War, between 1939 and 1946, during which time he was a prisoner of war for two years in Italy. On returning to the United Kingdom he specialised in obstetrics and gynaecology, with a special interest in infertility, and in 1951 finally achieved a consultant post at Oldham General Hospital, in the North of England. There he had a large National Health Service (NHS) practice and it was there that he pursued and developed his interest in laparoscopy. He had learned the technique from Frangenheim and Palmer in Europe and he further developed the technique, finally publishing the seminal textbook "Laparoscopy in Gynaecology" in 1967. During the early years of laparoscopy in the United Kingdom, this was the "bible", from which all young gynaecologists learned the technique of laparoscopy.

It was because of his ability to visualise the female pelvic organs during laparoscopy that he wrote his first major paper on "Laparoscopy and ovulation", published in The Lancet in 1967. He also discovered that it was possible to aspirate oocytes from follicles laparoscopically.

Robert Edwards was a young scientist working at Cambridge University in the 1960s. He had previously achieved a BSc in Cardiff in Wales and a PhD in Edinburgh. It was during a period of time he spent in London that he became interested in human oocyte development and the possibility of achieving *in vitro* fertilisation of human gametes. Edwards contacted Steptoe in 1968 with a view to collaborating, and they first met at the Royal Society of Medicine in London, where Patrick Steptoe was giving a lecture on laparoscopy, in which he showed the first laparoscopic photographs of ovaries in the female pelvis. Edwards approached Steptoe at the end of this meeting and introduced himself and suggested that they should collaborate; this suggestion was readily accepted by Steptoe.

From 1968 Steptoe and Edwards' early work was done in Dr Kershaw's cottage hospital at Royton, near Oldham, in the North of England. They

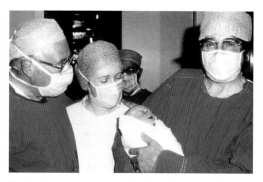

Fig. 1   Steptoe, Purdy and Edwards at the birth of Louise Brown 25 July 1978.

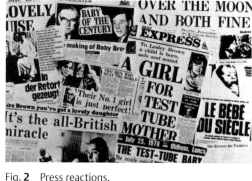

Fig. 2   Press reactions.

very soon started to produce important papers on early IVF, including: "Identification of the midpiece and tail of the spermatozoon during fertilisation of human eggs in vitro" (Journal of Reproduction and Fertility 1969), and "Laparoscopic recovery of pre-ovulatory human oocytes after priming of ovaries with gonadotrophins" (The Lancet 1970). They also carried out the first treatment cycles of oocyte recovery with tubal insemination (ORTI), which was much later developed by others, becoming known as gamete intra-fallopian transfer (GIFT). Other important papers included: "Control of human ovulation, fertilisation and implantation" (Proceedings of the Royal Society of Medicine, 1974) and "Induction of follicular growth, ovulation and luteinisation of the human ovary" (Journal of Reproduction and Fertility, 1975), and also "Normal and abnormal follicular growth in mouse, rat and human ovaries" (Journal of Reproduction and Fertility, 1977). All of these papers and others were produced during a time of intense activity in Oldham, with Edwards and Jean Purdy travelling hundreds of miles from Cambridge to Oldham on a regular basis.

During these early years there was much controversy and criticism of their work, especially when they started their first human embryo transfers in 1972. Difficult years followed in which none of their first 40 patients became pregnant, but in 1976 they did achieve their first IVF pregnancy, but suffered huge disappointment when it was discovered that this was an ectopic pregnancy. It is of interest to note that this pregnancy was achieved through a single blastocyst transfer! Finally, Mrs Leslie Brown was referred to Steptoe for infertility treatment in 1976 and, following a total of 102 failed embryo transfers in their series of patients, including the one ectopic

pregnancy, Leslie Brown became pregnant. This was achieved in a natural cycle IVF with one oocyte collected, fertilised and transferred as an 8 cell embryo. Mrs Brown suffered a stormy pregnancy but Louise Brown was finally delivered by caesarean section on Tuesday 25 July 1978. Much to the relief of everyone, she was a normal, fit and healthy baby (Fig. 1). This momentous achievement was announced with a simple publication in a letter to The Lancet (Lancet 1978; 2: 366) but was reported throughout the World with major headlines (Fig. 2). The arrival of Louise was heralded as "The Baby of the Century". Indeed, the achievement of this birth has been equated in importance with other major World firsts, such as the discovery of penicillin.

Steptoe and Edwards experienced euphoria at that time but they also suffered from criticism from a number of quarters. The Vatican said that this was "an event which can have very grave consequences for humanity" and Dr James Watson, of the DNA helix discovery, is quoted as saying: "This was dabbling with infanticide". The Archbishop of Liverpool said that it was "morally wrong". In spite of all this criticism, when Steptoe and Edwards presented the results of their work later in 1978 at the Royal College of Obstetricians and Gynaecologists in London, they received a standing ovation, which had never occurred before in the whole history of the College. At the American Fertility Society meeting in 1978 they also received a standing ovation at the end of their presentation.

On the 4 January 1979 they achieved the birth of their second baby, Alastair Macdonald, who was the world's first boy conceived by IVF. During the 2 years that followed, no institution in the United Kingdom would provide any support or funding for Steptoe and Edwards to continue their

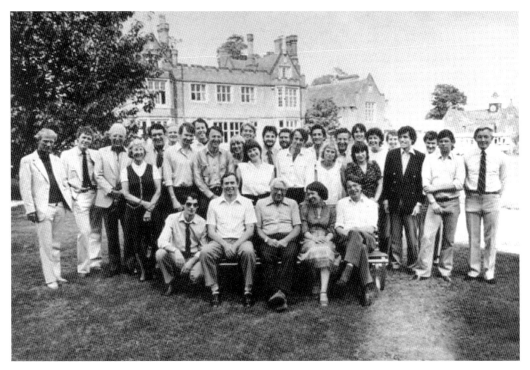

Fig. **3**   First World IVF Conference Bourn Hall 1982.

work. The NHS, the Universities and the Medical Research Council were all unwilling to help them to set up a clinic with Government funding, and so they were forced to set up a private clinic. This they did in Bourn, a village near to Cambridge, in a beautiful old manor house called Bourn Hall. Thus was started the world's first IVF clinic – Bourn Hall Clinic. Meanwhile, elsewhere work on human *in vitro* fertilisation was progressing and, in Melbourne, Australia, Candice Reed, the world's fourth test tube baby conceived through IVF was born as a result of the work of the team of Professor Carl Wood and Dr Alan Trounson; she was born in June 1980. The first child to be born in the United States as a result of IVF was, in fact, conceived in Bourn Hall, but the American pioneers Doctors Howard and Georgeanna Jones were successful in achieving the birth of Elizabeth Carr on 28 December 1981. Natalie Brown, a sister for Louise was born in 1982.

Bourn Hall Clinic opened its doors in September 1980. Steptoe and Edwards and their team continued their research, with a number of key publications including: "Current status of in vitro fertilisation and implantation of human embryos"

(The Lancet 1983), in which they reported the results of their first 1200 IVF cycles, and noted an increase in clinical pregnancy rates from 16.5% initially, to 30% by 1983.

In 1982 the world's first IVF conference was held at Bourn Hall Clinic, with many of the early pioneers of human IVF attending (Fig. **3**). A total of 30 clinicians and scientists took part in this very relaxed and informal exchange of information on the clinical and scientific aspects of human IVF.

By 1986, it was estimated that 2000 babies had been born worldwide, a 1000 of these were from Bourn Hall and the team at Bourn Hall Clinic published their observations on their first 500 births in Human Reproduction in 1986.

Patrick Steptoe and Robert Edwards were given a number of awards by the medical and scientific communities, and the Queen awarded them both the honour of a CBE. Of particular pride to Patrick Steptoe was his election to Fellowship of the Royal Society in 1988, an honour that has been afforded to very few clinicians in the past. It was unfortunate that, at the height of his achievements and fame, Patrick Steptoe fell ill with prostate cancer and finally died on 21 March 1988. Robert Edwards continued to work as Scientific Director at Bourn Hall and Editor of the journal "Human Reproduction" until 1994, when he left to start up a new journal "Reproductive Bio Medicine Online".

During the past 30 years of IVF there have been a number of major advances in the practice of IVF and the other assisted reproductive technologies (ARTs). Treatment is now available almost worldwide and many countries have introduced regulation of ART. The whole procedure of IVF with monitoring, stimulation, oocyte recovery and embryo transfer has been greatly simplified, with oocyte recovery now universally being carried out using the vaginal ultrasound technique, rather than the laparoscopic approach practiced by Steptoe 30 years ago.

Success rates have gradually increased, overall by about 1 percentage point per year over the last 30 years, brought about by advances and improvements in laboratory and clinical practices. We are now able to cryopreserve surplus embryos and, more recently, oocyte freezing has been increasingly practiced.

There have been changes in superovulation protocols over the years, from the earliest times when natural cycles were used through the use of clomiphene with urinary gonadotrophin. The recombinant gonadotrophins were developed in the 1990s and the use of gonadotrophin releasing hormone agonists, and now antagonists, are used almost universally in stimulation cycles.

In the early years of IVF practice, a large number of ethical concerns were perceived and addressed. Interestingly, Robert Edwards and David Sharpe addressed the issues as early as 1971 in a key paper titled: "Social values and research in human embryology" (Nature 1971; 231: 87–91). As a result of early concerns about a number of ethical issues, the United Kingdom Government commissioned a working party which subsequently reported in 1984, recommending that regulatory and licensing procedures be put in place for:

- All treatment involving the creation of human embryos outside the body
- All treatment involving donated gametes
- All storage of human gametes and embryos
- All research on human embryos

This was subsequently put into an Act of Parliament known as the "Human Fertilisation and Embryology Act 1990", and made the United Kingdom the first country to impose strict regulation of the practice of ART.

Over the years, a large number of ethical issues have been addressed, often by radically different approaches in different countries. The ability to select the sex of a child by sperm sorting was one of the early issues that was addressed in the UK and, following appropriate discussion and debate, is allowed for the prevention of inherited sex linked conditions, but not for social reasons. Other countries do allow sex selection for social reasons as well.

As the age of women starting their families has increased during the last 20 years, so has the age of women seeking help by ART, and the number of women over the age of 40 seeking treatment has increased greatly. Reports of women over the age of 50 having babies following ART and even over 60 have been recorded, for all of whom donor oocytes have been used. Single women are now able to have children using donor sperm and it is common for couples in same sex relationships to be helped to have children as well. Surrogacy has now become an accepted practice in a number of countries and has been successful in helping women with congenital or acquired absence of the uterus, recurrent miscarriage or repeated IVF failure to have their own genetic children with a help of a host surrogate.

Due to the imposition of severely restrictive regulation in some countries and relatively liberal regulation in others, more and more couples are now practising what has been termed "reproductive tourism". This is especially the case for women requiring egg donation, surrogacy or sex selection procedures. It is hoped that the introduction of pre-implantation genetic diagnosis (PGD) and aneuploidy screening (AS) will help to prevent the birth of children with severe genetic abnormalities and possibly to improve the chance of older women in particular, achieving pregnancies, without the increase in the incidence of having abnormal children that is expected with advanced age.

Accusations are made now that the technology is advancing too far and that "designer babies" will become common. Cloning also frequently appears as an issue in the media and success with animal cloning has shown that human cloning will soon be possible. This causes a great deal of concern to most workers in the field and to the general public. It is to be hoped that much more extensive research will be carried out before any attempts are made to clone humans. It is almost inevitable that it will happen sooner or later. Many countries have legislated to prevent cloning for reproductive purposes, but some, including the UK, have allowed the research to continue for therapeutic purposes.

The increased incidence of multiple pregnancies following ART has been a major complication and concern of ART practitioners for many years, with some 50% of all IVF births now being part of multiple births. Twin and high order multiple births are now considered to be a complication of IVF/ART and efforts are being made in many countries to reduce the incidence. There is move to pursuing single embryo transfer in selected patients and it has been shown that if 70% or more of women have single embryo transfer, the incidence of multiple pregnancy can be reduced to less than 10%.

One of the fundamental questions in ART today is "Why are we (ART practitioners) not better at what we do?" The fact remains that 50–70% or more of all couples fail at each attempt at IVF ART. Research on the factors affecting implantation of embryos is badly needed and methods of studying embryo culture media, the embryos themselves and the endometrium, by studying the genomic, proteomic and metabolomic profiles of these will hopefully in the future lead to much higher implantation and success rates.

Finally, the social implications of infertility throughout the world should not be underestimated. The effects on couples, both in developed and developing countries, are profound. The emotions experienced by infertile women, in particular, can be devastating. If the estimated 15% of couples wishing to conceive worldwide are unable to do so, the global problem becomes massive. The effects on women of the social changes that have occurred over the last two decades, in that women are waiting until later and later in their lives to start their families, also has profound implications. Women are now forced to decide between having a family or a career or struggling to achieve both at the same time. The consequent stresses that this places on women, their families and society should not be underestimated.

Looking to the future, it is likely that improved implantation rates will be achieved and single embryo transfer, probably at the blastocyst stage, will become the norm for the majority of patients. Embryo selection using techniques such as pre-implantation genetic diagnosis and aneuploidy screening will increasingly be used and factors affecting implantation determined by genomic and proteomic techniques will increasingly be practised. Cryopreservation of oocytes and ovarian tissue will become common, with *in vitro* maturation of primordial and immature oocytes.

Finally, in the year that we are celebrating the 30th anniversary of the birth of the World's first "test tube" baby, we should pay tribute to the early pioneers of IVF worldwide, but in particular, to Patrick Steptoe and Robert Edwards who, after ten years of research, failure and disappointment, finally achieved success. This early pioneering work has led to the development of thousands of IVF centres and estimates of between 4 and 8 million babies born worldwide as a result of this technology.

Session I

Aspects of Assisted Reproduction

Chairperson: J. Orgiazzi (Lyon)

1 Current Status of Assisted Reproductive Technology (ART) 30 Years after the First IVF Birth

A. Van Steirteghem

Centre for Reproductive Medicine, UZ Brussel, Laarbeeklaan 101, 1090 Brussels, Belgium

Abstract

Louise Brown, the first IVF baby, was born in Old-ham (UK) on 25 July 1978 which is 30 years ago. It is therefore appropriate to ask the following questions. (i) What have we achieved after almost three decades of clinical practice of ART? (ii) What are the challenges for the future? This chapter will include 1) an introduction to set the scene, 2) a summary of current achievements in applying conventional IVF and single sperm microinjection, including the outcome of these treatments as well as the combination of ART and genetic diagnosis on preimplantation embryos, i.e., preimplantation genetic diagnosis (PGD), and 3) two challenging items for the future, namely the prevention of the iatrogenic epidemic of multiple ART pregnancies and the derivation of embryonic stem cells from the inner cell mass of preimplantation embryos at the blastocyst stage.

1.1 Introduction

Infertility, in other words the impossibility of having children spontaneously after intercourse, is one of the most frequently occurring health problems for young adults during the most active period of their life. Unwilling childlessness is time-consuming, has a high cost and is a problem which concerns all social classes and all races.

Unwilling childlessness is a frequently occurring problem involving at least one of ten female patients aged 18 to 44 years. At least one out of four female patients in that age category has experienced difficulties in achieving spontaneous pregnancy. The male and female partners of these couples represent about 2% of the population in developed countries.

Epidemiological surveys at two different time periods (1960–1970 and 1980–1990) have indicated that the percentage of different aetiologies of infertility has remained quite constant over the years as well for unexplained infertility as female-factor and male-factor infertility (Fig. 1.1).

During the last fifty years a major milestone in reproductive medicine has occurred in each decade. In the 1960s reproductive endocrinology was at stake, especially because RIAs became available to measure reliably steroid and polypeptide hormones. In the 1970s surgery, and especially microsurgery, was applied in order to overcome tubal infertility. After the birth of Louise Brown on 25th July 1978 the introduction of *in vitro fertilisation and embryo transfer* was realised in many centres in the 1980s. IVF has been the standard procedure to overcome female-factor or idiopathic infertility. Conventional IVF was not successful to treat male-factor infertility. At the end of the 1980s several groups worked on assisted fertilisation procedures such as zona drilling, partial zona dissection and subzonal insemina-

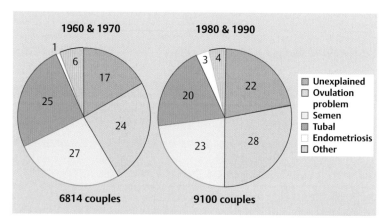

Fig. 1.**1**   Aetiology of infertility. Frequencies of aetiologies of infertility were similar during 1960–1970 (6814 couples) and 1980–1990 (9100).

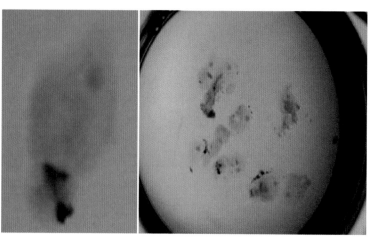

Fig. 1.**2**   Oocyte-cumulus complexes. Several cumulus-oocyte complexes are seen in the Petri dish (on the right side while on the left side a higher magnification of a cumulus-oocyte complex is shown). The oocyte and corona radiate are seen in the upper right corner of the left picture.

tion. All these procedures had inconsistent results. This resulted in the development of intracytoplasmic sperm injection (ICSI) at the Centre for Reproductive Medicine of the Vrije Universiteit Brussel, Belgium. ICSI has proved to be the procedure to alleviate (severe) male-factor infertility such as conventional IVF is for female-factor or idiopathic infertility.

In the 1990s *preimplantation genetic diagnosis* (PGD) was developed allowing the genetic diagnosis on one or two cells from an 8-cell embryo in couples who are at high risk for transmitting the genetic disease.

The current decade may well be the era where human embryonic stem cells are derived from human embryos donated for research.

1.2   Current Developments

1.2.1   IVF and ICSI

Both procedures have common steps except for the insemination procedure. This involves: patient selection for the ART procedure, controlled ovarian stimulation, the oocyte retrieval (Fig. 1.**2**), the semen preparation, insemination by conventional IVF or by ICSI, embryo culture, assessment of fertilisation and early embryo cleavage (Fig. 1.**3**), choice of embryo(s) for intrauterine transfer, cryopreservation of supernumerary embryos for eventual later use, and outcome of treatment cycle (successful implantation or not). Different types of embryo transfer catheters are now available. During the last decade the day of embryo transfer has become flexible: (day 1), day 2 or 3, (day 4) and day 5 or 6.

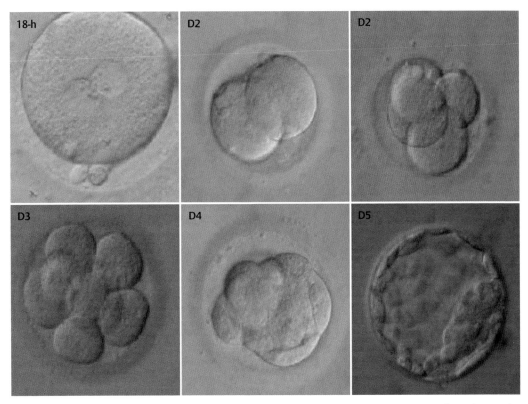

Fig. 1.**3**   Different stages of normal embryo development 18-h fertilised oocyte with two pronuclei and two polar bodies, D2 two-cell and four-cell embryo, D3 eight-cell embryo, D4 compacted morula and D5 expanded blasto-cyst with trophectoderm (periphery), inner-cell mass (right under) and blastocoelic cavity.

In the last decades the laboratory procedures have been professionalised extensively. Scientific societies such as the European Society for Human Reproduction and Embryology have established a recommended *code of practice for laboratory procedures*. Regulation has also been established at the national and international level. An example of the latter is the *European Tissue and Cell Directive (EUTCD)* which includes also reproductive cells.

As indicated in Fig. 1.**4**, conventional IVF can be applied to infertile couples with female-factor infertility as well as infertility of unknown origin (idiopathic infertility). When IVF was done for male-factor infertility it became obvious that cIVF was unsuitable for (severe) male-factor infertility. Failed fertilisation and impossibility to carry out embryo transfer occurred frequently when semen parameters were abnormal. Several procedures of assisted fertilisation were developed in the latter part of the 1980s: zona drilling, partial

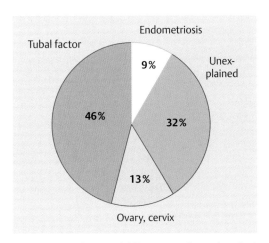

Fig. 1.**4**   Distribution of different aetiologies for which conventional IVF can be used successfully.

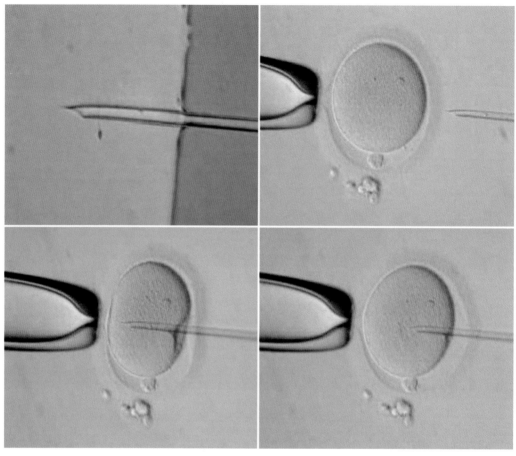

Fig. 1.**5**   Different steps in the ICSI procedure. 1) Upper left: a single spermatozoon is aspirated tail-first into a micropipette. 2) Upper right: a metaphase II oocyte is immobilised by a holding pipette, the injection pipette (right) is brought near to the zona pellucida. 3) Lower left: the injection pipette goes through the zona pellucida, the oolemna and the single spermatozoon is injected into the ooplasma of the oocyte. 4) Lower right: the injection pipette is then gently withdrawn from the oocyte.

zona dissection and subzonal insemination but none of them provided consistent success. Only intracytoplasmic sperm injection (ICSI) – the single sperm injection into the cytoplasm of an oocyte – has provided consistent results. It evolved from a serendipitous finding of a failed subzonal insemination into the standard treatment for all forms of severe male-factor infertility.

The different steps of ICSI are illustrated in Fig. 1.5. Since the first birth at the Vrije Universiteit Brussel on 14 January 1992, ICSI has been applied worldwide for male-factor infertility. It can be used with spermatozoa from the ejaculate in cases with severe oligo-astheno-teratozoospermia, with spermatozoa from epididymis in ob-

structive azoospermia and with spermatozoa from testis in obstructive and non-obstructive azoospermia. Figs. 1.6 and 1.7 illustrate how ICSI can be done using testicular spermatozoa (Devroey and Van Steirteghem, 2004).

1.2.2   Outcome IVF and ICSI

The only valid parameter to assess outcome of IVF and ICSI is the chance for an infertile couple to become parents of a healthy (singleton) child. Several surrogate, intermediate outcome parameters have been used but their practice should be abandoned. To increase the chance of pregnancy after IVF or ICSI more than one embryo is transferred.

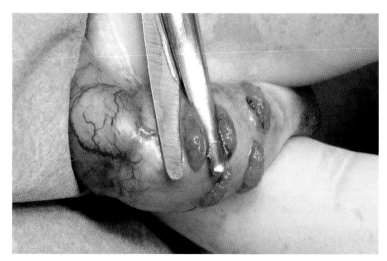

Fig. 1.**6** Testicular biopsy: in patients with azoospermia a small piece of testicular tissue can be removed surgically.

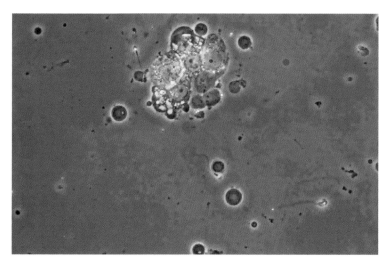

Fig. 1.**7** After mechanical shredding of testicular tissue a few spermatozoa can be isolated and used for ICSI in patients with obstructive and non-obstructive azoospermia.

The replacement of two, three or sometimes more than three embryos has increased indeed the chance of pregnancy; but as a side effect of transferring several embryos multiple pregnancies and deliveries have occurred. In the last decade the awareness of multiple ART pregnancies has resulted in replacing fewer embryos, especially in Europe and Australia, much less so in America and other parts of the world.

A meta-analysis (Jackson et al., 2004) and systematic review (Helmerhorst et al., 2004) on ART pregnancy complications have indicated that children born after IVF, with or without ICSI, have an increased risk for perinatal mortality, preterm or very preterm delivery, low and very low birth weight, small for gestational age, Caesarean sec-

tion and admission to the neonatal intensive care unit. The major congenital malformation rate after IVF and ICSI is higher than in spontaneously conceived children (Hansen et al., 2005). The comparison of IVF versus ICSI children does not indicate that the ICSI procedure represents significant additional risk of major birth defects than that involved in standard IVF.

So far studies of older ART children indicate that psychomotor development and health are similar to those of naturally conceived children. Follow-up studies at birth and later in life need to continue in the future to detect rare diseases such as genomic imprinting defects. The oldest ART children are now at an age that they will be able to have children themselves. Both male and female infertility may have some genetic factors involved and this may be transmitted to the children. Information on outcome that is as complete and reliable as possible is important in the counselling of prospective parents who need ART (Belva et al., 2007; Leunens et al., 2008).

1.2.3   Preimplantation Genetic Diagnosis – PGD

PGD involves the genetic diagnosis of an embryo before implantation of that embryo can occur. PGD is carried out on an *in vitro* embryo while conventional prenatal diagnosis is done on an *in vivo* foetus at about 10 or 16 weeks of gestation. PGD can be offered to couples with a high recurrence risk for carriers of specific genetic disease, carriers of a specific genetic disease, carriers of a sex-linked disease or carriers of chromosomal aberrations. PGD requires close collaboration between a Centre for Medical Genetics and a Centre for Reproductive Medicine (Fig. 1.**8**). The Centre for Medical Genetics is responsible for establishing a reliable diagnosis on a single cell (single blastomere of an eight-cell embryo) by using *fluorescent in situ hybridisation* (FISH) or *polymerase chain reaction* (PCR) techniques. The Centre for Reproductive Medicine performs the IVF-ICSI procedure, the embryo biopsy and the uterine replacement of an unaffected embryo. PGD can be considered as a novel option for couples with high recurrence risk. Especially couples requiring IVF-ICSI or objecting to pregnancy termination after prenatal diagnosis are interested in PGD. It is only possible if DNA mutations or chromosomal

abnormality are known and if a reliable diagnosis on a single cell (blastomere) is available (Sermon et al., 2004).

Since many preimplantation embryos are aneuploid, the hypothesis was put forward that IVF-ICSI results could be improved if embryos were screened for aneuploidy prior to transfer. The positive results of initial observational studies have not been confirmed by controlled studies comparing aneuploidy screening of embryos or not. PGS needs therefore still to be considered as clinical research.

For several years, the ESHRE PGD Consortium has collected data on PGD practice (and publishes every year the results of PGD cycles reported to the Consortium (Goossens et al., 2008). They have also published a *code of practice on PGD* (Thornhill et al., 2005).

1.3   Challenges for the Future

1.3.1   Prevention of all Multiple Births

It goes without any doubt that the major problem of all ART procedures is the occurrence of multiple births caused by the fact that several embryos are replaced into the uterus. It is estimated that several million children have been born after ART. This positive outcome is overshadowed by the fact that a large proportion of these children – not far from half of them – are not coming from singleton pregnancies but from twin, triplet and even higher order multiple gestations. It is obvious that multiple pregnancies including twins have a much higher inherent risk of complications (Fauser et al., 2005).

It is obvious that the only way to avoid the iatrogenic epidemic of multiple pregnancies including twins is to transfer a single embryo. This obvious knowledge is and has been there since the beginning of ART but it is only in the last decade that the practice of single embryo transfer (SET) has increased. It started with the initiative of a number of individual centres, especially in Northern Europe and in the Low Countries, above all in Belgium, and these centres should be recognised as the pioneers of elective SET. The adoption of elective SET by more and more centres may help to reduce the multiple pregnancy rates in those centres but experience has shown that the overall decrease in twinning in a certain country or region is not assured by such initiatives of individual centres. To illustrate this I want to describe both

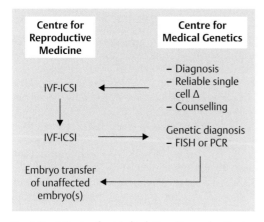

Fig. 1.**8**   A Centre for Medical Genetics and a Centre for Reproductive Medicine have specific tasks in Preimplantation Genetic Diagnosis.

as a privileged observer and participant what happened in Belgium. Since the mid-1980s there has been a voluntary registration of ART practice and this indicated that overall the delivery rate (slightly less than 20% per started cycle) indicated between 25 and 30% twin deliveries and 2–5% triplet deliveries. This remained constant over the years in spite of the fact that in the majority of transfers a shift from three to two embryos being transferred, occurred. The registration became mandatory in 1999 for all licensed ART centres (18 of them are fully licensed B centres, while a number of them – A centres – can do ART until oocyte retrieval). Notably, two centres in Belgium (Algemeen Ziekenhuis Middelheim and Universitair Ziekenhuis Gent) pioneered the practice of SET and were able to demonstrate that SET was working when a single top-quality embryo was transferred, especially in young patients. For these centres, the twinning rate decreased without any real impact on the number of twins being born in Belgium as a whole. Around that time a dialogue was started between the Belgian centres and the health authorities. Before this the B centres all agreed to propose a common policy. The health authorities were willing to provide a better reimbursement for ART on condition that the twinning rate would be reduced from 25–30% to 10% over a two-year period and that triplets would almost disappear. This reduction in twin and triplet births would reduce the cost of care for prematurely born babies and this money would be available for extra ART funding. A proposal, accepted by all centres, was finally put into a law in mid-2003 and involved the reimbursement of laboratory procedures for six cycles for patients up to the age of 43 years. Before 2003 the Belgian social security system reimbursed clinical procedures and fertility drugs but not the ART laboratory procedures, which were paid for out-of-pocket by patients. The number of embryos transferred had to be reduced for patients younger than 36 to one in the first two cycles and a maximum of two in the subsequent four cycles; for patients between 36 and less than 40 the number of embryos for transfer was two in the first two cycles and a maximum of three in the subsequent four cycles. There are no restrictions on the number of embryos transferred for patients between 40 and 43 years. One year after the introduction of this practice in Belgium (and after well over 10 000 treatment cycles) the twinning rate had fallen to about 10% (see Van Landuyt et al., 2006, for a description of the experi-

ence of the first year in the author's centre). This Belgian approach involved a mandatory, maximum number of embryos to transfer policy. In theory, the same could be achieved if all centres voluntarily adopted this practice, without legal requirements, although I personally doubt that this will work as well. I will illustrate this by another example of the Belgian practice. For patients under 36 there was an exception allowed in the regulation: if no top-quality embryo was available two embryos could be transferred in the second cycle. As a clinical embryologist with three decades of experience I think it is fair to say that this 'non-availability of at least one good-quality embryo' in this young group of patients would be very exceptional. However, this "exceptional" practice of transferring two embryos in young patients occurred in more than half of the second cycles, something I do not attribute to a sudden epidemic of bad-quality embryos in this age group! This illustrates that for public health measures to work one can, unfortunately I would say, not include exceptional measures. Although in theory I am in favour of retaining freedom of practice in medicine, rather strict regulation is sometimes needed for measures to be successful.

References

Belva F, Henriet S, Liebaers I et al. Medical outcome of 8-year-old singleton ICSI children (born ≥ 32 weeks' gestation) and a spontaneously conceived comparison group. Hum Reprod 2007; 22: 506–15.

Devroey P, Van Steirteghem A. A review of ten years experience of ICSI. Hum Reprod Update 2004; 10: 19–28.

Fauser BC, Devroey P, Macklon NS. Multiple birth resulting from ovarian stimulation for subfertility treatment. Lancet 2005; 365: 1807–16.

Goossens V, Harton G, Moutou C et al. ESHRE PGD Consortium data collection VIII. Cycles from January to December 2005 with pregnancy follow-up to October 2006. Hum Reprod 2008: Jul 18. Epub ahead of print

Hansen M, Bower C, Milne E, et al. Assisted reproductive technologies and the risk of birth defects – a systematic review. Hum Reprod 2005; 20: 328–38.

Helmerhorst FM, Perquin DA, Donker D et al. Perinatal outcome of singletons and twins after assisted conception: a systematic review of controlled studies. BMJ 2004; 328(7434): 261.

Jackson RA, Gibson KA, Wu YW et al. Perinatal outcomes in singletons following *in vitro* fertilization:

a meta-analysis. Obstet Gynecol 2004; 103: 551–63.

Leunens L, Celestin-Westreich S, Bonduelle M et al. Follow-up of cognitive and motor development of 10-year-old singleton children born after ICSI compared with spontaneously conceived children. Hum Reprod 2008; 23: 105–11.

Sermon K, Van Steirteghem A, Liebaers I. Preimplantation genetic diagnosis. Lancet 2004; 363: 1633–41.

Thornhill AR, deDie-Smulders CE, Geraedts JP et al. ESHRE PGD Consortium 'Best practice guidelines for clinical preimplantation genetic diagnosis (PGD) and preimplantation genetic screening (PGS)'. Hum Reprod 2005; 20: 35–48.

Van Landuyt L, Verheyen G, Tournaye H et al. New Belgian embryo transfer policy leads to sharp decrease in multiple pregnancy rate. Reprod Biomed Online 2006; 13: 765–71.

2 New Approaches to Ovarian Stimulation

N. S. Macklon

Department of Reproductive Medicine and Gynaecology, University Medical Centre Utrecht, Heidelberglaan 100, 3584 CX Utrecht, The Netherlands

Abstract

Due to the worldwide increased need for gonadotropin preparations, demands for postmenopausal urine have increased tremendously and adequate supplies can no longer be guaranteed. In addition, concern regarding the limited batch-to-batch consistency along with possibilities of urine contaminants have emerged. Through recombinant DNA technology and the transfection of human genes encoding for the common α and hormone specific β subunit of the glycoprotein hormone into Chinese hamster ovary cell lines, the large scale *in vitro* production of human recombinant FSH (recFSH) has been realised. The first pregnancies using this novel preparation in ovulation induction and in IVF were reported in 1992. Since then, numerous, large-scale, multicentre studies have been undertaken demonstrating their efficacy and safety. The recombinant products offer improved purity, consistency and large-scale availability. Because of its purity, recFSH can now be administered by protein weight rather than bioactivity and so-called "filled-by-mass" preparations are now available for clinical use. During recent years, recLH and rec hCG have also been introduced for clinical application. Moreover, a long-acting recFSH agonist (a chimeric hormone generated by the fusion of the carboxy-terminal peptide of hCG to the FSH-β chain) is undergoing clinical IVF trials, and the birth of the first healthy child using this preparation was reported in 2003. Recent studies have indicated that milder approaches to ovarian stimulation may improve outcomes in IVF, while reducing costs and side effects. The challenge now is to develop ways of individualising gonadotropin stimulation treatment to optimise outcomes for each woman.

2.1 Introduction

Ovarian stimulation is a central component of many infertility therapies. It is important to emphasise that two different concepts of ovarian stimulation exist. These approaches differ in both the starting point (i.e., the type of patients) and end-points (i.e., the aim of the medical intervention). Ovulation induction is the type of ovarian stimulation for anovulatory women aimed at restoring normal fertility by generating normoovulatory cycles (i.e., to mimic physiology and induce single dominant follicle selection and ovulation). In contrast the aim of ovarian stimulation in ovulatory women is to induce ongoing development of multiple dominant follicles and to mature many oocytes in order to improve chances for conception either *in vivo* [empirical ovarian hyperstimulation with or without intra-uterine insemination (IUI)] or *in vitro* with *in vitro* fertilization (IVF). This chapter will focus on recent development in the application of gonadotropins in IVF.

2.2 Concepts of Ovarian Stimulation in IVF

The general aim of ovarian hyperstimulation in this clinical context is to induce the development of multiple dominant follicles in order to be able to retrieve many oocytes to allow for inefficiencies in subsequent fertilization *in vitro*, embryo culture, embryo selection for transfer and implantation (Macklon et al., 2006). Hence, multiple embryos can be transferred in the great majority of patients and often spare embryos can be cryopreserved to allow for subsequent chances of pregnancy without the need for repeated ovarian stimulation and oocyte retrieval (Macklon et al., 2006). The paradigm of so-called "controlled" ovarian hyperstimulation by high doses of exogeneous gonadotropins and GnRH agonist long-protocol co-treatment for IVF has constituted the gold standard for clinicians throughout the world since the early 1990s. It appears that large numbers of developing follicles are still considered a useful surrogate marker of successful IVF, whereas their significance in relation to the chance of achieving a pregnancy and birth of a healthy baby is in doubt (van der Gaast et al., 2006; Heijnen et al., 2004; Heijnen et al., 2007). The ovarian stimulation protocols required to produce large number of follicles have become extremely complex and costly over the years (Macklon et al., 2006; Huirne et al., 2004) creating considerable side effects, risks of complications, and the need for intense monitoring of ovarian response (Fauser et al., 1999).

Physicians appear to be in control of ovarian stimulation due to their ability to adjust the gonadotropin doses or the type of preparation on the basis of ovarian response monitoring. However, the major individual variability in response is outside the doctor's control and is an extremely important determining factor for both success and complications of IVF treatment (Kligman et al., 2001). A good ovarian response to standard stimulation indicates normal ovarian function and a good prognosis for successful IVF. A low ovarian response suggests ovarian ageing and is therefore associated with poor IVF outcome. A low response can to some extent be predicted by chronological age and endocrine and ultrasound ageing parameters assessed before the initiation of treatment, as will be discussed later (van Rooij et al., 2002; Broekmans et al., 2007). However, the widely applied approach to increase gonadotropin doses administered in case of insufficient ovarian response has very little scientific foundation (Tarlatzis et al., 2003). The occurrence of a severe hyperresponse comes as a surprise in most cases and therefore cannot be predicted (Delvigne and Rozenberg, 2002; ASRM Practice Committee, 2006). Severe OHSS is induced by hCG and is therefore associated with pregnancy. This can be prevented from happening by refraining from embryo transfer in the cycle at risk and cryopreserving all available embryos for transfer in another cycle.

Slowly ovarian hyperstimulation protocols have shifted from the use of HMG to urinary FSH and to recombinant FSH (Zwart-van Rijkom et al., 2002). In recent years several groups have focussed on the potential significance of late follicular phase LH levels for clinical IVF outcome. In-

deed, it has been shown that dominant follicle development can be stimulated exclusively by LH rather than FSH opening new possibilities for therapeutic interventions (Filicori et al., 2002), as discussed in more detail later.

Despite the fact that the first child born after IVF was conceived in a spontaneous menstrual cycle, natural cycle IVF has received little attention. The major focus has been the improvement of complex ovarian stimulation regimens. Natural cycle IVF offers major advantages such as negligible complications (arising from multiple pregnancy or OHSS), reduced patient discomfort and a low cost. The efficacy of natural cycle IVF is hampered, however, by high cancellation rates due to premature ovulation or luteinisation. A systematic review of 20 selected studies involving a total of 1800 cycles showed a 7.2% overall pregnancy rate per started cycle, and 16% per embryo transfer (Pelinck et al. 2002). Cumulative pregnancy and live birth rates over 4 cycles of 42% and 32%, respectively, have been reported (Nargund et al., 2001). Despite the relatively high failure rate, the approach of natural cycle may still be cost-effective. In one study, it was calculated that natural cycle IVF could be offered at 23% of the cost of a stimulated cycle (Nargund et al., 2007).

More recently a 'modified' natural cycle (Nargund et al., 2007) has been proposed, in which GnRH antagonists are instituted to prevent premature ovulation, and low-dose exogenous gonadotropin cotreatment is given as an add-back to prevent a GnRH antagonist-induced involution of follicle development. Using this approach which, like natural cycle IVF, aims to achieve monofollicular development, cumulative pregnancy rates of 44% have been reported over 9 cycles of treatment (Pelinck et al., 2007).

2.2.1   Gonadotropin Preparations

Gonadotropin preparations have been used for ovarian stimulation since the early days of IVF and were originally developed in the USA (Cohen et al., 2005). The daily administration of these preparations is usually efficacious in the induction and maintenance of growth of multiple dominant follicles, allowing for the retrieval of many oocytes for IVF. Preparations initially used were HMG (containing both LH and FSH bioactivity), followed by purified urinary (u) FSH and more recently recombinant (rec) FSH. No general consensus exists with regard to starting day and doses of gonadotropins. In conclusion, although higher gonadotropin doses may result in the retrieval of 1–2 more oocytes, improved clinical outcomes in terms of pregnancy rates could not be demonstrated.

A chimeric FSH agonist (so-called recFSH-CTP), generated by the fusion of the carboxy-terminal peptide of hCG (responsible for its prolonged metabolic clearance compared to LH) with the FSH-β chain has recently been undergoing phase 3 studies in IVF. The birth of a first healthy baby was reported in 2003 following the single injection of this novel compound in the early follicular phase of the cycle and a 7-day medication-free period (Beckers et al., 2003). Phase 2 (Devroey et al., 2004) and phase 3 studies are establishing the optimal dose and the clinical efficacy of this preparation in comparison to recFSH. It is anticipated that this latter development is going to represent a step forward in rendering stimulation regimens more patient friendly, but it is not to be expected that clinical outcome will improve.

The type, duration and dosing of GnRH analogue co-treatment to suppress endogenous pituitary gonadotropin release may also affect the preferred gonadotropin preparation. Classical principles teach us that both LH and FSH are required for adequate ovarian oestrogen biosynthesis and follicle development. Theca cell-derived androgen production (which is under LH control) is mandatory as a substrate for the conversion to oestrogens by FSH-induced aromatase activity of granulosa cells (Macklon et al., 2006). A number of studies have indicated that excessively suppressed late follicular phase LH concentrations may be detrimental for clinical IVF outcome (Westergaard et al., 2000; Fleming et al., 2000). Under these circumstances the use of urinary preparations containing both LH and FSH activity or the addition of rec LH or rec hCG next to exogeneous FSH may be useful (Macklon et al., 2006). It is uncertain as yet, however, for which patients this approach may be beneficial. Recent meta-analyses failed to show clinically relevant differences in relation to late follicular phase LH concentrations (Kilibianakis et al., 2007), or when cycles with or without the addition of exogenous LH are compared (Baruffi et al., 2007).

Recently the concept that exogenous LH is capable of selectively stimulating the development of the more mature dominant follicles has been developed. A shift from FSH to LH preparations during stimulation may therefore be useful in order to stimulate a more homogeneous cohort of follicles for IVF (Filicori et al., 2002; Sullivan et al., 1999).

2.2.2   Treatment Regimens

To allow for the clinical introduction of recombinant FSH, large-scale, multi-centre, comparative trials in IVF were published from 1995 onwards (Out et al., 1995). It should be noted, however, that these studies, including several hundreds of women, were sponsored by pharmaceutical companies. The results should therefore be interpreted with an appropriate degree of caution. For instance, it was arbitrarily chosen for all initial studies that rec FSH would only be compared with u FSH and not HMG, although the latter preparation was still considered to be the gold standard by the majority of clinicians. Several independent comparative trials have been published since then, but the sample size of these single-centre studies was usually insufficient to allow for the detection of relatively small differences. An early meta-analysis (Daya, 2002) as well as health economics studies (Daya et al., 2001; Sykes et al., 2001) indicate a slightly improved outcome for rec FSH compared to u FSH. In addition, a meta-analysis involving a limited number of IVF studies comparing rec FSH versus HMG suggested comparable outcomes (Afrawal et al., 2000). However, recently published multi-centre, company-sponsored trials reported similar clinical outcomes comparing u FSH versus rec FSH, or HMG versus rec FSH (Andersen et al., 2006).

Many different regimens are applied with little if any proof of their efficacy and safety. Different starting days and doses are applied worldwide along with incremental or decremental doses. In case of imminent OHSS resulting from the development of too many follicles, the possibility of complete cessation of gonadotropin administration (also referred to as 'coasting') has been advocated by several investigators (Delvigne and Rotenberg, 2002). Studies on the efficacy of this approach thus far undertaken have been limited and inconclusive. Adequate doses for gonadotropin preparations may also vary depending on whether GnRH agonist or antagonist co-treatment is used (Al-Inany and Abouighar, 2002). Major individual differences in body weight may also determine response (Mannaerts et al., 1993). Because endogenous gonadotropins are suppressed by GnRH antagonists for a limited period of time (as will be discussed later), less exogenous FSH is required. The ideal day of initiation of gonadotropin therapy is another variable which has been poorly characterised so far, and may also vary depending on GnRH agonist or antagonist co-treatment. It is surprising to conclude that very few of the above-mentioned questions with regard to applied dose regimens can be answered on the basis of scientific evidence by properly designed studies.

Usually starting doses vary between 100 and 300 IU/d and doses are often altered depending on the observed individual ovarian response. A typical daily starting dose would currently be 150–225 IU in Europe and 225–300 IU in the USA. Only few randomised studies regarding dose regimens can be found in the literature. A single-centre randomised controlled trial from Rotterdam showed that a doubling of the HMG dose in low responders after a 225 IU/d dose for 5 days is not efficacious compared to continuation of similar doses (van Hooff et al., 1993). Moreover, an RCT in which higher versus standard doses of FSH were administered to expected poor responders showed no difference in pregnancy rates (Klinkert et al., 2005).

2.3   Gonadotropin-Releasing Hormone Agonist Co-Treatment

During initial studies with HMG stimulation of multiple follicle development for IVF it became apparent that a premature LH peak occurred in around 20 to 25% of cycles, due to positive feedback activity by high serum E_2 levels during the mid-follicular phase of the stimulation cycle (Macklon et al., 2006). This advanced exposure to high LH resulted in premature luteinisation of follicles and either cycle cancellation due to follicle maturation arrest or severely compromised IVF outcome. The clinical development of GnRH agonists in the early 1980s (Huirne and Lambalk, 2001) allowed for the complete suppression of pituitary gonadotropin release during ovarian stimulation protocols for IVF (Macklon et al., 2006). Induced pituitary down-regulation indeed resulted in significantly reduced cancellation rates and improved overall IVF outcome (Smitz et al., 1988; Hughes et al., 1992). Moreover, the approach of GnRH agonist co-treatment did facilitate scheduling of IVF and timing of oocyte retrieval. Frequently used preparations include buserelin, triptorelin, nafarelin and leuprorelin.

Due to the intrinsic agonist activity of the compound, pituitary down-regulation is preceded by an initial stimulatory phase (referred to as the 'flare' effect) which lasts for around 2 weeks. In this 'long-protocol', GnRH agonist treatment therefore usually commences in the luteal phase in the preceding cycle and is continued until hCG administration. Stimulation with gonadotropins is started when pituitary and ovarian quiescence has been achieved. Moreover, it is uncertain whether ovarian response to exogenous stimulation is affected by GnRH agonist co-treatment (Hughes and Cedrin, 1998). Some women suffer from serious hypo-oestrogenic side effects, such as mood changes, sweating and flushes. Alternative approaches include the 'short' (and sometimes 'ultrashort') protocols where the initial flare effect of GnRH agonist treatment is used to stimulate the ovaries. Attempts to discontinue GnRH agonist administration during the ovarian stimulation phase (Beckers et al., 2000; Pantos et al., 1994) have not shown beneficial effects. Reported clinical results of these alternative clinical protocols remain variable, and the GnRH agonist long-protocol has remained the standard of care for over a decade (Macklon et al., 2006).

2.4   Gonadotropin-Releasing Hormone Antagonist Co-Treatment

Two third-generation GnRH antagonists (cetrorelix, and ganirelix) became available for large-scale clinical studies around 1995. Previous generations of the antagonist suffered from problems with pharmaceutical formulation and related bioavailability along with the local or systemic induction of histamine release. The potential advantage of a GnRH antagonist is that pituitary gonadotropin secretion is suppressed immediately after initiation of therapy. Therefore the co-treatment with GnRH antagonists can be restricted to the time in the cycle at risk for a premature rise in LH, i.e., the mid- to late-follicular phase of the cycle (Macklon et al., 2006).

Both single, high-dose and multiple, low-dose GnRH antagonist regimens have been described. Multiple, daily dose regimens are most widely used at present. Initial dose finding studies suggested that a daily injection of 0.25 mg represents the minimal effective dose to suppress a premature LH rise in most patients. In all phase 3 comparative trials of the daily GnRH antagonist co-treatment regimen, it was initiated on cycle day 6. However, in principle, GnRH antagonists need only be given when there is follicular development and rising E_2 levels which might give rise to a premature elevation in pituitary LH release due to positive feedback mechanisms. However, a meta-analysis of 4 studies comparing fixed with flexible regimens showed a trend towards lower pregnancy rates following the flexible protocol (odds ratio: 0.70, 95 % CI: 0.47 – 1.05) (Al-Inany et al., 2005). The first meta-analysis published comparing outcomes following co-treatment with GnRH antagonist versus GnRH agonist (Al-Inany and Aboulghar, 2002) based on 5 multicentre RCTs concluded that the GnRH antagonist is as efficient as the GnRH agonist in preventing a premature LH surge in IVF (odds ratio: 1.76, 95 % CI: 0.75 – 4.16). However, a small but significant reduction in pregnancies was observed per started cycle (OR: 0.79, 95 % CI: 0.63 – 0.99). Since then, protocols have been refined, and a recent meta-analysis of later studies has shown no difference in live-birth rates (Kolibianakis et al., 2006).

Concerns have been raised regarding the possibility of direct effects of GnRH antagonists on the embryo. However, no adverse effects were observed on the freeze-thaw embryos of GnRH antagonist cycles (Kol et al., 1999). Possible detrimental effects of GnRH antagonists at the endometrial level and on follicle development have not been confirmed (Macklon et al., 2006). Moreover, recent studies have indicated that gonadotropin regimens do not need to be adjusted when GnRH antagonists are commenced (Aboulghar et al., 2004; Propst et al., 2006). Furthermore, exogeneous LH is probably not required next to FSH (Kolibainakis et al., 2007; Baruffi et al., 2007; Kolibianakis et al., 2004).

Despite improving outcomes the debate regarding the advantages and disadvantages compared with GnRH agonists continues (Tariatzis et al., 2006).

2.5   Adverse Effects and Complications

Complications related to invasive IVF procedures such as oocyte retrieval and embryo transfer, predominantly involve infection and bleeding along with anaesthesia problems (Schenker and Ezra, 1994). The drawbacks associated with profound ovarian stimulation for IVF include considerable patient discomfort such as weight gain, headache, mood swings, breast tenderness, abdominal pain and sometimes diarrhoea and nausea. In this respect it is important to comprehend that after a first unsuccessful IVF attempt, around 25 % of patients refrain from a second cycle, even in countries where costs are covered by health insurance companies (Osmanagaoglu et al., 1999).

OHSS is a potentially life-threatening complication characterised by ovarian enlargement, high serum sex steroids and extravascular fluid accumulation, primarily in the peritoneal cavity. Mild forms of OHSS constitute around 20 – 35 % of IVF cycles, moderate forms 3 – 6 % of cycles along with 0.1 – 0.2 % severe forms (Delvigne and Rozenberg, 2002; Anoulghar and Mansour, 2003). To some extent, patients at risk of developing OHSS may be recognised by the following features: young age, PCOS, profound hyperstimulation protocols with GnRH agonist long-protocol co-treatment, large numbers of pre-ovulatory Graafian follicles, high serum E_2 levels, a high (> 5000 IU) bolus dose of hCG to induce final oocyte maturation, the use of hCG for luteal phase supplementation, and finally the occurrence of pregnancy. In fact, the incidence of OHSS is directly related to hCG concentrations with a 2- to 5-fold increased incidence in case of multiple pregnancy.

Preventive strategies in case of imminent OHSS include cessation of exogeneous gonadotropins for several days (referred to as "coasting"), follicular aspiration, prevention of pregnancy during the stimulation cycle by cryopreserving all embryos, or the prophylactic infusion of glucocorticoids or albumen. The risk of OHSS may also be lowered by using alternative strategies to induce oocyte maturation, such as inducing an endogenous LH surge by administration of a single bolus dose of GnRH agonist or the short half-life preparation recLH instead of hCG.

The most important complication related to IVF treatment is multiple pregnancy. Between the years of 1980 and 2000, twin birth rates in the USA increased by 75 %, and currently represent around 3 % of total births (Fauser et al., 2005). Similar trends have been reported in European countries (Verberg et al., 2007). Although an association between increased female age and multiple gestation is clearly established, the delay in childbearing accounts for no more than 30 % of the observed overall increase in multiple pregnancies (Fauser et al., 2005). Although the available data indicate that the majority of twin births are still unrelated to infertility therapies (Fauser et al., 2005), up to 80 % of higher order multiple births are considered to be due to ovarian stimulation and ART. Births resulting from infertility therapies account for around 1 – 3 % of all singleton live births, 30 – 50 % of twin births and more than 75 % of higher order multiples.

Pregnancy complications include increased risk of miscarriage, pre-eclampsia, growth retardation and pre-term delivery. Perinatal mortality rates are at least 4-fold higher in twin, and at least 6-fold higher in triplet births compared with singleton births. Moreover, the risks of prematurity in twin and higher order multiple birth are increased 7- to 40-fold, and for low birth weight 10- to 75-fold, respectively. Adverse outcomes among children conceived through IVF are largely associated with multiple gestation.

Recent data are reassuring with respect to possible long-term health consequences such as ovarian cancer, breast cancer or advanced menopausal age (Mahdavi et al., 2006).

2.6   New Approaches to Mild Ovarian Stimulation for IVF

After the initial years of IVF, profound ovarian stimulation became the rule for more than two decades. The stimulation of the growth of large numbers of follicles and the retrieval of many oocytes has been viewed as an acceptable marker of successful IVF treatment. Medication regimens to achieve profound ovarian stimulation are extremely complex and expensive, take many weeks of frequent injections and intense monitoring. Moreover, patient discomfort and chances for serious side effects and complications are considerable. In addition, this profound stimulation gives rise to greatly abnormal luteal phase endocrinology, and its impact on endometrial receptivity and therefore IVF success is mostly unknown.

Attitudes towards profound ovarian stimulation are changing (Fauser et al., 1999; Edwards et al., 1996), particularly given the growing tendency to transfer a reduced number of embryos. It has previously been demonstrated on the basis of the UK national database that reducing the number of embryos transferred from 3 to 2 does not diminish chances of birth despite a reduction in risk of multiple birth (Templeton and Morris, 1998). In Europe, an increasing number of centres are carrying out single transfers in younger women. Emphasis may therefore now be directed towards the development of more simple mild stimulation protocols (Macklon et al., 2006; Fauser et al., 1999; Nargund et al., 2007; Pennings and Ombelet, 2007) or the improvement of natural cycle IVF outcomes (Pelinck et al., 2002; Nargund et al., 2001; Pelinck et al., 2007). The increasing quality of embryo cryopreservation programmes will serve to encourage the transfer of one embryo at a time (Lundin and Bergh, 2007).

Previous studies in normo-ovulatory female volunteers (Schipper et al., 1998; Hohmann et al., 2001) confirmed that the development of multiple dominant follicles can be induced by interfering with decremental FSH concentrations during the mid- to late-follicular phase. As shown previously, this decrease is required for the selection of a single dominant follicle (Pache et al., 1990; van Santbrink et al., 1995). These observations are in agreement with previous findings in the monkey model (Zeleznik et al., 1985; Zeleznik and Kubik, 1986). We were subsequently able to demonstrate that the initiation of exogeneous FSH (fixed dose, 150 IU/d, GnRH antagonist co-treatment) as late as cycle day 5 results in a comparable clinical IVF outcome, despite a reduced duration of stimulation (number of ampoules used) and increased cancellation rates (Hohmann et al., 2003). To test the efficacy of this mild stimulation protocol in standard practice, a large randomised effectiveness study has been performed to analyse whether a strategy including the mild stimulation protocol in combination with single embryo transfer (SET) would lead to a similar outcome assessed over a one year interval after initiation of treatment, while reducing patients' discomfort, multiple pregnancies, and costs compared with standard treatment (Heijnen et al., 2007). The study included a total of 404 patients and observed that due to the shorter duration of treatment per cycle, less medication needed and a reduction in twin pregnancies, the mild approach led to an equal chance of live birth after a year of treatment while reducing the total costs.

Apart from clinical efficacy and costs (see later), emotional stress should be considered an important negative side effect associated with IVF treatment. Following mild stimulation, patients reported fewer side effects and stress related to hormone treatment and cycle cancellation compared with conventional stimulation (de Klerk et al., 2006). Treatment-related stress has been found to be the most important reason why patients drop out of IVF treatment (Filicori et al., 1999). The early drop-out of treatment deprives the couple of an optimal cumulative chance of achieving pregnancy, and therefore also impacts on the success of the respective IVF programme. Mild stimulation might therefore have a positive impact on cumulative treatment success rates as it positively affects the chance that patients are willing to continue treatment following a failed attempt.

Other novel protocols under investigation include the replacement of FSH by LH; an approach based on the acquired LH responsiveness of granulosa cells of dominant follicles. Besides the expected reduction of gonadotropin usage, this ovarian stimulation approach might also reduce the number of small, less mature follicles, conceivably reducing the chance of OHSS, because smaller ovarian follicles are unlikely to be responsive to LH (Filicori et al., 1999). Three randomised controlled trials (Filicori et al., 2005; Koichi et al., 2006; Serafini et al., 2006) have shown that this approach can result in a significant reduction in FSH needed and in the number of small follicles at final oocyte maturation. Pregnancy rates do not appear to be compromised. More extensive studies are required to determine the critical threshold for FSH replacement by LH stimulation and the most appropriate dosage of LH or hCG.

There are indications that the degree of ovarian stimulation affects both the morphological embryo quality and the chromosomal constitution of the developed embryos (Munne et al., 1997; Katz-Jaffe et al., 2005). This phenomenon could be the result of interference with the natural selection of good quality oocytes or the exposure of growing follicles to the potentially negative effects of ovarian stimulation. A randomised trial concerning the chromosomal analysis of human embryos following mild ovarian stimulation for IVF showed a significantly higher proportion of euploid embryos compared to conventional ovarian stimulation, suggesting that through maximal stimulation the surplus of obtained oocytes result in chromosomally abnormal and inferior embryos (Baart et al., 2007).

2.7   Individualising Treatment

In recent years a number of prediction models for calculating individual chances of spontaneous conception in subfertile couples have been published (Eimers et al., 1994; Collins et al., 1995; Hunault et al., 2005). The chance of conception over a given time-frame can be calculated from the results of a number of fertility investigations and patient parameters such as age and duration of infertility. Caution is, however, required when applying a prediction model developed elsewhere to one's own patient population. Before a prediction model can be introduced into everyday clinical practice, prospective external validation is required. Furthermore, knowledge of the develop-

ment cohort is important when selecting a model for application in one's own setting. The mean duration and degree of subfertility in a primary care population is less than in a tertiary population. As a result, the conclusions derived from a model developed in academic centres may have limited relevance for primary subfertility management and vice versa (Evers, 2002).

The majority of women undergoing ovulation induction have WHO class 2 anovulation. Although this is a highly heterogeneous group, the treatment for these women is the same (Laven et al., 2002). The identification of patient characteristics predictive of ovulation induction outcome would not only allow the design of individual treatment regimens, but would also provide useful information regarding the factors which determine the extent of ovarian dysfunction (Laven et al., 2002). In recent years a number of studies addressing these issues have been published. In one study the criteria which could predict the response of women with WHO class 2 anovulation to treatment with CC were identified (Imani et al., 2000). Following multivariate analysis, the free androgen index (FAI), body mass index (BMI), presence of amenorrhoea (as opposed to oligomenorrhoea) and ovarian volume were found to be independent predictors of ovulation. The area under the receiver operating curve in a prediction model using these factors was 0.82. By adding additional endocrine factors, the AUC increased to 0.86 (Imani et al., 2000). In a subsequent study, those factors which could predict conception following ovulation were studied. Multivariate analysis of a number of clinical, endocrine and ultrasound characteristics revealed lower age and the presence of amenorrhoea to be the only significant parameters for predicting conception.

When gonadotropin therapy for ovulation induction is selected, the duration of treatment, the amount of gonadotropins administered, the associated risks of cycle-to-cycle variability, multifollicular development, OHSS and multiple pregnancy might all be reduced if the starting doses were individualised. This would require a means to reliably predict the dose of FSH at which a given individual will respond by way of monofollicular selection to dominance, in other words, the individual FSH threshold for stimulation. A prediction model has recently been developed which may be used to determine the individual FSH response dose (which is presumably closely related to the FSH threshold) (Imani et al., 2002). Women about to undergo low-dose step-up ovulation induction with recombinant FSH, were subject to a standard clinical, sonographic and endocrine screening. The measured parameters were analysed for predictors of the FSH dose on the day of ovarian response. In multivariate analysis, body mass index (BMI), ovarian response to preceding clomiphene citrate (CC) medication (CC resistant anovulation [CRA], or failure to conceive despite ovulatory cycles), initial free insulin-like growth factor-I (free IGF-I) and serum FSH levels were included in the final model (Imani et al., 2002). In a subsequent analysis of women with PCOS who had undergone ovulation induction with the step-down regimen, a correlation was observed between the predicted individual FSH response dose and the number of treatment days before dominance was observed (van Santbrink et al., 2002). Application of this model may enable the administration of the lowest possible daily dose of exogeneous gonadotropins to surpass the individual FSH threshold of a given patient and achieve follicular development and subsequent ovulation. Refining ovulation induction therapy in this way offers the prospect of improving safety, reducing the risk of multiple pregnancies and improving the efficiency of gonadotropin ovulation induction.

2.8   Conclusions

Any form of ovarian stimulation increases the chances of pregnancy per cycle but at the expense of increased complication rates, most importantly multiple pregnancies and OHSS. This holds especially true for ovarian hyperstimulation aiming at maturing multiple dominant follicles for fertilisation either *in vivo* (following intercourse or IUI) or *in vitro* by IVF. With IVF, the incidence of occurring multiple pregnancies can be controlled by the number of embryos transferred. Moreover, various strategies may significantly reduce the chances for OHSS. In skilful hands and with proper ovarian response monitoring, the chances for complications are lowest for ovulation induction. The aim of this intervention is to mimic physiological circumstances in anovulatory women and, hence, single dominant follicle development and ovulation.

Milder forms of ovarian hyperstimulation (or indeed none at all) may be considered for empirical treatment of unknown infertility (with or without IUI) due to the inherent risk of higher order multiple pregnancies. In general, however, the price to pay is a slightly lower pregnancy rate per cycle. Overall, assessment of cumulative pregnancy rates over a given period of time (which may involve multiple cycles) may be similar.

Individualising ovarian stimulation in order to optimise outcomes between risks and desired outcomes is likely to improve in the future with the development of pharmacogenetics. Clinical studies have shown that FSH receptor gene polymorphisms can influence the ovarian response to stimulation in women undergoing IVF (Grebb et al., 2005). Genotyping of patients prior to treatment may therefore aid in tailoring FSH doses dependent on individual ovarian sensitivity (Fauser et al., 2008).

References

Aboulghar MA, Mansour RT, Serour GI, Al-Inany HG, Amin YM, Aboulghar MM. Increasing the dose of human menopausal gonadotrophins on day of GnRH antagonist administration: randomized controlled trial. Reprod Biomed Online 2004; 8: 524–7.

Aboulghar MA, Mansour RT. Ovarian hyperstimulation syndrome: classifications and critical analysis of preventive measures. Hum Reprod Update 2003; 9: 275–89.

Agrawal R, Holmes J, Jacobs HS. Follicle-stimulating hormone or human menopausal gonadotropin for ovarian stimulation in *in vitro* fertilization cycles: a meta-analysis. Fertil Steril 2000; 73: 338–43.

Al-Inany H, Aboulghar M. GnRH antagonist in assisted reproduction: a Cochrane review. Hum Reprod 2002; 17: 874–85.

Al-Inany H, Aboulghar MA, Mansour RT, Serour GI. Optimizing GnRH antagonist administration: meta-analysis of fixed versus flexible protocol. Reprod Biomed Online 2005; 10: 567–70.

Andersen AN, Devroey P, Arce JC. Clinical outcome following stimulation with highly purified hMG or recombinant FSH in patients undergoing IVF: a randomized assessor-blind controlled trial. Hum Reprod 2006; 21: 3217–27.

ASRM Practice Committee. Ovarian hyperstimulation syndrome. Fertil Steril 2006; 86 (5 Suppl): S178–S183.

Baart EB, Martini E, Eijkemans MJ, Van OD, Beckers NG, Verhoeff A et al. Milder ovarian stimulation for *in-vitro* fertilization reduces aneuploidy in the human preimplantation embryo: a randomized controlled trial. Hum Reprod 2007; 22: 980–8.

Baruffi RL, Mauri AL, Petersen CG, Felipe V, Martins AM, Cornicelli J et al. Recombinant LH supplementation to recombinant FSH during induced ovarian stimulation in the GnRH-antagonist protocol: a meta-analysis. Reprod Biomed Online 2007; 14: 14–25.

Beckers NG, Laven JS, Eijkemans MJ, Fauser BC. Follicular and luteal phase characteristics following early cessation of gonadotrophin-releasing hormone agonist during ovarian stimulation for *in-vitro* fertilization. Hum Reprod 2000; 15: 43–9.

Beckers NG, Macklon NS, Devroey P, Platteau P, Boerrigter PJ, Fauser BC. First live birth after ovarian stimulation using a chimeric long-acting human recombinant follicle-stimulating hormone (FSH) agonist (recFSH-CTP) for *in vitro* fertilization. Fertil Steril 2003; 79: 621–3.

Broekmans FJ, Knauff EA, te Velde ER, Macklon NS, Fauser BC. Female reproductive ageing: current knowledge and future trends. Trends Endocrinol Metab 2007; 18: 58–65.

Cohen J, Trounson A, Dawson K, Jones H, Hazekamp J, Nygren KG et al. The early days of IVF outside the UK. Hum Reprod Update 2005; 11: 439–59.

Collins JA, Burrows EA, Wilan AR. The prognosis for live birth among untreated infertile couples. Fertil Steril 1995; 64: 22–8.

Daya S, Ledger W, Auray JP, Duru G, Silverberg K, Wikland M et al. Cost-effectiveness modelling of recombinant FSH versus urinary FSH in assisted reproduction techniques in the UK. Hum Reprod 2001; 16: 2563–9.

Daya S. Updated meta-analysis of recombinant follicle-stimulating hormone (FSH) versus urinary FSH for ovarian stimulation in assisted reproduction. Fertil Steril 2002; 77: 711–4.

de Klerk C, Heijnen EM, Macklon NS, Duivenvoorden HJ, Fauser BC, Passchier J et al. The psychological impact of mild ovarian stimulation combined with single embryo transfer compared with conventional IVF. Hum Reprod 2006; 21: 721–7.

Delvigne A, Rozenberg S. Epidemiology and prevention of ovarian hyperstimulation syndrome (OHSS): a review. Hum Reprod Update 2002; 8: 559–77.

Devroey P, Fauser BC, Platteau P, Beckers NG, Dhont M, Mannaerts BM. Induction of multiple follicular development by a single dose of long-acting recombinant follicle-stimulating hormone (FSH-CTP, corifollitropin alfa) for controlled ovarian stimulation before *in vitro* fertilization. J Clin Endocrinol Metab 2004; 89: 2062–70.

Edwards RG, Lobo R, Bouchard P. Time to revolutionize ovarian stimulation. Hum Reprod 1996; 11: 917–9.

Eimers JM, te Velde ER, Gerritse R, Vogelzang ET, Looman CW, Habbema JD. The prediction of the chance to conceive in subfertile couples. Fertil Steril 1994; 61: 44–52.

Evers JL. Female subfertility. Lancet 2002; 151–9.

Fauser BC, Devroey P, Macklon NS. Multiple birth resulting from ovarian stimulation for subfertility treatment. Lancet 2005; 1807–16.

Fauser BC, Devroey P, Yen SS, Gosden R, Crowley WF, Jr., Baird DT et al. Minimal ovarian stimulation for IVF: appraisal of potential benefits and drawbacks. Hum Reprod 1999; 14: 2681–6.

Fauser BC, Diedrich K, Devroey P. Predictors of ovarian response: progress towards individualized treatment in ovulation induction and ovarian stimulation. Hum Reprod Update 2008; 14: 1–14.

Filicori M, Cognigni GE, Gamberini E, Parmegiani L, Troilo E, Roset B. Efficacy of low-dose human chorionic gonadotropin alone to complete controlled ovarian stimulation. Fertil Steril 2005; 84: 394–401.

Filicori M, Cognigni GE, Samara A, Melappioni S, Perri T, Cantelli B et al. The use of LH activity to drive folliculogenesis: exploring uncharted territories in ovulation induction. Hum Reprod Update 2002; 8: 543–57.

Filicori M, Cognigni GE, Taraborrelli S, Spettoli D, Ciampaglia W, de Fatis CT et al. Luteinizing hormone activity supplementation enhances follicle-stimulating hormone efficacy and improves ovulation induction outcome. J Clin Endocrinol Metab 1999; 84: 2659–63.

Fleming R, Rehka P, Deshpande N, Jamieson ME, Yates RW, Lyall H. Suppression of LH during ovarian stimulation: effects differ in cycles stimulated with purified urinary FSH and recombinant FSH. Hum Reprod 2000; 15: 1440–5.

Greb RR, Grieshaber K, Gromoll J, Sonntag B, Nieschlag E, Kiesel L et al. A common single nucleotide polymorphism in exon 10 of the human follicle stimulating hormone receptor is a major determinant of length and hormonal dynamics of the menstrual cycle. J Clin Endocrinol Metab 2005; 90: 4866–72.

Heijnen EM, Eijkemans MJ, de KC, Polinder S, Beckers NG, Klinkert ER et al. A mild treatment strategy for *in-vitro* fertilisation: a randomised non-inferiority trial. Lancet 2007; 743–9.

Heijnen EM, Macklon NS, Fauser BC. What is the most relevant standard of success in assisted reproduction? The next step to improving outcomes of IVF: consider the whole treatment. Hum Reprod 2004; 19: 1936–8.

Hohmann FP, Laven JS, de Jong FH, Eijkemans MJ, Fauser BC. Low-dose exogenous FSH initiated during the early, mid or late follicular phase can induce multiple dominant follicle development. Hum Reprod 2001; 16: 846–54.

Hohmann FP, Macklon NS, Fauser BC. A randomized comparison of two ovarian stimulation protocols with gonadotropin-releasing hormone (GnRH) antagonist cotreatment for *in vitro* fertilization commencing recombinant follicle-stimulating hormone on cycle day 2 or 5 with the standard long GnRH agonist protocol. J Clin Endocrinol Metab 2003; 88: 166–73.

Hughes EG, Fedorkow DM, Daya S, Sagle MA, Van de KP, Collins JA. The routine use of gonadotropin-releasing hormone agonists prior to *in vitro* fertilization and gamete intrafallopian transfer: a meta-analysis of randomized controlled trials. Fertil Steril 1992; 58: 888–96.

Hugues JN, Cedrin DI. Revisiting gonadotrophin-releasing hormone agonist protocols and management of poor ovarian responses to gonadotrophins. Hum Reprod Update 1998; 4: 83–101.

Huirne JA, Lambalk CB, van Loenen AC, Schats R, Hompes PG, Fauser BC et al. Contemporary pharmacological manipulation in assisted reproduction. Drugs 2004; 64: 297–322.

Huirne JA, Lambalk CB. Gonadotropin-releasing-hormone-receptor antagonists. Lancet 2001; 1793–803.

Hunault CC, Laven JS, van R, I, Eijkemans MJ, te Velde ER, Habbema JD. Prospective validation of two models predicting pregnancy leading to live birth among untreated subfertile couples. Hum Reprod 2005; 20: 1636–41.

Imani B, Eijkemans MJ, de Jong FH, Payne NN, Bouchard P, Giudice LC et al. Free androgen index and leptin are the most prominent endocrine predictors of ovarian response during clomiphene citrate induction of ovulation in normogonadotropic oligoamenorrheic infertility. J Clin Endocrinol Metab 2000; 85: 676–82.

Imani B, Eijkemans MJ, Faessen GH, Bouchard P, Giudice LC, Fauser BC. Prediction of the individual follicle-stimulating hormone threshold for gonadotropin induction of ovulation in normogonadotropic anovulatory infertility: an approach to increase safety and efficiency. Fertil Steril 2002; 77: 83–90.

Imani B, Eijkemans MJ, te Velde ER, Habbema JD, Fauser BC. Predictors of patients remaining anovulatory during clomiphene citrate induction of ovulation in normogonadotropic oligoamenorrheic infertility. J Clin Endocrinol Metab 1998; 83: 2361–5.

Katz-Jaffe MG, Trounson AO, Cram DS. Chromosome 21 mosaic human preimplantation embryos predominantly arise from diploid conceptions. Fertil Steril 2005; 84: 634–43.

Kligman I, Rosenwaks Z. Differentiating clinical profiles: predicting good responders, poor responders, and hyperresponders. Fertil Steril 2001; 76: 1185–90.

Klinkert ER, Broekmans FJ, Looman CW, Habbema JD, te Velde ER. Expected poor responders on the basis of an antral follicle count do not benefit from a higher starting dose of gonadotrophins in IVF treatment: a randomized controlled trial. Hum Reprod 2005; 20: 611–5.

Koichi K, Yukiko N, Shima K, Sachiko S. Efficacy of low-dose human chorionic gonadotropin (hCG) in a GnRH antagonist protocol. J Assist Reprod Genet 2006; 23: 223–8.

Kol S, Lightman A, Hillensjo T, Devroey P, Fauser B, Tarlatzis B et al. High doses of gonadotrophin-releasing hormone antagonist in *in-vitro* fertilization cycles do not adversely affect the outcome of subsequent freeze-thaw cycles. Hum Reprod 1999; 14: 2242–4.

Kolibianakis EM, Collins J, Tarlatzis BC, Devroey P, Diedrich K, Griesinger G. Among patients treated for IVF with gonadotrophins and GnRH analogues, is the probability of live birth dependent on the type of analogue used? A systematic review and meta-analysis. Hum Reprod Update 2006; 12: 651–71.

Kolibianakis EM, Kalogeropoulou L, Griesinger G, Papanikolaou EG, Papadimas J, Bontis J et al. Among patients treated with FSH and GnRH analogues for *in vitro* fertilization, is the addition of recombinant LH associated with the probability of live birth? A systematic review and meta-analysis. Hum Reprod Update 2007; 13: 445–52.

Kolibianakis EM, Zikopoulos K, Schiettecatte J, Smitz J, Tournaye H, Camus M et al. Profound LH suppression after GnRH antagonist administration is associated with a significantly higher ongoing pregnancy rate in IVF. Hum Reprod 2004; 19: 2490–6.

Laven JS, Imani B, Eijkemans MJ, Fauser BC. New approach to polycystic ovary syndrome and other forms of anovulatory infertility. Obstet Gynecol Surv 2002; 57: 755–67.

Lundin K, Bergh C. Cumulative impact of adding frozen-thawed cycles to single versus double fresh embryo transfers. Reprod Biomed Online 2007; 15: 76–82.

Macklon NS, Stouffer RL, Giudice LC, Fauser BC. The science behind 25 years of ovarian stimulation for *in vitro* fertilization. Endocr Rev 2006; 27: 170–207.

Mahdavi A, Pejovic T, Nezhat F. Induction of ovulation and ovarian cancer: a critical review of the literature. Fertil Steril 2006; 85: 819–26.

Mannaerts B, Shoham Z, Schoot D, Bouchard P, Harlin J, Fauser B et al. Single-dose pharmacokinetics and pharmacodynamics of recombinant human follicle-stimulating hormone (Org 32489*) in gonadotropin-deficient volunteers. Fertil Steril 1993; 59: 108–14.

Munne S, Magli C, Adler A, Wright G, de BK, Mortimer D et al. Treatment-related chromosome abnormalities in human embryos. Hum Reprod 1997; 12: 780–4.

Nargund G, Fauser BC, Macklon NS, Ombelet W, Nygren K, Frydman R. The ISMAAR proposal on terminology for ovarian stimulation for IVF. Hum Reprod 2007; 22: 2801–4.

Nargund G, Waterstone J, Bland J, Philips Z, Parsons J, Campbell S. Cumulative conception and live birth rates in natural (unstimulated) IVF cycles. Hum Reprod 2001; 16: 259–62.

Olivius K, Friden B, Lundin K, Bergh C. Cumulative probability of live birth after three in vitro fertilization/intracytoplasmic sperm injection cycles. Fertil Steril 2002; 77: 505–10.

Osmanagaoglu K, Tournaye H, Camus M, Vandervorst M, Van SA, Devroey P. Cumulative delivery rates after intracytoplasmic sperm injection: 5 year follow-up of 498 patients. Hum Reprod 1999; 14: 2651–5.

Out HJ, Mannaerts BM, Driessen SG, Bennink HJ. A prospective, randomized, assessor-blind, multicentre study comparing recombinant and urinary follicle stimulating hormone (Puregon versus Metrodin) in in-vitro fertilization. Hum Reprod 1995; 10: 2534–40.

Pache TD, Wladimiroff JW, de Jong FH, Hop WC, Fauser BC. Growth patterns of nondominant ovarian follicles during the normal menstrual cycle. Fertil Steril 1990; 54: 638–42.

Pantos K, Meimeth-Damianaki T, Vaxevanoglou T, Kapetanakis E. Prospective study of a modified gonadotropin-releasing hormone agonist long protocol in an in vitro fertilization program. Fertil Steril 1994; 61: 709–13.

Pelinck MJ, Hoek A, Simons AH, Heineman MJ. Efficacy of natural cycle IVF: a review of the literature. Hum Reprod Update 2002; 8: 129–39.

Pelinck MJ, Vogel NE, Arts EG, Simons AH, Heineman MJ, Hoek A. Cumulative pregnancy rates after a maximum of nine cycles of modified natural cycle IVF and analysis of patient drop-out: a cohort study. Hum Reprod 2007; 22: 2463–70.

Pennings G, Ombelet W. Coming soon to your clinic: patient-friendly ART. Hum Reprod 2007; 22: 2075–9.

Propst AM, Bates GW, Robinson RD, Arthur NJ, Martin JE, Neal GS. A randomized controlled trial of increasing recombinant follicle-stimulating hormone after initiating a gonadotropin-releasing hormone antagonist for in vitro fertilization-embryo transfer. Fertil Steril 2006; 86: 58–63.

Schenker JG, Ezra Y. Complications of assisted reproductive techniques. Fertil Steril 1994; 61: 411–22.

Schipper I, Hop WC, Fauser BC. The follicle-stimulating hormone (FSH) threshold/window concept examined by different interventions with exogenous FSH during the follicular phase of the normal menstrual cycle: duration, rather than magnitude, of FSH increase affects follicle development. J Clin Endocrinol Metab 1998; 83: 1292–8.

Serafini P, Yadid I, Motta EL, Alegretti JR, Fioravanti J, Coslovsky M. Ovarian stimulation with daily late follicular phase administration of low-dose human chorionic gonadotropin for in vitro fertilization: a prospective, randomized trial. Fertil Steril 2006; 86: 830–8.

Smitz J, Devroey P, Camus M, Khan I, Staessen C, Van WL et al. Addition of buserelin to human menopausal gonadotrophins in patients with failed stimulations for IVF or GIFT. Hum Reprod 1988; 3 (Suppl 2): 35–8.

Sullivan MW, Stewart-Akers A, Krasnow JS, Berga SL, Zeleznik AJ. Ovarian responses in women to recombinant follicle-stimulating hormone and luteinizing hormone (LH): a role for LH in the final stages of follicular maturation. J Clin Endocrinol Metab 1999; 84: 228–32.

Sykes D, Out HJ, Palmer SJ, van LJ. The cost-effectiveness of IVF in the UK: a comparison of three gonadotrophin treatments. Hum Reprod 2001; 16: 2557–62.

Tarlatzis BC, Fauser BC, Kolibianakis EM, Diedrich K, Rombauts L, Devroey P. GnRH antagonists in ovarian stimulation for IVF. Hum Reprod Update 2006; 12: 333–40.

Tarlatzis BC, Zepiridis L, Grimbizis G, Bontis J. Clinical management of low ovarian response to stimulation for IVF: a systematic review. Hum Reprod Update 2003; 9: 61–76.

Templeton A, Morris JK. Reducing the risk of multiple births by transfer of two embryos after in vitro fertilization. N Engl J Med 1998; 339: 573–7.

van der Gaast MH, Eijkemans MJ, van der Net JB, de Boer EJ, Burger CW, van Leeuwen FE et al. Optimum number of oocytes for a successful first IVF treatment cycle. Reprod Biomed Online 2006; 13: 476–80.

van Hooff MH, Alberda AT, Huisman GJ, Zeilmaker GH, Leerentveld RA. Doubling the human menopausal gonadotrophin dose in the course of an in-vitro fertilization treatment cycle in low responders: a randomized study. Hum Reprod 1993; 8: 369–73.

van Rooij, IA, Broekmans FJ, te Velde ER, Fauser BC, Bancsi LF, de Jong FH et al. Serum anti-Mullerian hormone levels: a novel measure of ovarian reserve. Hum Reprod 2002; 17: 3065–71.

van Santbrink EJ, Eijkemans MJ, Macklon NS, Fauser BC. FSH response-dose can be predicted in ovulation induction for normogonadotropic anovulatory infertility. Eur J Endocrinol 2002; 147: 223–6.

van Santbrink EJ, Hop WC, van Dessel TJ, de Jong FH, Fauser BC. Decremental follicle-stimulating hormone and dominant follicle development during the normal menstrual cycle. Fertil Steril 1995; 64: 37–43.

Verberg MF, Macklon NS, Heijnen EM, Fauser BC. ART: iatrogenic multiple pregnancy? Best Pract Res Clin Obstet Gynaecol 2007; 21: 129–43.

Westergaard LG, Laursen SB, Andersen CY. Increased risk of early pregnancy loss by profound suppression of luteinizing hormone during ovarian stimulation in normogonadotrophic women undergoing assisted reproduction. Hum Reprod 2000; 15: 1003–8.

Zeleznik AJ, Hutchison JS, Schuler HM. Interference with the gonadotropin-suppressing actions of estradiol in macaques overrides the selection of a single preovulatory follicle. Endocrinology 1985; 117: 991–9.

Zeleznik AJ, Kubik CJ. Ovarian responses in macaques to pulsatile infusion of follicle-stimulating hormone (FSH) and luteinizing hormone: increased sensitivity of the maturing follicle to FSH. Endocrinology 1986; 119: 2025–32.

Zwart-van Rijkom JE, Broekmans FJ, Leufkens HG. From HMG through purified urinary FSH preparations to recombinant FSH: a substitution study. Hum Reprod 2002; 17: 857–65.

3 The Psychological Burden of the Subfertile Couple

J. Boivin

School of Psychology, Cardiff University, Psychology Building, Cardiff CF10 3 AT, Wales, U.K.

Abstract

The psychological burden of infertility is due to the childlessness itself and the steps taken to resolve it (mainly medical treatment). The challenges of medical treatment are varied. At the start of treatment, not knowing when to get medical help and fear or misconceptions about what can be done to help people with fertility problems are the main psychological issues to be addressed. In treatment the major challenges are to cope with the uncertainty of whether treatment will be effective and to stay in treatment long enough to achieve success. Staying in treatment mainly depends on effective stress management and coping skills. Treatment failure is associated with significant emotional distress and decisional conflict about what to do next with respect to the project of having a child. Decision-making and support interventions would be usefully applied here. Although the transition to parenthood is somewhat different for people with previous infertility the differences are minor. The cognitive, emotional and physical development of children conceived with medical interventions is not appreciably different from that of naturally conceived children. Couples who do not conceive with treatment will experience a transition period to non-parenthood and this period can be emotionally demanding for the individual and taxing to the couple relationship. However, once couples feel they have done enough to achieve a pregnancy, they can usually end unsuccessful treatment with "peace of mind" and move on to other life pursuits and achieve good life satisfaction.

3.1 Introduction

The discovery of a fertility problem is a major psychological challenge to most people because most want to have children at some point in their lives (Lampic et al., 2006). Infertility secondary to thyroid disease is no different from infertility due to reproductive disease and empirical findings from other infertile couples will help to understand reactions and psychological processes people affected by thyroid disease could face. The psychological burden of infertility consists of challenges due to childlessness itself and (where applicable) to fertility medical interventions. As the field of psychological aspects of infertility is substantial, this review is neither exhaustive nor comprehensive but is sufficient to show the major challenges people with thyroid disease are likely to face with some guidance about interventions that can minimise distress and help people face these challenges. For more in-depth reviews the reader is directed to other sources (Bovin, 2003; Greil, 1997; Eugster and Vingerhoets, 1999; Hahn, 2001; Verhaak et al., 2007).

3.2 Impact of Childlessness

Becoming a parent is a major life goal and a key framework for the organisation of one's life. Most people want and eventually do have children (Lampic et al., 2006), most do so in their mid to late twenties (United Nations, 2007) and most report deep satisfaction at having reached this developmental life goal (van Balen et al., 1997). Although the demographics of parenting are changing both in the later timing of parenthood (Bakeo, 2004) and the fewer number of children per couple (United Nations, 2007), nevertheless most still plan their lives around the project to have a family, for example, in their choice of life mate (Robinson et al., 1987), timing of specific life events (career changes, travel) and expectations of what will happen to them later in life (e.g., spending time with grandchildren; having children take care of them) (van Balen, 2005). Discovering a fertility problem is therefore not only a threat to the deeply desired goal of parenting but also to how people envisaged structuring their lives.

There is a multitude of studies showing that any diagnosis of infertility is associated with significant emotional distress in the form of depressive symptoms, grief reactions and anger and frustration (Greil, 1997). Childlessness can also put significant strain on social relationships either because others do not understand what the couple is going through (Peronace et al., 2007) or because the couple eventually isolate themselves from fertile family and friends (Wischmann, 2008). Partnerships are affected in a variety of ways. Most studies show that going through the experience of infertility brings the couple closer together and strengthens marital commitment (Hammarberg et al., 2001). However, there will be times of significant disagreement, mainly about treatment decisions (Daniluk, 2001b) and strain caused by gender differences in how men and women cope with emotional and threatening life events (Berg et al., 1991). Although the individual and couple will go through a period of great turmoil, couples eventually do survive these experiences (Verhaak et al., 2007) and most not only achieve a high life satisfaction (Hammarberg et al., 2001) but also find benefit in having gone through this experience, mainly in recognising their own strength and that of their partnership (Brew, 2002).

3.3   Psychological Challenges of Initiating Medical Treatment

Entering and staying in medical interventions long enough to conceive is a complex psychological undertaking. Given that most people want children at some point in their lives one would expect that most would also seek medical advice if they suspected a fertility problem. In reality only about 55% of couples currently experiencing infertility (i.e., at least 12 months unprotected intercourse without conception) seek any kind of medical advice about failure to conceive and, importantly, this percentage remains constant irrespective of access to care or financial resources (Boivin et al., 2007). Although some research shows that attempts to conceive could be thwarted by ambivalence toward having children (Stoleru et al., 1993) this is not the main reason for poor uptake of medical interventions.

Two factors interact to produce unexpectedly low rates of treatment seeking (Bunting and Boivin, 2007). First, individuals need to perceive that they are at risk for a fertility problem but they have no easy way of knowing that. In most areas of health, risk awareness is dependent on symptoms or signs of disease, for example, finding a breast lump or experiencing significant chest pain, and these symptoms act as cues to action. The main symptom of fertility problems is not conceiving after trying for a period of time. There is ambiguity as people are not clear about how long they should wait before the lack of conception is indicative of a genuine fertility problem that warrants medical attention (Bunting and Boivin, 2007). The lack of clear signs and symptoms makes it difficult for people to know when they ought to get help. In a recent online study of well-educated women, 20% had not yet sought medical advice even though they had been trying for more than 24 months and they did not feel very confident that they could conceive on their own (Bunting and Boivin, 2007).

A second factor that contributes to lower than expected seeking of medical advice is fear (Bunting and Boivin, 2007). People who do suspect a fertility problem are fearful about being given this diagnosis. From the online research one could not say what this fear was about but the pattern of results suggested that people were fearful they would be told that nothing could be done to help them conceive since one difference with those who had sought advice was greater faith that medical intervention could redress any problem detected. These results would be in line with those found in other health contexts that suggest that delay in seeking help is often due to misconceptions about the effectiveness of treatment (see Rosenstock, 1990). Fear could additionally be due to the significant stigma attached to having a diagnosis of infertility, as perceived by oneself or others. If great meaning is attached to having children in relation to ones identity and ones place in the community (United Nations, 2007) then a diagnosis of infertility could be so threatening that one would prefer not discovering it at all.

3.4   Psychological Aspects of Undergoing Medical Intervention

Couples are likely to undergo different forms of treatment from first-stage therapies of ovulation induction and/or intrauterine insemination (IUI) to more complex interventions of *in vitro* fertilisation/intracytoplasmic sperm injection (hereafter referred to as IVF). Treatments may also be differentiated according to whether individuals and couples need a donor or gestational surrogate for conception. All these factors determine the fine detail of psychological issues and what can be done to minimise the burden of treatment. In this section the focus is on psychological reactions to IVF using own gametes as this concerns by far the people most commonly sampled in research but these findings are more or less applicable to other treatments. However, for more detailed information on psychological aspects and counselling in third party reproduction the reader is referred to Boivin and Kentenich (2002) and Covington and Hammer-Burns (2006) for guidelines in infertility counselling.

There are well-established findings concerning reactions to fertility treatment. First, emotional, physical and social reactions to fertility treatment vary across the cycle in line with the practical demands and psychological challenges of each stage of treatment (Boivin and Takefman, 1996). Thus fatigue is highest when practical demands are highest (i.e., during stimulation, when attending for scans or blood tests); physical reactions are highest when fertility drugs exert their greatest influence (i.e., peak breast tenderness and ovarian pain at oocyte retrieval); optimism is highest when people feel they have a good chance or opportunity to conceive (i.e., initiation of treatment, embryo transfer); need for social support is greatest when people expect results and/or feel distressed (i.e., just before the pregnancy test, after a failed cycle). In general there is a cyclic pattern to stress reactions with a gradual anticipatory increase just before results of a treatment stage are given (just before retrieval, embryo transfer, pregnancy test) with a gradual decrease when couples know whether it was successful (or conversely increase if unsuccessful). The two-week implantation period and finding out that IVF was not successful are rated as the most stressful (Connolly et al., 1993).

A second consistent finding is that unsuccessful treatment is associated with an acute period of depression, elevated anxiety, anger and frustration and a variety of other reactions, including suicidal thoughts (Newton et al., 1990) that can persist for more than 5 weeks in about 20% of patients (Litt et al., 1990). Despite these negative effects, an important percentage of women report that participation in the IVF program did bring some benefits, especially with regard to satisfaction that they had tried all medical options available ["for later peace of mind" (Daniluk, 2001b)] and greater closeness to their spouse (Brew,

2002). Third, results converge to show that the main difference in reactions between men and women is in intensity of reactions to IVF rather than in kind since men have a similar pattern of reactions (Boivin et al., 1998). Finally, an emerging finding is that psychological factors are a principle cause of premature dropout in IVF (Smeenk et al., 2004). People who start IVF with higher levels of depression and those who find treatment a psychological burden tend to end treatment prematurely despite having the resources to access treatment and a good prognosis (Olivius et al., 2004).

3.5 The Experience of Pregnancy and Parenting in Couples Conceiving with Assisted Reproductive Techniques

Concern about the long-term development of children born following IVF has been expressed for a number of reasons, including effects due to: obstetric risks linked to IVF (e.g., increased multiple birth rate, prematurity and low birth weight); psychological issues (e.g., difficulties in the transition to parenthood, over-protectiveness, effects of secrecy in the use of donor gametes); effects due to the IVF process itself (e.g., use of culture media, cryopreservation) and so on. Causes of concern have not materialised into actual problems for the children and families.

As a 'hard-to-achieve-pregnancy', previously infertile couples consider their pregnancy as an exceptional event (Sandelowski et al., 1991). Previously infertile women tend to worry more about events that may threaten the pregnancy and a live birth (e.g., miscarriage, labour complications) compared to never infertile women who worry more about the effect of pregnancy on body shape and attractiveness (Leiblum et al., 1990). In addition, previously infertile women tend to delay telling others about the pregnancy and delay preparing the home for the arrival of the child so as not to 'jinx' the pregnancy (Olshansky, 1990). In this respect, previously infertile women are similar to other women whose pregnancy is high risk for other reasons (e.g., genetic conditions) (Reading et al., 1989). However, such cautiousness does not appear to affect the maternal-foetal bond since previously infertile women do not differ from other women in their attachment to the foetus (McMahon et al., 1997). Men are less affected by prior fertility status than are women although they too consider the pregnancy as a more exceptional event than do never infertile men (McMahon et al., 1997).

3.6   Parenting Style and Child Development in Couples Conceiving with Assisted Reproductive Techniques

During infancy (up to 18 months after the birth of the child) previously infertile men and women report some differences in their experiences compared to couples who had conceived naturally but there are no consistent findings of deficits and differences mainly concerning higher levels of anxiety about taking up the parenting role in IVF mothers (Golombok, 2002). Follow-up studies with children of older age, 4 to 8 years old, show that previously infertile women as compared to their never infertile counterparts show less negative affect and parenting stress and show more maternal confidence than their fertile counterparts (Abbey et al., 1994). Moreover, they have more frequent interactions with their children and tend to be warmer and more emotionally involved with their children (Golombok et al., 1996). There are fewer differences between previously and never infertile fathers although previously infertile men report greater home stress and less intimacy with their partner (Abbey et al., 1994).

There is almost universal agreement that child development is not affected by IVF technology or knowledge that conception has taken place using this technique (Rice, 2006). Children show the same psychological and intellectual development as age-matched control children conceived naturally or conceived with other non-IVF fertility treatments. School performance among IVF children is also comparable to children conceived naturally. Children conceived with IVF could not be distinguished from other children on emotional development, behaviour or in their relationship with parents in a large study (Golombok, 2002).

3.7   Long-Term Adjustment in Couples that do not Conceive with Medical Intervention

Research shows that couples who do not conceive with treatment fare well; they can achieve a contented life and can interpret their infertility experience in terms of its positive impact on their life, for example, on their commitment as a couple and personal psychological growth (Brew, 2002; Daniluk, 2001b). Despite this positive growth, the sadness of infertility is not entirely forgotten and this traumatic life experience does continue to have effects. For example, studies have shown that many years post-treatment women still report intrusive thoughts about their fertility (Sundby, 1992) and still report fertility problem stress (Abbey et al., 1994), even though their overall life satisfaction is good (Verhaak et al., 2007).

Concern over being able to achieve a contented life after medical intervention can impact on decision-making about when to end treatment. The hope produced by being in treatment keeps at bay the full sorrow of never having your own children. Daniluk (2001a) proposed that one of the main factors preventing couples from ending treatment is the fear that such feelings will be overwhelming and impossible to cope with. Although the transition to non-parenthood is distressing, it is manageable and couples will move from being certain that they want further treatments, to being ambivalent about the biological, psychological, social and financial costs, to eventually being comfortable in their decision to end treatment. The acceptability of ending treatment will vary as a function of where couples find themselves in this transition process.

A further concern is that for many couples the basis for committing to a relationship is the eventuality of forming a family with children. The end of treatment may cause people to question the basis for their marriage. Furthermore, the diagnosed partner may have fears that their partner may not wish to continue in a childless relationship. Strauss et al. (1998) found that couples that felt their union would be threatened by a lack of children were the ones most likely to persist with treatment and/or be reluctant to end treatment. Thus, the end of treatment may trigger marital issues that have lain dormant or threaten the viability of the marriage. However, positive marital growth is one of the most commonly reported benefits of the experience and hardship of infertility, suggesting that contrary to popular fear most relationships are made stronger as a result of this negative life event (Hammarberg et al., 2001).

3.8   Interventions for Infertile Couples

Given the significant distress couples can experience prior to, during and after IVF, the use of psychological interventions seems warranted. In fact, the code of practice developed by the Human Fertilisation and Embryology Authority (HFEA) that regulates IVF in the U.K. stipulates that psychosocial counselling *must* be offered to any patient seeking IVF and such legislation has been adopted in other countries too (e.g., Canada). As described in the HFEA code of practice, the purpose of counselling is to provide IVF patients with emotional support in times of crisis and to help patients come to terms with their infertility and cope with its effect on their lives. In the early days of *in vitro* fertilisation pre-screening for psychological robustness was advocated but as IVF becomes part of the mainstream approach to reproductive medicine, most practitioners shy away from taking a gatekeeper role.

Different types of psychological interventions have been proposed and evaluated (Boivin, 2003; de Liz and Strauss, 2005). Couple interventions are devoted to help express reactions to infertility and discuss the effect of infertility on various domains of well-being, for example, the impact of infertility on marital and sexual relations. Group interventions are more comprehensive and use structured programmes that provide methods for emotional expression, new ways of thinking about fertility problems, relaxation training, nutrition and exercise, and group support – all as they apply to infertility (e.g., Domar et al., 2002). Finally brief coping interventions focus on providing very specific skills to cope with infertility, for example increasing active coping skills or increasing autonomy through the acquisition of treatment specific information.

The main task of the mental health professional embedded in fertility clinics is to maximise goodness-of-fit among patient need, the demands of the situation and available psychological interventions. The psychological challenges for a couple facing permanent childlessness after years of medical treatment are substantially different from those of a young couple beginning their first course of treatment or a couple wondering whether they have a problem in the first place and, accordingly, will require different types of interventions. Maximising goodness of fit is relevant because it may make the difference between producing a psychological effect or not and of positively influencing health outcomes (pregnancy) and avoiding premature treatment dropout.

References

Abbey A, Andrews FM, Halman LJ. Infertility and parenthood: Does becoming a parent increase well-being? J Consul Clin Psychol, 1994; 62: 398 – 403.

Bakeo AC. Trends in live births by mother's country of birth and other factors affecting low birthweight in England and Wales, 1983 – 2001. Health Stat Q 2004; 23: 25 – 33.

Berg BJ, Wilson JF, Weingartner PJ. Psychological sequelae of infertility treatment: The role of gender and sex-role identification. Soc Sci Med 1991; 33: 1071 – 80.

Boivin J. A review of psychosocial interventions in infertility. Soc Sci Med 2003; 57: 2325 – 41.

Boivin J, Andersson L, Shoog-Svanberg A, Hjelmstedt A, Collins A, Bergh T. Psychological reactions during *in vitro* fertilization (IVF): Similar response pattern in husbands and wives. Hum Reprod 1998; 13: 3262 – 7.

Boivin J, Bunting L, Collins JA, Nygren K. An international estimate of infertility prevalence and treatment-seeking: Potential need and demand for infertility medical care. Hum Reprod 2007; 22: 1506 – 12.

Boivin J, Kentenich H. ESHRE Monographs: Guidelines for counselling in infertility. London: Oxford University Press: 2002.

Boivin J, Takefman J. The impact of the *in-vitro* fertilization-embryo transfer (IVF-ET) process on emotional, physical and relational variables. Hum Reprod 1996; 11: 903 – 7.

Brew T. Benefit finding in women's lives following unsuccessful infertility treatment. Dissertation. Cardiff: Cardiff University, 2002.

Bunting L, Boivin J. Decision-making about seeking medical advice in an internet sample of women trying to get pregnant. Hum Reprod 2007; 22: 1662 – 8.

Connolly KJ, Edelmann RJ, Bartlett H, Cooke ID, Lenton E, Pike S. An evaluation of counselling for couples undergoing treatment for *in-vitro* fertilization. Hum Reprod 1993; 8: 1332 – 8.

Covington SN, Hammer-Burns L. Infertility counselling: a comprehensive handbook for clinicians. 2nd edition. Cambridge University Press; 2006.

Daniluk JC. The Infertility Survival Guide. California: New Harbinger Publications, 2001a.

Daniluk JC. Reconstructing their lives: A longitudinal, qualitative, analysis of the transition to biological childlessness for infertile couples. J Counsel Devel 2001b; 79: 439 – 49.

de Liz TM, Strauss B. Differential efficacy of group and individual/couple psychotherapy with infertile patients. Hum Reprod 2005; 20: 1324–32.

Domar AD, Clapp D, Slawsby EA, Dusek J, Kessel B, Freizinger M. Impact of group psychological interventions. Fertil Steril 2002; 73: 805–11.

Eugster A, Vingerhoets AJJM. Psychological aspects of *in vitro* fertilisation: A review. Soc Sci Med 1999; 48: 575–89.

Golombok S. Parenting and the psychological development of the child in ART families. In Vayena E, Rowe PJ, Griffin PD (Eds.). Current practices & controversies in assisted reproduction: Report of a WHO meeting, 2001: Geneva, Switzerland, 2002.

Golombok S, Brewaeys A, Cook R, Giavazzi MT, Guerra D, Mantovani A, van Hall E, Crosignani PG, Dexeus S. The European study of assisted reproduction families: family functioning and child development. Hum Reprod 1996; 11: 2324–31.

Greil AL. Infertility and psychological distress: A critical review of the literature. Soc Sci Med 1997; 45: 1679–704.

Hahn S-C. Review: Psychosocial well-being of parents and their children born after assisted reproduction. J Pediatr Psychol 2001; 26: 525–38.

Hammarberg K, Astbury K, Baker HWG. Women's experience of IVF: A follow-up study. Hum Reprod, 2001; 16: 374–82.

Lampic C, Svanberg AS, Karlström P, Tydén T. Fertility awareness, intentions concerning childbearing, and attitudes towards parenthood among female and male academics. Hum Reprod 2006; 21: 558–64.

Leiblum SR, Kemmann E, Taska L. Attitudes toward multiple births and pregnancy concerns in infertile and non-infertile women. J Psychosom Obstet Gynaecol 1990; 11: 197–210.

Litt MD, Tennen H, Affleck G, Klock S. Coping and cognitive factors in adaptation to *in vitro* fertilization failure. J Behav Med 1990; 15: 171–87.

McMahon CA, Ungerer JA, Tennant CC, Saunders, DM. Psychosocial adjustment and the quality of the mother-child relationship at four months postpartum after conception by *in vitro* fertilisation. Fertil Steril 1997; 68: 492–500.

Newton CR, Hearn MT, Yuzpe AA. Psychological assessment and follow-up after *in vitro* fertilization: Assessing the impact of failure. Fertil Steril 1990; 54: 879–86.

Olivius C, Friden B, Borg G, Bergh B. Why do couples discontinue *in vitro* fertilization treatment? A cohort study. Fertil Steril 2004; 81: 258–61.

Olshansky EF. Psychosocial implication of pregnancy after infertility. Clin Issue Perinat Womens Health Nurs 1990; 1: 342–7.

Peronace LA, Boivin J, Schmidt L. Patterns of suffering and social interactions in infertile men: 12 months after unsuccessful treatment. J Psychosom Obstet Gynaecol 2007; 28: 105–14.

Reading AE, Chang LC, Kerin JF. Attitudes and anxiety levels in women conceiving through *in vitro* fertilization and gamete intrafallopian transfer. Fertil Steril 1989; 52: 95–9.

Rice F. Follow-up of children conceived with fertility treatment. Paper presented at the 22nd Annual Meeting of the European Society for Human Reproduction and Embryology. What is new? Where are we going? Special Interest Group Psychology and Counselling. June 2006; Prague.

Robinson GE, Garner DM, Gare DJ, Crawford B. Psychological adaptation to pregnancy in childless women more than 35 years of age. Am J Obstet Gynecol 1987; 156: 328–33.

Rosenstock I The health belief model: explaining health behavior through expectancies. In: Health Behavior and Health Education. Edited by Glanz K, Lewis FM, Rimers B, San Francisco, CA, Jossey-Bass 1990.

Sandelowski M, Harris BG, Holditch-Davis D. Amniocentesis in the context of infertility. Health Care Women Int 1991; 12: 167–178

Smeenk JMJ, Verhaak CM, Stolwijk AM, Kremer JAM, Braat DDM. Reasons for dropout in an *in vitro* fertilization/intracytoplasmic sperm injection program. Fertil Steril 2004; 81: 262–8.

Stoleru S, Teglas JP, Fermanian J, Spira A. Psychological factors in the aetiology of infertility: a prospective cohort study. Hum Reprod 1993; 8: 1039–1046.

Strauss B, Hepp U, Staeding G, Mettler L. Psychological characteristics of infertile couples: Can they predict pregnancy and treatment persistence. J Comm Appl Soc Psychol 1998; 8: 289–301.

Sundby JS. Long-term psychological consequences of infertility: a follow-up study of former patients. J Women Health 1992; 1: 209–217.

United Nations, Department of Economic and Social Affairs, Population Division (2007). World Population Prospects: The 2006 Revision, Highlights, Working Paper No. ESA/P/WP.202.

van Balen F, Verdurmen J, Ketting E. Choices and motivations of infertile couples. Patient Educ Couns 1997; 31: 19–27.

van Balen F. Late parenthood among subfertile and fertile couples: motivations and educational goals. Patient Educ Couns 2005; 59: 276–282.

Verhaak CM, Smeenk JMJ, Evers AWM, Kremer JAM, Kraaimaat FW, Braat DDM. Women's emotional adjustment to IVF: a systematic review of 25 years of research. Hum Reprod Update 2007; 13: 27–36.

Wischmann T. Implications of psychosocial support in infertility – a critical appraisal. J Psychosom Obstet Gynaecol 2008; 29: 83–90.

4   Thyroid Function and Assisted Reproduction

K. Poppe[1]*, D. Glinoer[2], H. Tournaye[3], P. Devroey[3], J. Schiettecatte[3], B. Velkeniers[1]

[1] Department of Endocrinology, Universitair Ziekenhuis Brussel, Free University Brussels (VUB), Laarbeeklaan 101, 1090 Brussels-Belgium
[2] Department of Endocrinology, Université Libre de Bruxelles, CHU Saint-Pierre; Hoogstraat, 322; 1000 Brussels, Belgium
[3] Centre for Reproductive Medicine, Universitair Ziekenhuis Brussel (VUB) and Biostatistics (VUB) Laarbeeklaan 101, 1090 Brussels, Belgium

Abstract

Thyroid hormones are in continuous interaction with other (mainly sexual) hormones to preserve a normal menstrual pattern. An optimal thyroid function is thus necessary to obtain normal fertility, but despite this, 10 to 15 % of women remain childless after one year of unprotected intercourse. After the work-up of the infertility cause (s), a proposal for treatment is given to the couple, with a realistic prognosis regarding the outcome. Only when ovulation induction (OI), endoscopic alleviation of tubal obstruction or endometriosis and intrauterine insemination fails, will assisted reproduction technology (ART) be proposed. The preparation for an ART procedure is the so-called controlled ovarian hyperstimulation (COH) which leads to high oestradiol levels before and during the very early stages of pregnancy. This increase in oestradiol levels depends on the type and the duration of COH and leads on its turn to an increase in thyroxine-binding globulin (TBG) levels. The alteration in thyroid function after COH is persistent in women with associated thyroid autoimmunity (TAI) compared to that in women without. Thyroid hormonal changes after COH are comparable according to the outcome of the assisted pregnancies, when women are free of thyroid diseases. When COH becomes pathological it is called an ovarian hyperstimulation syndrome (OHSS); this is characterised by even higher oestradiol levels compared to those obtained in a normal COH setting. When OHSS occurs in a woman with TAI the changes in thyroid function are very important, necessitating an important adjustment in LT_4 dosage. Since thyroid function has an impact on normal reproduction, COH has an impact on thyroid function and the essential role of thyroid function during pregnancy, we advise to screen systematically for thyroid function and autoimmunity in women of infertile couples. Furthermore, follow-up of these parameters is advised when TAI was initially present.

4.1   Introduction

Thyroid hormones are in close interplay with both oestrogens and progesterone to preserve a normal uterine receptivity, and maturation of the oocytes. The impact of thyroid hormones has been reported to be direct through thyroid hormone receptors on the ovaries and indirect through an impact on the secretion of SHBG, PRL and LHRH. Sufficient levels of thyroid hormones and a normaly functioning immune system are thus necessary to obtain normal fertility (Jones et al., 2004). Thyroid autoimmunity (TAI) is the most frequent cause of hypothyroidism in women of reproductive age and links thus both the immunological and the endocrine systems in it (Hollowell et al., 2002). Isolated TAI has been associated with an increased risk of first trimester miscarriage and women with hypothyroidism can experience menstrual irregularities, infertility and increased pregnancy morbidity (Poppe et al., 2007; Krassas, 2000).

Infertility is the absolute inability to conceive after 1 year of regular intercourse without contraception; the prevalence of infertility is estimated to range from 10 % to 15 % and seems to have remained stable over the past few decades (Mosher and Pratt, 1991). The cause of infertility is in 35 % of the couples a female factor (ovulatory dysfunction, endometriosis and tubal occlusion); in 30 % a male factor; in 20 % a combination of both and in

15% no cause (idiopathic infertility) can be detected (Healy et al., 1994, Schenken and Guzick, 1997; Lunenfeld and Insler, 1974). Two types of ART are currently used for infertility: in vitro fertilization (IVF) or intracytoplasmic sperm injection (ICSI) (Rosene-Montella et al., 2000; Braude and Rowell, 2003). After one cycle of ART, the live birth rate among women aged 30–35 years ranges from 25% to 30% (Osmanagaoglu et al., 2002).

COH is the preparation for an ART procedure and combines a treatment to down-regulate the pituitary gonadal axis [gonadotropin-releasing hormone (GnRH) agonists or antagonists], and stimulation of the ovaries with (r)-FSH to obtain multiple cumulus-oocyte complexes. When three or more large follicles are seen on echography, GnRH and FSH injections are discontinued and 10 000 units of hCG are given to induce ovulation (OI). Depending on the used protocol, oestradiol levels become very high and are comparable to those in the second trimester of spontaneous pregnancies (4000–6000 ng/L). The marked rise in oestrogen levels induces an additional strain on the hypothalamic-pituitary-thyroid axis and could, therefore, significantly impair thyroid hormone distribution and kinetics, especially in women with concomitant TAI (Muller et al., 2000; Poppe et al., 2004).

In about 5% of the COH procedures, this will be complicated by an ovarian hyperstimulation syndrome (OHSS). This varies clinically from a slight abdominal discomfort over abdominal and pleural effusion to a collapse (Golan et al., 1989; Papanikolaou et al., 2005). OHSS is biologically characterized by – even – higher oestradiol levels ($E_2 \geq 5000$ ng/L) before and during early pregnancy, compared to those obtained in women after an uncomplicated COH procedure. The exact aetiology of OHSS remains unknown to date.

During pregnancy, TBG levels double, which markedly increases the number of T_4 binding sites and since TBG binds around 75% of circulating T_4, thyroid hormone production will therefore be increased (Glinoer, 1997). In pregnant women with a low iodine intake, a history of TAI or thyroidectomy, the required increase in thyroid hormone production cannot always be met and can potentially lead to the development of hypothyroidism. Two studies identified the need for a rapid increase in T_4 concentrations in weeks 4–6 of pregnancy among women who had been treated previously for hypothyroidism. The timing of this need was earlier and more pronounced when

conception was achieved by ART (Davis et al., 2007; Alexander et al., 2004).

The present paper discusses the impact of high E_2 levels after COH on thyroid function in women with and without TAI, in correlation with the ART pregnancy outcome and in case of OHSS.

4.2   Impact of High E_2 Levels

In recent years several papers have been published on the essential role of maternal T_4 hormones in the placental physiology, in the early foetal development and especially in the first trimester when foetal thyroid is not yet functioning (Glinoer and Delange, 2000; Haddow et al., 1999; Morreale et al., 2004; De Felice and Di lauro, 2004). Data on thyroid hormone levels in the earliest gestational stages (i.e., before the first trimester) remain scarce. The optimal setting to investigate this is in women undergoing an ART procedure, in which the biochemical stage of pregnancy can be precisely determined.

Muller et al. (2000) were the first to perform such a study by measuring thyroid function in the period immediately after COH. They showed that, compared to the pre-COH levels, serum TSH significantly increased (2.3 ± 0.3 vs. 3.0 ± 0.4 mIU/L; $p < 0.0001$) and FT_4 decreased (14.4 ± 0.2 vs. 12.9 ± 0.2 pmol/L; $p < 0.0001$) after COH. The authors explained these changes in thyroid function by a rapid increase in oestrogen levels (359.3 ± 25.9 pmol/L vs. 3491.8 ± 298.3 pmol/L; $p < 0.0001$); and in turn TBG levels and hypersialylation (25.2 ± 0.7 vs. 33.9 ± 0.9 mg/L; $p < 0.0001$). Long-term follow-up of the thyroid hormones was not performed in this study, nor did the authors mention the timing of thyroid hormone measurement in relation to the OI, the thyroid autoimmune status or pregnancy outcome. Following this initial study, our group investigated the impact of COH on thyroid hormones during the first weeks of assisted pregnancies and compared it between women with – or without – AITD (Poppe et al., 2004). We prospectively analysed data in 35 clinically proven pregnant women, who all received the same COH procedure. Thyroid function tests (serum TSH and FT_4) and the antibody status (determined by TPO-Ab) were determined before COH and every 20 days after OI during the first trimester of pregnancy. Nine women (27%) were TAI positive. This study also showed an significant increase in serum TSH and

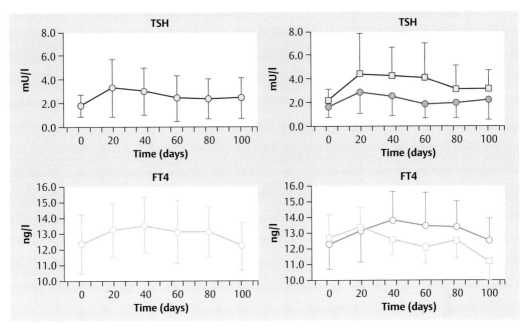

Fig. 4.**1** Evolution of thyroid function in infertile women after COH. Pattern of change over time for the TSH and FT$_4$ serum values (mean ± SD) collected before COH (time 0), and at days 20, 40, 60, 80, and 100 after OI. *Left panels*: among all patients, a significant difference exists in the TSH and FT$_4$ measured over time (TSH and FT$_4$, $p < 0.001$ and $p = 0.005$, respectively). *Right panels:* the pattern of change over time is different for TPO positive (□) and TPO negative (○) (TSH and FT$_4$, $p = 0.010$ and $p = 0.020$, respectively) patients. Modified with permission from Poppe et al. (2004).

FT$_4$ at day 20 after OI, compared with baseline values (3.3 ± 2.4 vs. 1.8 ± 0.9 mIU/L; $p < 0.0001$ and 13.2 ± 1.7 vs. 12.4 ± 1.9 ng/L; $p = 0.005$). The AUC for TSH among TAI positive women was significantly higher compared with that in TAI negative women ($p = 0.010$) and the opposite was observed for the FT$_4$ curve ($p = 0.020$); see Fig. 4.**1**.

It should be noted that already before the COH procedure, the serum TSH levels were slightly – although not significantly – higher in TAI-positive women compared to those in TAI-negative women (2.2 ± 0.9 vs. 1.6 ± 0.9 mIU/L). We concluded that COH in preparation for ART places an important strain on the maternal thyroid and also that during the first trimester (i.e., the period associated with the higher incidence of abortions) serum FT$_4$ levels are always lower in the women with TAI compared to women without TAI. In contrast to the Muller study, we could not show a drop in serum FT$_4$ two weeks after implantation. A possible explanation for this discordance might be related to differences in oestradiol levels after oocyte pick-up due to the timing of thyroid hormone measurements.

The present study supports the systematic screening of TSH, FT4, and TPO-Ab in infertile women before a COH procedure and subsequently after COH and during pregnancy when TAI was initially present.

The early pregnancy surge in FT$_4$ is mediated partially by increasing hCG levels after implantation and may therefore represent an example of a control by the endocrine system. Lower T$_4$ levels (even in the presence of normal serum TSH) could disrupt the local availability of T$_3$ to placental and foetal thyroid hormone receptors. If thyroid function is further impaired, steroid – and cytokines – actions may fail to sustain further normal early pregnancy. However, the dosage of FT$_4$ during pregnancy remains difficult, and thus the definition of what normal cut-off value is therefore difficult too. One hypothesis is thus that low T$_4$ levels may cause miscarriage and that this occurs more frequently when TAI is present.

Due to the clinical setting in both the study by Muller and that by Poppe, it was impossible to determine whether the TAI status or low FT$_4$ levels were the main determinant of the pregnancy outcome after ART. We therefore performed a prospective study in 77 women free of thyroid disorders, in order to compare thyroid function before and 2, 4 and 6 weeks after ART in a group of women with ongoing pregnancies (n = 45) and one with clinical miscarriages (n = 32; median period of miscarriage 6.7 weeks) (Poppe et al., 2005). Mean age and number of transferred embryos were similar in both groups. Free of thyroid disorders was defined as women who were not taking any thyroid hormones or antithyroid drugs and who had no TAI. Compared with baseline values, serum TSH and FT_4 increased significantly 2 weeks after ART in both the ongoing pregnancy group (TSH 2.5 ± 1.3 vs. 1.6 ± 0.8 mIU/L and FT4 13.8 ± 1.4 vs. 12.4 ± 1.8 ng/L; p < 0.0001) and in the miscarriage group (TSH 2.1 ± 1.0 vs. 1.5 ± 0.7 mIU/L and FT4 14.2 ± 2.0 vs. 12.4 ± 1.9 ng/L; p < 0.0001). When the data were analysed according to the pregnancy outcome, both the AUC for serum TSH and FT_4 were comparable even when serum hCG levels dissociated significantly 4 weeks after ART between both groups (p = 0.003). Important to note in this study is that in both outcome groups serum TSH levels (before and after ART) were always < 2.5 mIU/L. This study indirectly indicates (because all patients were TAI-negative) that it is probably the presence of TAI that primarily leads to changes in thyroid hormones after ART and potentially influences the pregnancy outcome.

Therefore, in women free of thyroid disorders no particular follow-up of thyroid function after COH is warranted, in contrast to women with TAI.

In a third part we wanted to show by means of a case report, that, when extremely high oestradiol levels are present (as it is by definition the case in the OHSS) in association with TAI, the impact on thyroid function can be extremely important as if there was an addition of both strains on thyroid function (Poppe et al., 2008).

The report relates to a 37-year-old woman with autoimmune hypothyroidism taking 125 µg LT_4 daily scheduled to undergo COH for reason of idiopathic infertility. Before COH, her serum TSH was at the upper limit of normality (3.5 mIU/L; reference value: 0.27 – 4.2) and FT_4 was normal (11.1 ng/L; reference value: 9.3 – 17.2). She was advised to increase her dose of LT_4 to 150 µg daily for at least 4 weeks before starting COH, but the patient refused this recommendation. COH consisted of 6 days orgalutran followed by 8 days treatment with Menopur 1125 IE and for the OI she received 10 000 U hCG. She developed a grade

2 (moderate) OHSS with pertinent features of abdominal discomfort and nausea. An ultrasound image showing multicystic ovaries with diameters > 10 cm and very high E_2 levels of 5.549 ng/L. The patient's pregnancy, based on hCG levels of 360 IU/L was established 14 days after hCG injection. At that moment thyroid function tests were performed, revealing a severe but asymptomatic hypothyroidism; serum TSH 41.5 mIU/L and FT_4 7.7 ng/L. The patient's LT_4 dose was increased to 200 µg daily and serum TSH decreased to 3.1 mIU/L 6 weeks after OI and to 0.1 mIU/L 8 weeks later. At the time the TSH was 0.1 mIU/L, serum hCG levels were 35 340 IU/L and the oestradiol levels declined to 1900 ng/L. The patient delivered a healthy boy to end a pregnancy of normal term length.

This increase in serum TSH can be variable according to the type and the duration of COH and is more pronounced in case of associated TAI as shown in the present case report. In a recent paper by Davis et al. (2007) for pregnant women treated with LT_4, it was advised to increase their dosage by a mean of 32 % after fertility treatment. Further studies are, however, needed to determine the exact increment in LT_4 according to that in E_2 levels.

This case report and the data on the impact of high oestrogens on thyroid function add some arguments in favour of lowering the upper TSH limit in particular clinical settings such as infertility, this in order to anticipate the possible development of clinical hypothyroidism after COH (Brabant et al., 2006). In a paper from Negro et al. (2005) it was shown that, when LT_4 was given to TAI positive women undergoing ART procedures, they had a lower serum TSH at one month of their pregnancies compared to that in women not treated and that this led to a better pregnancy outcome in terms of less miscarriages. The results were, however, not statistically significantly different, probably due to the low number of TAI-positive women included in the study. In an other paper by the same group they proved that the higher the serum TSH levels were before ART pregnancies, the more miscarriages occurred later on during pregnancy. Women with TAI had significantly higher serum TSH levels compared to women without TAI in that study Negro et al., 2007).

However, it has not been shown so far that systematically lowering the upper limit of serum TSH could have a favourable impact on the pregnancy outcome of all women undergoing an ART procedure.

Based on the data in literature and our own studies, we propose screening for thyroid function and autoimmunity in infertile women as shown in Fig. 4.**2**.

4.3 Conclusions

Thyroid function is important to maintain normal reproductive functions by interactions through several pathways. Women undergoing a COH procedure have an important increase in their oestradiol levels, leading to an additional strain on the thyroid, already before or in the very earliest stages of pregnancy. When thyroid autoimmunity is present, the impact of COH on thyroid function is more severe compared to that in women without autoimmunity. The impact on thyroid function can lead to borderline normal values of thyroid hormones depending on those before COH. The changes in thyroid hormones after COH are independent of the outcome of ART, when women do not have concomitant thyroid autoimmunity. When OHSS occurs in women with thyroid autoimmunity, tremendous changes in thyroid function leading to hypothyroidism can be observed.

We advise to screen infertile women for thyroid function and autoimmunity before a COH procedure and further during pregnancy, when TAI was initially present.

Acknowledgements

Financial support to perform all studies was provided by the Willy Gepts fonds UZ Brussel VUB.

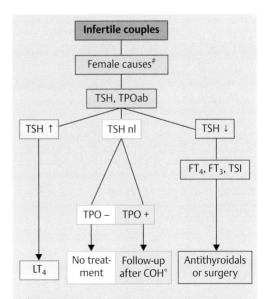

consider screening in other causes of infertility when suspicion of thyroid disorder
° consider treatment with LT4 before controlled ovarian hyperstimulation (COH), when TSH is high normal (> 2.5 mIU/l)

Fig. 4.**2** Algorithm for the screening of thyroid dysfunction and autoimmunity in infertile women. Modified with permission from Poppe et al. (2007).

References

Alexander EK Marqusee E, Lawrence J et al. Timing and magnitude of increases in levothyroxine requirements during pregnancy in women with hypothyroidism. N Engl J Med 2004; 351: 241–49.

Brabant G, Beck-Peccoz P, Jarzab B et al. Is there a need to redefine the upper normal limit of TSH? Eur J Endocrinol 2006; 154: 633–7.

Braude P, Rowell P. Assisted conception. II – in vitro fertilization and intracytoplasmic sperm injection. BMJ 2003; 327: 852–5.

Davis LB, Lathi RB, Dahan MH. The effect of infertility medication on thyroid function in hypothyroid women who conceive. Thyroid 2007; 17: 773–7.

De Felice M, Di Lauro R. Thyroid development and its disorders: genetics and molecular mechanisms. Endocr Rev 2004; 25: 722–46.

Glinoer D. The regulation of thyroid function in pregnancy: pathways of endocrine adaptation from physiology to pathology. Endocr Rev 1997; 18: 404–33.

Glinoer D, Delange F. The potential repercussions of maternal, fetal, and neonatal hypothyroxinemia on the progeny. Thyroid 2000; 10: 871–7.

Golan A, Ron-El R, Herman A et al. Ovarian hyperstimulation syndrome: an update review. Obst Gyn Survey 1989; 44: 430–40.

Haddow JE, Palomaki GE, Allan WC et al. Maternal thyroid deficiency during pregnancy and subsequent neuro-psychological development of the child. N Engl J Med 1999; 341: 549–55.

Healy DL Trounson AO, Andersen AN. Female infertility: causes and treatment. Lancet 1994; 343: 1539–44.

Hollowell JG, Staehling NW, Flanders WD et al. Serum TSH, T_4, and thyroid antibodies in the United States population (1988 to 1994): National Health and Nutrition Examination Survey (NHANES III). J Clin Endocrinol Metab 2002; 87: 489–99.

Jones RL, Hannan NJ, Kaitu'u TJ et al. Identification of chemokines important for leukocyte recruitment to the human endometrium at the times of embryo implantation and menstruation. J Clin Endocrinol Metab 2004; 89: 6155–67.

Krassas GE. Thyroid disease and female reproduction. Fertil Steril 2000; 74: 1063–70.

Lunenfeld B, Insler V. Classification of amenorrhoeic states and their treatment by ovulation induction. Clin Endocrinol 1974; 3: 223–37.

Morreale GM, Obregon MJ, Escobar del Rey FE. Maternal thyroid hormones early in pregnancy and fetal brain development. Best practice and research. J Clin Endocrinol Metab 2004; 18: 225–48.

Mosher WD, Pratt WF. Fecundity and infertility in the United States: incidence and trends. Fertil Steril 1991; 56: 192–3.

Muller AF, Verhoeff A, Mantel MJ et al. Decrease of free thyroxine levels after controlled ovarian hyperstimulation. J Clin Endocrinol Metab 2000; 85: 545–8.

Negro R, Formoso G, Coppola L et al. Euthyroid women with autoimmune disease undergoing assisted reproduction technologies: the role of autoimmunity and thyroid function. J Endocrinol Invest 2007; 30: 3–8.

Negro R, Mangieri T, Coppola L et al. Levothyroxine treatment in thyroid peroxidase antibody-positive women undergoing assisted reproduction technologies: a prospective study. Hum Reprod 2005; 20: 1529–33.

Osmanagaoglu K Tournaye H, Kolibianakis E et al. Cumulative delivery rates after ICSI in women aged > 37 years. Hum Reprod 2002; 17: 940–4.

Papanikolaou EG, Tournaye H, Verpoest W et al. Early and late ovarian hyperstimulation syndrome: early pregnancy outcome and profile. Hum Reprod 2005; 20: 636–41.

Poppe K, Glinoer D, Tournaye H et al. Impact of ovarian hyperstimulation on thyroid function in women with and without thyroid autoimmunity. J Clin Endocrinol Metab 2004; 89: 3808–12.

Poppe K, Glinoer D, Tournaye H et al. Impact of the ovarian hyperstimulation syndrome on thyroid function Thyroid 2008; 18: 801–2

Poppe K, Glinoer D, Tournaye H et al. Thyroid function after assisted reproductive technology in women free of thyroid disease. Fertil and Steril 2005; 83: 1753–7.

Poppe K, Velkeniers B, Glinoer D. Thyroid disease and female reproduction. Clin Clin Endocrinol (Oxf) 2007; 66: 309–21.

Rosene-Montella K, Keely E, Laifer SA et al. Evaluation and management of infertility in women: the internists' role. Ann Intern Med 2000; 132: 973–81.

Schenken RS, Guzick DS. Revised endometriosis classification: 1996. Fertil Steril 1997; 67: 815–6.

Session II

Thyroid Function and Pregnancy

Chairperson: G. J. Kahaly (Mainz)

5 Epidemiology and Iodine Status

M. Vanderpump

Department of Endocrinology, Royal Free Hampstead NHS Trust, London NW3 2QG, U.K.

Abstract

Pregnancy has variable effects on thyroid hormone concentrations throughout gestation as well as being associated with goitre. The latter is largely preventable by ensuring optimal iodine intake of at least 200 µg/day. Hypothyroidism in pregnancy, usually characterised by a high serum TSH value, has been found to occur in around 2–3% of otherwise normal pregnancies with the prevalence of overt hypothyroidism estimated to be up to 0.5%. On a worldwide basis the most important cause of thyroid insufficiency remains iodine deficiency whilst in iodine-replete communities the cause is usually chronic autoimmune thyroiditis. Untreated hypothyroidism may lead to obstetric complications, such as preterm delivery and foetal loss. Women who are taking thyroxine at conception will require an increase in the dose during the pregnancy. Epidemiological data suggest that the children of women with hypothyroxinaemia may have psychoneurological deficits. In classic areas of iodine deficiency, a similar range of deficits in children has been described where maternal hypothyroxinaemia rather than high thyrotrophin (TSH) is the main biochemical abnormality. In these areas, maternal iodine intake is often substantially less than the 200 µg/day currently recommended. Even in areas previously thought to be iodine sufficient, there is now evidence of substantial gestational iodine deficiency, which may lead to low maternal circulating thyroxine concentrations. Hyperthyroidism is found in 0.1–0.4% of all pregnancies. It is usually caused by Graves' disease and characterised by TSH receptor stimulating antibodies (TSHRAb), which usually decrease in titre throughout pregnancy. Maternal complications include miscarriage, placenta abruption, pre-eclampsia and preterm delivery. High titres of TSHRAb if present at 36 weeks of gestation, predict a high risk of neonatal thyrotoxicosis. Postpartum Graves' disease also develops in predisposed women, although the prevalence of TSHRAb during gestation is much less than that of antithyroid peroxidase antibodies (TPOAb). Thyroid antibodies, particularly TPOAb, occur in 10% of women at 14 weeks of gestation. A proportion of these women will have subclinical hypothyroidism with a high serum TSH, but most will be euthyroid. However, after delivery thyroid dysfunction will develop in 50% of TPOAb-positive women, as ascertained in early gestation, clinically apparent as postpartum thyroiditis. In addition to the childhood neuropsychological problems relating to low thyroxine values, there is evidence from a retrospective study that maternal TPOAb may result in intellectual impairment even when there is normal thyroid function. The value of screening for thyroid dysfunction in relation to pregnancy was considered in the recent Endocrine Society Guidelines. Case finding of at-risk women is recommended but ongoing studies may alter this recommendation. Further data are required to determine which screening tests, their exact timing and whether outcomes are improved following treatment.

5.1   Introduction

The endocrine changes and metabolic demands during pregnancy result in major alterations in the biochemical parameters of thyroid function including:
- Increase in serum thyroxine-binding globulin levels.
- A marginal decrease in free thyroid hormone concentrations that is greater when there is iodine restriction or overt iodine deficiency.
- A trend toward a slight rise in basal serum TSH values between the first trimester and term.
- A transient stimulation of the maternal thyroid gland by elevated levels of human chorionic gonadotropin (hCG) resulting in a rise in free thyroid hormones and decrement in serum TSH concentrations during the first trimester (Glinoer, 2005).

Thyroid disorders are amongst the most prevalent of medical conditions in pregnancy. Their manifestations vary considerably and are determined principally by the availability of iodine in the diet. The problems encountered in epidemiological studies of thyroid disorders in pregnancy are those of definition, for example, overt hypothyroidism and subclinical hypothyroidism, gestation-related reference ranges for thyroid hormones (Panesar et al., 2001; Soldin et al., 2004), the selection criteria used, the influence of age, sex, environmental factors and the different techniques used for the measurement of thyroid hormones. Longitudinal studies are necessary to determine incidence rates, aetiological risk factors and the natural history of the disease process (Tunbridge and Vanderpump, 2000).

5.2   Impact of Iodine Status

For healthy pregnant women with iodine sufficiency, the maternal thyroid gland adjusts the thyroid hormone output in order to achieve the new equilibrium state, and thereafter maintain the equilibrium until term. This cannot easily be reached during pregnancy when the functional capacity of the thyroid gland is impaired because of iodine deficiency.

The ideal dietary allowance of iodine recommended by World Health Organization (WHO) is 200 µg of iodine per day for pregnant women. Many people are still deficient in iodine, despite major national and international efforts to increase iodine intake, primarily through the voluntary or mandatory iodination of salt. The WHO estimates that two billion people including 285 million school-age children still have iodine deficiency, defined as a urinary iodine excretion of less than 100 µg per litre (de Benosi et al., 2004; WHO). Mild to moderate iodine deficiency occurs in areas that are not immediately recognised as iodine deficient. In southwest France, 75% of pregnant women had a urinary iodine excretion levels less than 100 µg per litre (Caron et al., 1997). The severity of iodine deficiency correlated with thyroid enlargement in pregnancy and iodine supplements prevented this enlargement. National efforts to implement the mandatory use of iodised salt in Switzerland over many years eventually corrected a mild iodine deficiency. When the concentration of iodine in table salt was increased from 15 to 20 mg/kg, the median iodine excretion in a Berne population sample was documented to increase from 138 µg to 249 µg per litre in surveys of pregnant women in 1999 and 2004 (Als et al., 2000; Zimmerman et al., 2005). The iodine intake may also vary markedly within a country because of significant variations in the natural iodine content of food and water. This was demonstrated in Denmark where pregnant women without iodine supplements had a median iodine excretion level of 66 µg/g creatinine in Copenhagen and 33 µg/g creatinine in East Jutland (Nøhr et al., 1993; Pedersen et al., 1999).

In countries such as the United States of America (USA) which have been previously considered to be iodine sufficient, iodised salt is used in about 70% of households. However, recent data have shown that the median urinary iodine excretion in adults declined from 320 µg per litre in 1971–1974 to 145 µg per litre in 1988–1994, and was more recently measured at 168 µg per litre in 2001–2002 (Caldwell et al., 2005; Hollowell et al., 1998). According to the WHO, a median urinary iodine excretion of 100 to 199 µg per litre indicates that the iodine intake is adequate, so according to these data the iodine status of the USA should now be considered as marginal. This US survey also showed that as many as 15% of women in childbearing age, and almost 7% of them during a pregnancy, had iodine excretion levels into the range of moderate iodine deficiency, namely below 50 µg per litre (Glinoer, 2005; Hollowell et al., 1998).

Epidemiological studies have demonstrated that reduced iodine intake during pregnancy leads to goitrogenesis (Caron et al., 1997; Glinoer, 2005). Iodine deficiency has also been shown to lower free T_4 concentrations in pregnant women in Sudan, compared with unaltered free T_4 concentrations in pregnant women in Sweden (Elnager et al., 1998). Iodine deficiency resulted in increased serum TSH in pregnant women from one area with iodine deficiency in Sicily, compared with iodine-sufficient pregnant women from another Sicilian area (Vermiglio et al., 1999).

In summary the main change in thyroid function associated with the pregnant state is therefore the requirement for an increased production of thyroid hormone that depends directly upon the adequate availability of dietary iodine and the underlying integrity of the thyroid. Physiological adaptation can take place when the iodine intake is adequate. When iodine intake is deficient, pregnancy can reveal an underlying iodine restriction. Severe iodine deficiency may be associated with impairment in the psychoneurological outcome in the progeny because both mother and offspring are exposed to iodine deficiency during gestation (and the postnatal period). Particular attention is therefore required to ensure that pregnant women receive an adequate iodine supply, by administering multivitamin tablets containing iodine supplements, in order to achieve the ideal recommended dietary allowance of 200–250 µg iodine/day. As maternal thyroxine is crucial to foetal nervous system maturation, even modest states of iodine deficiency could be deleterious. The small risks of chronic iodine excess are outweighed by the substantial hazards of iodine deficiency (Teng et al., 2006).

5.3 Epidemiological Studies of Autoimmune Thyroid Disease in Women of Reproductive Age

In epidemiological studies of iodine-replete communities, the prevalence of spontaneous hypothyroidism in women of reproductive age is approximately 1% (Canaris et al., 2000; Hollowell et al., 2002; Spencer et al., 2007; Tunbridge and Vanderpump, 2000). The cause is either chronic autoimmune disease [atrophic autoimmune thyroiditis or goitrous autoimmune thyroiditis (Hashimoto's thyroiditis)] or destructive treatment for hyperthyroidism which may account for up to one-third of cases of hypothyroidism in the community. The term subclinical hypothyroidism or mild thyroid failure is used to describe the finding

Table 5.**1** The effect of environmental iodine intake on the prevalence of subclinical thyroid disease (Spencer et al., 2007).

Iodine Status	Subclinical Hypothyroidism	Subclinical Hyperthyroidism
Deficient	1–4%	6–10%
Replete	4–9%	1–2%
Excess	18–14%	<1%

of a raised serum TSH but a normal free thyroxine (T_4). The most common aetiology of subclinical hypothyroidism in the community is chronic autoimmune thyroiditis. In women of reproductive age, the prevalence of evidence of mild thyroid failure is approximately 5% (Canaris et al., 2000; Hollowell et al., 2002) and the majority have thyroid autoantibodies (Spencer et al., 2007). A slightly lower prevalence of subclinical hypothyroidism is seen in iodine deficient communities (see Table 5.**1**). Subclinical hypothyroidism is found at higher frequency in areas where iodine intake is high but most cases are not of autoimmune origin (Teng et al., 2006; Tunbridge and Vanderpump, 2000).

The most common causes of hyperthyroidism in iodine-replete communities are Graves' disease, followed by toxic multinodular goitre, whilst rarer causes include an autonomously functioning thyroid adenoma or thyroiditis. The prevalence of hyperthyroidism in women is between 0.5–2% (Tunbridge and Vanderpump, 2000). Subclinical hyperthyroidism is defined as a low serum TSH concentration in the presence of normal serum T_4 concentrations, and the absence of hypothalamic or pituitary disease, non-thyroidal illness, or ingestion of drugs that inhibit TSH secretion. In cross-sectional studies approximately 2% of the population have a subnormal serum TSH and 1% have an undetectable serum TSH of whom half are on thyroxine therapy (Canaris et al., 2000; Hollowell et al., 2002). The prevalence of subnormal serum TSH (detection limit 0.01 mU/L and excluding those on thyroxine therapy) is significantly higher in iodine-deficient communities due to functional autonomy from nodular goitres. Subclinical hyperthyroidism is rare in iodine-rich regions (Table 5.**1**). An increased incidence of autoimmune thyroiditis is seen in communities following an increased dietary iodine intake (Teng et al., 2006; Tunbridge and Vanderpump, 2000).

A large number of patients on replacement thyroid hormone therapy are biochemically hypothyroid or hyperthyroid, including women who are pregnant or at reproductive age, emphasising the importance of monitoring thyroid function in these groups. In the National Health and Nutrition Examination Survey (NHANES III) (1988–1994), only 63% of individuals with self-reported thyroid disease or taking thyroid-replacement medications had serum TSH within the reference range (Hollowell et al., 2002). A more recent analysis (NHANES 1999–2002) reported that among pregnant women and those of reproductive age, 7% and 3%, respectively, were hypothyroid and 3% and 0.5%, respectively, were hyperthyroid (Aoki et al., 2007). Only 209 pregnant women were included in this survey and some of those classified as hyperthyroid were not likely to have thyroid disease since decreased serum TSH often occurs during pregnancy.

5.3.1   Hypothyroidism

Hypothyroidism in pregnancy usually characterised by a high serum TSH value has been found to occur in around 2–3% of otherwise normal pregnancies with the prevalence of overt hypothyroidism estimated to be up to 0.5% (Lazarus, 2002). On a worldwide basis the most important cause of thyroid insufficiency remains iodine deficiency whilst in iodine-replete communities the cause is usually chronic autoimmune thyroiditis. Thyroid antibodies, particularly TPOAb, occur in approximately 10% of women at 14 weeks of gestation. A proportion of these women will have subclinical hypothyroidism with a high serum TSH, but most will be euthyroid. A prospective population study in the USA of 9742 pregnant women, in whom serum TSH was measured during the second trimester, found evidence of hypothyroidism in 2.2%. Autoimmune thyroiditis was present in 55% of those with mild thyroid failure and more than 80% in women with overt hypothyroidism (Allan et al., 2000). Untreated hypothyroidism is associated with obstetric complications and neonatal risk such as preterm delivery and foetal loss (Glinoer, 2005). Women who are taking thyroxine at conception usually require an increase in the dose during the pregnancy (Alwexander et al., 2004).

Data from the USA and Netherlands suggest that the children of women with hypothyroxinaemia may have psychoneurological deficits. In a study by Haddow et al. (1999) 62 children aged approximately eight years born to mothers retrospectively found to have a high serum TSH during pregnancy (but normal T_4 values) were compared with 124 control children whose mothers had normal TSH. The main finding was that 19% of the first group had an intellectual quotient (IQ) less than 85 compared with 5% of the control group which was a highly significant difference. In this study 77% of the hypothyroid mothers were thyroid antibody positive. Pop et al. (1995) have also suggested that there was an association with a lower IQ in children at five years born to thyroid antibody positive mothers when compared with thyroid antibody negative controls. The Dutch group subsequently performed a prospective follow-up study of pregnant women and their infants up to the age of two years (Pop et al., 2003). The women selected in this study had a low serum free T_4 – below the lowest 10th percentile of control pregnant women – but with a normal serum TSH. The infants born to mothers with isolated hypothyroxinaemia at 12 weeks gestation (n = 63) had delayed mental and motor function both at the ages of one and two years when compared with control infants (n = 62). This correlates with the studies in classic areas of iodine deficiency where a range of psychological and neurological deficits in children has been described during the past century, but in many of the mothers it is the maternal hypothyroxinaemia rather than high TSH that is the clear abnormality (Hollowell et al., 2002; Lazarus, 2002).

5.3.2   Hyperthyroidism

The reported prevalence of hyperthyroidism ranges from 0.1% – 0.4%, with Graves' disease accounting for the vast majority of cases (Marx et al., 2008). TSH receptor stimulating antibodies (TSHRAb) usually decrease in titre throughout pregnancy. Maternal complications include miscarriage, placenta abruption, and preterm delivery. The risk of pre-eclampsia is significantly higher in women with poorly controlled hyperthyroidism. In addition, if high titres of TSHRAb are present at 36 weeks of gestation there is a high risk of neonatal thyrotoxicosis which, although transient, may cause considerable neonatal morbidity if unrecognised. Between 2–10% of neonates of mothers with Graves' disease have neonatal hyperthyroidism (Marx et al., 2008). There is a greater frequency of recurrence or exacerbation of Graves' disease in the mother postpartum. In a Japanese cohort 40% of all new cases of Graves' disease occurred postpartum (Hidaka et al., 1994) but this has not been confirmed in other populations (Glinoer, 2005).

Mild or subclinical hyperthyroidism (suppressed serum TSH alone) has not been specifically associated with adverse pregnancy outcomes. A recent US study of 25 765 women who underwent thyroid screening identified 433 (1.7%) with serum TSH values at or below the 2.5th percentile for gestational age and normal free T_4 levels (Casey et al., 2006). There was no difference in pregnancy complications and perinatal morbidity and mortality were not increased in these women when compared with those in women whose serum TSH levels were between the 5th and 95th percentiles.

5.3.3 Gestational Thyrotoxicosis

Gestational thyrotoxicosis is defined as a non-autoimmune hyperthyroidism of variable severity that occurs in women with a normal pregnancy, typically in association with hyperemesis (Marx et al., 2008). Prospective studies have indicated that it occurs in approximately 2–3% of all pregnancies which is ten-fold more frequent than hyperthyroidism resulting from Graves' disease. The prevalence of gestational thyrotoxicosis can vary from as low as 0.3% in Japan to as high as 11% in Hong Kong with no obvious explanation for such a discrepancy in frequency (Glinoer, 2005).

5.3.4 Postpartum Thyroiditis

The development of hyperthyroidism, hypothyroidism, or both, around 13–19 weeks postpartum occurs in 5–9% of women, and is strongly associated with the presence of TPOAb (Lazarus, 2002). Of the 10% of women who are found to be TPOAb-positive in early gestation, 50% will develop postpartum thyroid dysfunction (PPTD), whereas the other 50% will remain euthyroid but still have TPOAb. The condition is transient, but 20–30% will develop permanent hypothyroidism. Long-term follow-up studies show that 50% of those whose thyroid function recovers after an episode of PPTD will become hypothyroid at seven years, compared with about 5% of antibody positive patients who were PPTD-negative (that is, euthyroid postpartum) (Lazarus, 2004).

There is a higher rate of postpartum psychiatric symptomatology in all TPOAb-positive women compared with controls (Lazarus, 2004). There is also considerable morbidity associated with the hypothyroid phase of PPTD. However, thyroxine treatment results in a satisfactory clinical state. Although the sensitivity of TPOAb measured during early pregnancy is only 50% for postpartum thyroid dysfunction, there is evidence that the gestational titre of antibody is also predictive of disease. Proponents of screening for PPTD argue that it is relatively common, causes considerable morbidity, and can be diagnosed with freely available tests that are inexpensive. Effective treatment is available if required. There is a lack of consensus about the timing of screening or the screening test for PPTD prediction. Opponents of screening cite the lack of good prospective cost-benefit analyses to support their view. A review of published data on PPTD prediction using thyroid antibodies in different population groups reveals several reasons for this lack of consensus, such as variability of the antibody measured (microsomal or TPOAb), variations in assay methodology, and different times of screening during pregnancy and the postpartum period. Although TPOAb measurement remains the leading candidate for PPTD screening, the sensitivity, specificity, and positive predictive value are highly variable. A targeted screening of individuals at the highest risk of developing PPTD, such as those with type 1 diabetes or previous PPTD, and those with a family history of thyroid autoimmunity would seem appropriate until further data is available (Lazarus, 2004).

5.4 Conclusions

The value of screening for thyroid dysfunction in relation to pregnancy was considered in the recent Endocrine Society Guidelines (Abalovich et al., 2007). Targeted case-finding of at-risk women is advised but ongoing studies may alter this recommendation. Further data are required to determine which screening tests, their exact timing and whether maternal and progeny outcomes are improved following intervention. The best medical care for the sake of mother and child are preventive measures such as awareness of trimester-related reference range and iodine status, knowledge of the local iodine status, population-based measures such as iodisation of salt, increasing iodine supply to pregnant and lactating women to 200–250 µg per day, early correction of maternal hypothyroxinaemia and screening of high-risk women for thyroid dysfunction pre-conception and postpartum.

References

Abalovich M, Amino N, Barbour LA et al. Management of thyroid dysfunction during pregnancy and postpartum: an Endocrine Society Clinical Practice Guideline. J Clin Endocrinol Metab 2007; 92 (Suppl 8): S1 – S47.

Alexander EK, Arqusee E, Lawrence J et al. Timing and magnitude of increases in levothyroxine requirements during pregnancy in women with hypothyroidism. N Engl J Med 2004; 351: 292 – 4.

Allan WC, Haddow JE, Palomaki GE et al. Maternal thyroid deficiency and pregnancy complications: implications for population screening. J Med Screen 2000; 7: 1271 – 30.

Als C, Keller A, Minder C et al. Age- and gender-dependent urinary iodine concentrations in an area-covering population sample from the Bernese region in Switzerland. Eur J Endocrinol 2000; 143: 629 – 37.

Aoki Y, Belin RM, Clickner R et al. Serum TSH and total T_4 in the United States population and their association with participant characteristics: National Health and Nutrition Examination Survey (NHANES 1999 – 2002). Thyroid 2007; 17: 1211 – 23.

Caldwell KL, Jones R, Hollowell JG et al. Urinary iodine concentration: United States National Health and Nutrition Examination Survey 2001 – 2002. Thyroid 2005; 15: 692 – 9.

Canaris GJ, Manowitz NR, Mayor G et al. The Colorado Thyroid Disease Prevalence Study. Arch Int Med 2000; 160: 526 – 34.

Caron P, Hoff M, Bazzi S et al. Urinary iodine excretion during normal pregnancy in healthy women living in the south-west of France: correlation with maternal thyroid parameters. Thyroid 1997; 7: 749 – 754.

Casey BN, Dashe JS, Wells CE et al. Subclinical hyperthyroidism and pregnancy outcomes. Obstet Gynecol 2006; 107: 337 – 41.

de Benoist B, Andersson M, Egil I et al. Iodine status worldwide: WHO global database on iodine deficiency. Geneva: World Health Organisation, 2004.

Elnager B, Eltom A, Wide L et al. Iodine status, thyroid function and pregnancy: study of Swedish and Sudanese women. Eur J Clin Nutr 1998; 86: 2360 – 3.

Glinoer D. Thyroid disease during pregnancy. In "Werner and Ingbar's The Thyroid: A Fundamental and Clinical Text", 9/E. (Ed.LE Braverman and RD Utiger). JB Lippincott-Raven, Philadelphia, 2005, pp 1086 – 108.

Haddow JE, Palomaki GE, Allan WC et al. Maternal thyroid deficiency and subsequent neuropsychological development of the child. N Engl J Med 1999; 341: 549 – 55

Hidaka Y, Tamaki H, Iwatani Y et al. Prediction of postpartum Graves' thyrotoxicosis by measurement of thyroid stimulating antibody in early pregnancy. Clin Endocrinol 1994; 41: 15 – 20.

Hollowell JG, Staehling NW, Flanders WD et al. Serum TSH, T_4, and thyroid antibodies in the United States population (1988 to 1994): National Health and Nutrition Examination Survey (NHANES III). J Clin Endocrinol Metab 2002; 87: 489 – 99.

Hollowell JG, Staehling NW, Hannon WH et al. Iodine nutrition in the United States. Trends and public health implications: iodine excretion data from national health and nutrition examination surveys I and III (1971 – 1974 and 1988 – 1994). J Clin Endocrinol Metab 1998; 83: 3401 – 8.

Lazarus JH. Epidemiology and prevention of thyroid disease in pregnancy. Thyroid 2002; 12: 861 – 5.

Lazarus JH, Premawardhana LDKE. Best Practice No 184. Screening for thyroid disease in pregnancy. J Clin Pathol 2004; 14: 610 – 5

Marx H, Amin P, Lazarus JH. Hyperthyroidism and pregnancy. BMJ 2008; 336: 663 – 7.

Nøhr SB, Laurberg P, Borlum K-G et al. Iodine deficiency in Denmark: regional variations and frequency of individual iodine supplementation. Acta Obstet Gynecol Scand 1993; 72: 350 – 3.

Panesar NS, Li CY, Rogers MS. Reference intervals for thyroid hormones in pregnant Chinese women. Ann Clin Biochem 2001; 38: 329 – 32.

Pedersen KM, Laurberg P, Nøhr S et al. Iodine in drinking water varies by more than 100-fold in Denmark: importance for iodine content of infant formulas. Eur J Endocrinol 1999; 140: 400 – 3.

Pop VJ, Brouwers EP, Vader HL et al. Maternal hypothyroxinaemia during early pregnancy and subsequent child development: a 3-year follow-up study. Clin Endocrinol 2003; 59: 282 – 8.

Pop VJ, de Vries E, van Baar AL et al. Maternal thyroid peroxidase antibodies during pregnancy: a marker of impaired child development? J Clin Endocrinol Metab 1995; 80: 3561 – 6.

Soldin OP, Tractenberg RE, Hollowell JG et al. Trimester-specific changes in maternal thyroid hormone, TSH and thyroglobulin concentrations during gestation: trends and associations across trimesters in iodine sufficiency. Thyroid 2004; 14: 1084 – 90.

Spencer CA, Hollowell JG, Kazarosyan M et al. National Health and Nutrition Examination Survey III. Thyroid-stimulating hormone (TSH)-thyroperoxidase antibody relationships demonstrate that TSH upper reference limits may be skewed by occult thyroid dysfunction. J Clin Endocrinol Metab 2007; 92: 4236 – 40.

Teng W, Shan Z, Teng X et al. Effect of iodine intake on thyroid diseases in China. New Engl J Med 2006; 354: 2783 – 2793.

Tunbridge WMG, Vanderpump MPJ. Population screening for autoimmune thyroid disease. Endocrinol Metab Clin North Am 2000: 29; 239–53.

Vermiglio F, Lo Presti VP, Castagna MG et al. Increased risk of maternal thyroid failure with pregnancy progression in an iodine deficient area with major iodine deficiency disorders. Thyroid 1999; 9: 9–24.

WHO global database on iodine deficiency. Geneva: World Health Organisation. http://www3.who.int/whosis/micronutrient.

Zimmerman MB, Aeberli I, Torresani T et al. Increasing the iodine concentration in the Swiss iodized salt program markedly improved iodine status in pregnant women and children: a 5-y prospective national study. Am J Clin Nutr 2005; 82: 388–392.

6 Thyroidal and Immune Adaptation to Pregnancy: Focus on Maternal Hypo- and Hyperthyroidism

D. Glinoer

University Hospital Saint Pierre, Division of Endocrinology, 322 rue Haute, 1000 Brussels, Belgium

Abstract

The review provides an overview of our present understanding of thyroidal and immune adaptation to pregnancy. The maternal immune system must adapt to prevent recognition of the foetus as a foreign body, leading to miscarriage. The common perception that the maternal immune response is suppressed is a (over)simplistic way to explain maternal tolerance, not supported by actual evidence. A series of protective factors have been recognised that play a pivotal role in maternal immune tolerance. The main focus concerns autoimmune thyroid disorders (AITD), namely hypo- and hyperthyroidism. In non-pregnant women AITD often remains asymptomatic, while during pregnancy the thyroid may become unable to compensate for the required increments in thyroid hormone production, hence leading to subclinical (SH) or overt hypothyroidism (OH). Both SH and OH are detrimental for maternal health and development of progeny. The overall prevalence of AITD in pregnancy is 7.8% (range: 5% – 20%). With regard to pregnant women with hypothyroidism, AITD represents the main cause with a mean prevalence of 46%, 5-fold more frequent than in euthyroid AITD-positive pregnancies. Thyroid antibodies (Th-Ab) decrease by ≥50% during gestation. This marked fall in Th-Ab is important, as it has an impact on screening programmes. Women with AITD have a significant risk of developing hypothyroidism as gestation progresses. Because early hypothyroxinaemia might affect more severely the course and outcome of pregnancy, early screening is recommended. Hyperthyroidism complicates approximately 0.1 – 0.4% of pregnancies, with 85% of cases due to Graves' disease (GD). In pregnant women with GD, the pattern of TSH-receptor auto-antibodies (TSHR-Ab) fluctuates and generally reflects the clinical course of the disease. During the 2nd and 3rd trimesters, GD patients often undergo apparent remission of hyperthyroidism, which has been attributed to the immunosuppressive effect of pregnancy. In women with active GD, TSHR-Ab titres decrease by 20% to 60%. Good control of thyrotoxicosis by treatment with ATD is directly correlated with pregnancy outcome. The risk of foetal/neonatal thyroid dysfunction can reach up to 16% in mothers with past or present GD, and is related to TSHR-Ab titres and the doses of ATD given to the mother. In conclusion, pregnancy has profound effects on the regulation of thyroid function in healthy women and in patients with thyroid disorders. These effects need to be recognised, precisely assessed, clearly interpreted, and correctly managed in order to drastically reduce the detrimental effects of thyroid dysfunction on pregnancy outcome.

6.1 Introduction

The purpose of this review is to provide an overview of our present understanding of thyroidal and immune adaptation to pregnancy. After reviewing briefly the overall changes in immune surveillance occurring after conception, the principal focus is on autoimmune thyroid disorders (AITD), mainly those diseases associated with hypothyroidism and hyperthyroidism in the pregnant state. There is also some discussion on possible strategies currently proposed for the systematic detection of these disorders by screening procedures, both before and during pregnancy.

6.2 Immunology of Normal Pregnancy

After a woman becomes pregnant, her immune system must adapt to prevent the body from recognising her foetus as a foreign entity – since the latter represents a semi-allogeneic graft – and rejecting it, hence leading to miscarriage. Not only

Table 6.**1**   Factors recognised to be pivotal in immune tolerance.

Factor	Function
Mechanical barrier	There is a mechanical barrier constituted by the membranes surrounding the embryo and attached to the placenta. These are directly exposed to maternal blood and tissues but acquire a remarkable ability to protect themselves from maternal immune cell attack.
Altered HLA expression	Trophoblastic cells do not express MHC class Ia (HLA-A, HLA-B, HLA-C) and class II molecules (HLA-DP, HLA-DQ, HLA-DR): this prevents mounting an immune response against paternal antigens. Furthermore, there is a unique pattern of expression of 'non-classical' MHC class Ib molecules (HLA-E, HLA-G). Their exact function is not known, but they seem to play an important role in the immunological acceptance of the foetus. HLA-G expression by trophoblast populations contributes to immune tolerance by reducing NK cell function and activating suppressor (CD8⁺) T cells.
Complement proteins	Several important proteins are expressed locally, that play a role in inhibiting complement activation.
Apoptosis	If immune cells should still become activated, the trophoblast cells are able to induce apoptosis in these activated immune cells, through the expression of apoptosis-inducing ligands, such as Fas ligand and "TRAIL" (TNF-related apoptosis-inducing ligand).
Shift from Th1 to Th2	In addition to immune responses within the fetal tissues, maternal helper T cells shift from Th1 to Th2 cytokine response, presumably under the influence of high estrogen and progesterone levels. High levels of T helper-2 (Th2)-type cytokines are typical of pregnancy.

does immunological tolerance take place at the maternal-foetal interface but, in addition, a combination of foetal and maternal immunological factors conspires to allow – and perhaps encourage – the conceptus to evolve and grow. Several mechanisms have been described to account for such changes in immune surveillance while, at the same time, the mother's general immune surveillance must remain intact to preserve maternal health. The common clinical perception that the maternal immune response is suppressed during pregnancy is a simplistic way to explain maternal tolerance, and is not supported by the evidence. In reality, there is no clear trend towards either general suppression or enhancement of the maternal systemic immune function during pregnancy (Hunt, 2006; Veenstra van Nieuwenhoven et al., 2003; Moffett and Loke, 2004; Aagaard-Tillery et al., 2006; Dosiou and Giudice, 2005). Table 6.**1** lists the main 'protective' factors that have been recognised to play a pivotal role in immune tolerance during normal gestation.

6.3 Prevalence of Thyroid Autoantibodies in Pregnancy

The changes in immune surveillance, briefly alluded to above, help protect the foetus from rejection. An added benefit is that some autoimmune diseases may also benefit from amelioration and/or remission during pregnancy (Smallridge, 2000; Badenhoop, 2007). With regard to the thyroid, thyroid autoimmunity should be considered as a 'thyroid stressor', acting as an additional burden on the necessary adaptation of thyroidal economy during pregnancy. In a non-pregnant young woman, thyroid autoimmune features are often asymptomatic, but during pregnancy the thyroid gland may become unable to fully compensate for the required increment in thyroid hormone production, hence leading progressively to subclinical or overt hypothyroidism (Glinoer, 1997). There is mounting evidence that both subclinical (SH) and overt hypothyroidism (OH) are detrimental for maternal health and for the neuropsychological development of the progeny, and our purpose is to review first the prevalence of – and the changes in – thyroid autoimmunity in preg-

Table 6.2 Prevalence of thyroid autoimmunity during pregnancy.

Type of study[a]	Country[b]	Population screened (N)	Timing of screening during gestation	Prevalence of positive thyroid antibodies[c]	First author (Year)
P	Italy	100	12 weeks	13% (Tg-Ab and/or TPO-Ab)	D'Armiento (1980)
P	Sweden (1981–1982)	460	1st trimester	9.6% (TPO-Ab)	Jansson (1984)
P	U.K. (1983–1985)	901	1st prenatal visit	13% (Tg-Ab and/or TPO-Ab)	Fung (1988)
P	U.S.A. (1985–1986)	1034	2 days postpartum	7% (Tg-Ab and/or TPO-Ab)	Hayslip (1988)
P	U.S.A.	552	< 13 weeks	19.6% (Tg-Ab and/or TPO-Ab)	Stagnaro-Green (1990)
P	Belgium (1988–1990; 1990–1992)	2565	1st prenatal visit	6.2–6.5% (Tg-Ab and/or TPO-Ab)	Glinoer (1991 and 1994)
P	U.S.A.	2000	15–18 weeks	11% (TPO-Ab)	Klein (1991)
P	Canada	1376	at delivery	8.2% (TPO-Ab)	Walfish (1992)
R	The Netherlands (1988–1990; 1994)	291; 293	12 weeks and/or 32 weeks	10%; 9% (TPO-Ab)	Pop (1995 and 1999)
P	Japan	1179	6–14 weeks	10.6% (TPO-Ab)	Iijima (1997)
R	USA (1987–1990)	124	17 weeks	14% (TPO-b), 10% (Tg-Ab)	Haddow (1999); Mitchell (2003)
P	Denmark (1999)	1284	11 weeks	9.1% (TPO-Ab)	Nøhr (2000)
R	USA (1990–1992)	9194	15–18 weeks	9% (Tg-Ab and/or TPO-Ab)	Allan (2000)
P	U.K.	1248	16 weeks	11.6% (TPO-Ab)	Premawardhana (2000)
P	Turkey (1998–2001)	876	12 weeks and/or 32–36 weeks	12.3% (Tg-Ab and/or TPO-Ab)	Bagis (2001)
P	Brazil	534	5–12 weeks	5% (TPO-Ab)	Sieiro Netto (2004)
P	Italy (2002–2004)	984	5–25 weeks	11.7% (TPO-Ab)	Negro (2006)
R	U.S.A. (2000–2003)	16842	< 20 weeks	5.3% (TPO-Ab)	Casey (2007)

[a] **Type of study**: prospective (P)/retrospective (R).
[b] **Country** where the study was performed (in parentheses, the period during which the study was conducted, when available).
[c] **TPO-Ab:** thyroperoxidase autoantibodies (or microsomal autoantibodies); **Tg-Ab:** thyroglobulin autoantibodies.

nant women in general, and more specifically in pregnant women with a diagnosis of hypothyroidism.

Thyroid autoimmunity is relatively frequent in the female population in the reproductive period. It is therefore not surprising that thyroid auto-antibodies (Th-Ab) can be found in a significant fraction of women during pregnancy. Table 6.**2** collates the main results from 18 studies conducted over the past 3 decades in 10 countries, where the prevalence of Th-Ab was determined during pregnancy. In this analysis, we tried to consider only studies where Th-Ab were measured in apparently healthy pregnant women, although precise epidemiological data were not systematically provided by the authors, even after a careful scrutiny of the original articles. A large majority of these studies (14/18) corresponded to prospective cohort investigations and, altogether, Th-Ab was determined in ~42000 pregnancies (D'Armiento et al., 1980; Jansson et al., 1984; Fung et al., 1988; Hayslip et al., 1988; Stagnaro-Green et al., 1990; Glinoer et al., 1991; Glinoer et al., 1994; Klein et al., 1991; Walfish et al., 1992; Pop et al., 1995; Pop et al., 1999; Iijima et al., 1997; Haddow et al., 1999; Mitchell et al., 2003; Nohr et al., 2000; Allan et al., 2000; Premawardhana et al., 2000; Bagis et al., 2001; Sieiro Netto et al., 2004; Negro et al., 2006; Casey et al., 2007). The weighed mean prevalence of positive Th-Ab reached 7.8%, with between-study frequencies varying between 5% – 20%. Various factors may have influenced the final prevalence of a positive antibody status in these studies. Besides possible geographical differences in the absolute frequency of thyroid autoimmunity ('ethnic-related' and/or 'iodine-related'), we must keep in mind that the techniques used to measure Th-Ab evolved over time and differed between studies. Most importantly, timing of screening varied widely from as early as 5 weeks to as late as 25 – 36 weeks of the estimated gestational age in 16 studies, while screening was carried out at delivery (or immediately thereafter) in 2 studies.

6.4 Thyroid Autoimmunity in Hypothyroid Pregnant Women

With regard to thyroid autoimmunity in women with a diagnosis of hypothyroidism, it is currently admitted that AITD represents the major cause of hypothyroidism during pregnancy, at least when women reside in areas with adequate iodine in-take (Abalovich et al., 2007). Several other possible causes must obviously also be kept in mind and, among these, hypothyroidism that is the consequence of the radical cure of pre-existing hyperthyroidism (by surgery or radioactive iodine administration) as well as surgery for thyroid cancer or a voluminous goitre.

In Table 6.**3**, the readers will find detailed information from a series of published studies that have investigated the prevalence of Th-Ab in pregnant women with a diagnosis of hypothyroidism. Ten studies were analysed, of which 6 were retrospective (Klein et al., 1991; Haddow et al., 1999; Allan et al., 2000; Sieiro Netto et al. 2004; Casey et al., 2007; Leung et al., 1993; Glinoer, 1995, Fukushi et al., 1999; Abalovich et al., 2002; Stagnaro-Green et al., 2005). The overall prevalence of hypothyroidism varied between 2.2% – 3.4%, depending on the study design. While some studies encompassed women already known to be hypothyroid, other studies based the diagnosis on serum TSH screening, usually carried out before 20 weeks gestation. It is important to note that the cut-off level for an abnormal serum TSH differed in the studies (from $> 3 \mu U/mL$ to $> 6 \mu U/mL$). Interestingly, in the recent study by Casey et al. (2007) where the lowest serum TSH cut-off limit was employed, the highest prevalence of gestational hypothyroidism was observed. Another variable was related to variable timing in serum TSH measurements (between 5 – 20 weeks), a factor that may have impacted on the final prevalence. Altogether, the analysis of the data showed that Th-Ab was present in 25% – 77% of the cases, with a weighed mean prevalence of 45.6% (581/1275 hypothyroid pregnant women). In studies where epidemiological information was available on adequate control groups, the data confirmed that thyroid autoimmunity was 5.2-fold more prevalent in women with a diagnosis of hypothyroidism, compared with euthyroid controls (mean of 48.5% *vs.* 9.2%). It should also be mentioned that the prevalence of Th-Ab in hypothyroid pregnant women depends on the severity of thyroid dysfunction. In the study by Allan et al. (2000), for instance, the prevalence of positive Th-Ab was 55% among women with only a modest serum TSH elevation $(6 - 10 \mu U/mL)$, while the prevalence reached 80% among women with a markedly elevated serum TSH level $(10 - 200 \mu U/mL)$. In summary, the evidence confirms that chronic thyroiditis is the main cause of hypothyroidism during pregnancy, but evidently AITD is not the only cause, even in

Table 6.**3**   Thyroid autoimmunity in pregnant women with a diagnosis of hypothyroidism.

Type of study[a]	Country[b]	Hypothyroid pregnant women (N)[c]	Timing of screening (weeks)	Prevalence of thyroid antibodies[d]	First Author (Year)
R	U.S.A.	49/2000 (2.5%) (TSH: > 6 mU/L)	15–18	58% (TPO-Ab) (*vs.* 11% in C)	Klein (1991)
R	U.S.A. (1981–1990)	68 (TSH: > 5 mU/L)	Before pregnancy and/or at 1st prenatal visit	37% (MIC-Ab)	Leung (1993)
P	Belgium (1990–1992)	41/1.900 (2.2%) (TSH: > 4 mU/L)	First prenatal visit	40% (TG-Ab and/or TPO-Ab) (*vs.* 6.4% in C)	Glinoer (1995)
P	Japan (1986–1998)	102 (TSH: >?) (not specified)	12	66% (TG-Ab and/or TPO-Ab)	Fukushi (1999)
R	U.S.A. (1987–1990)	62 (TSH: > 5 mU/L)	Before or during pregnancy	77% (TPOAb) (*vs.* 14% in C)	Haddow (1999)
R	U.S.A. (1990–1992)	209/9403 (2.2%) (TSH: > 6 mU/L)	15–18	60% (TG-Ab and/or TPO-Ab) (*vs.* 9% in C)	Allan (2000)
R	Argentina (1987–1999)	114 (TSH: > 5 mU/L)	Diagnosis made before pregnancy	69% (TG-Ab and/or TPO-Ab)	Abalovich (2002)
P	Brazil	16 (TSH: > 3.6 mU/L)	5–12	25% (TG-Ab and/or TPO-Ab)	Sieiro Netto (2004)
P	U.S.A. (1996–2002)	16 (TSH: ≥ 3 mU/L)	15.5	25% (TG-Ab and/or TPO-Ab) (*vs.* 11% in C)	Stagnaro-Green (2005)
R	U.S.A. (2000–2003)	598/17298 (3.4%) (TSH: ≥ 3 mU/L)	< 20	31% (TPO-Ab) (*vs.* 4% in C)	Casey (2007)

[a]   **Type of study:** prospective (P)/retrospective (R).
[b]   **Country** where the study was performed (in parentheses, the period during which the study was conducted, when available).
[c]   **Hypothyroid pregnant women:** number of women with a diagnosis of hypothyroidism (prevalence is indicated when available), and serum TSH cut-off limit used for the diagnosis.
[d]   **Prevalence of thyroid antibodies** given in percent with indication of the type of antibody measured (when available); when available, the prevalence of Th-Abs in control pregnant women (*vs.* C) is also indicated.

the studies that carefully excluded women with a prior-to-pregnancy diagnosis of hypothyroidism. This argument can be used, in turn, to further consolidate the notion that screening for thyroid dysfunction should include both measurements of serum TSH (+ free T_4) and determination of Th-Ab (Glinoer, 1998).

6.5   Pattern of Thyroid Autoantibody Changes during Pregnancy

A limited number of studies have investigated changes in Th-Ab titres occurring during pregnancy. Indirect information can also be gathered from studies dealing with postpartum thyroid dysfunction, where the authors have measured Th-Ab at different time points before parturition (Jansson et al., 1984; Fung et al., 1988; Hayslip et al., 1988; Walfish et al., 1992; Premawardhana et al., 2000; Fukushi et al., 1999). Globally, the decrease in Th-Ab titres during gestation reaches at least 50%, corresponding to the immunosuppressive effect of pregnancy (Glinoer et al., 1994; Smyth et al., 2005; Panesar et al., 2006). This marked fall in antibody titres is important for several reasons: a) it indicates an amelioration of the immune aspect of AITD during pregnancy (but we will show below that this is paradoxical); b) Th-Ab may become negative in many women as gestation progresses and this has a clear impact on the temporal organisation of screening programmes; and finally c) in women with AITD who develop postpartum thyroid dysfunction, the pregnancy-associated dampening in Th-Ab is most often followed by a major Th-Ab rebound in the months following delivery. These facts are illustrated in Fig. 6.**1**. In addition to the changes that occur in humoral immunity, there is also regulation of peripheral T-lymphocyte subsets during normal pregnancy, characterised by a decrease in helper (CD4$^+$) T-cells and increase in suppressor (CD8$^+$) T-cells, thus causing a significant fall in the CD4$^+$/CD8$^+$ ratio in late pregnancy (Stagnaro-Green et al., 1992).

The apparent paradox of maternal thyroid insufficiency in the context of AITD can easily be explained. Despite the marked decrease in Th-Ab titres during gestation, women with AITD have a significantly increased risk of developing hypothyroidism with progression of gestation (Glinoer, 1994; Negro et al., 2006; Glinoer, 2003). This risk is therefore mainly ascribed to the diminished functional reserve of the maternal thyroid machinery. In women with AITD, the capacity to adapt to the necessary changes in thyroidal economy that are associated with the pregnant state is less than adequate and is not counterbalanced by the decrease in the antibody titres.

6.6 Screening for Thyroid Antibodies and Dysfunction during Pregnancy

Should thyroid antibodies be determined before or in the pregnant state? When determined before pregnancy, positive Th-Ab provides an indicator of the risk of infertility and/or early miscarriage after conception (spontaneous or medically-assisted) (Abalovich et al., 2007; Poppe and Glinoer, 2003). As already discussed, positive Th-Ab – even in the context of apparent euthyroidism – is associated with a significantly greater risk of developing hypothyroidism during gestation, a risk that is associated with increased obstetric

morbidity and that can be alleviated by adequate treatment with thyroxine (Negro et al., 2006). Positive Th-Ab discovered during pregnancy is also associated with a high risk of postpartum thyroid dysfunction (~50%): the higher the autoantibody titres during early and late gestation, the greater the risk of thyroid dysfunction after delivery (Premawardhana et al., 2000). Finally as shown in the study by Haddow et al. (1999), a majority of pregnant women with AITD have a significant risk of developing permanent hypothyroidism later on in life. Therefore, advance knowledge of the presence of thyroid autoimmune features – even when women remain euthyroid during pregnancy without treatment – is an effective way of delineating a subgroup of women for whom thyroid function ought to be regularly monitored.

The best time to measure thyroid autoimmune markers remains controversial. Since Th-Ab titres tend to decrease with the progression of gestation, it would be logical to consider that the earlier the screening the more accurate the information gained (i.e., at 1st prenatal visit). Conversely, since hypothyroidism tends to develop progressively during late gestation in women with positive Th-Ab who remained euthyroid near conception, measuring serum TSH at a later stage (i.e., after mid-gestation) would appear more beneficial. Finally, both for practical reasons and because early hypothyroxinaemia might affect more severely the course and outcome of pregnancy as well as the adequate development of the foetus, it is logical to recommend early screening (Abalovich et al., 2007; Glinoer, 1998). In the Clinical Guidelines recently edited by The Endocrine Society, our international *ad hoc* committee was not in a position to advocate unanimously universal screening for thyroid dysfunction during pregnancy, because of a lack of evidence-based information to prove beyond doubt the benefits of universal screening. A compromise was therefore to propose targeted screening in high-risk groups of women (Abalovich et al., 2007). However, it was recently shown in the study by Vaidya et al. (2007) that by screening only so-called high-risk women, there was a risk of missing a significant fraction of pregnant women with hypothyroidism (see Fig. 6.**2**).

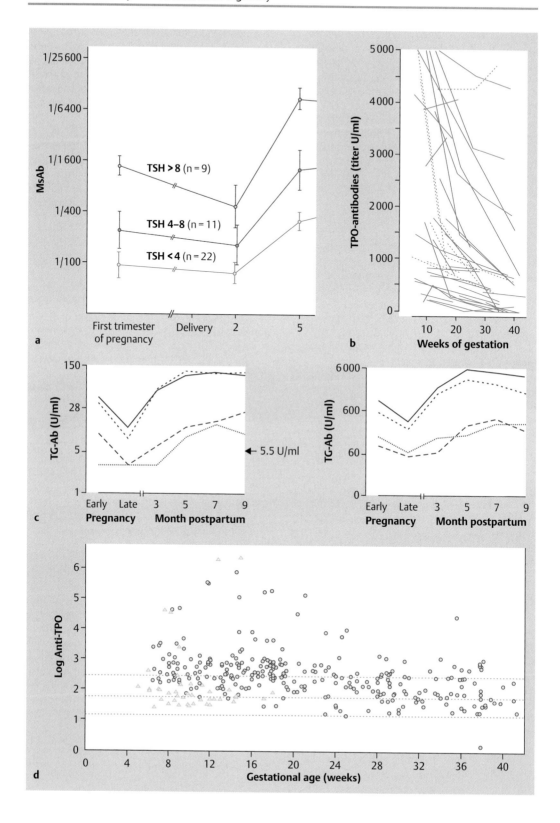

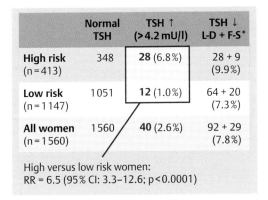

	Normal TSH	TSH ↑ (>4.2 mU/l)	TSH ↓ L-D + F-S*
High risk (n=413)	348	**28** (6.8%)	28 + 9 (9.9%)
Low risk (n=1147)	1051	**12** (1.0%)	64 + 20 (7.3%)
All women (n=1560)	1560	**40** (2.6%)	92 + 29 (7.8%)

High versus low risk women:
RR = 6.5 (95% CI: 3.3–12.6; p<0.0001)

Fig. 6.2 A study carried out in 2002–2003 in the U.K., with a total of 1560 consecutive pregnant women screened for an elevated serum TSH (>4.2 µU/mL) between 6–22 weeks gestation (median: 9 weeks). High-risk women were defined on the basis of a personal history of thyroid disorders (including women already treated for hypothyroidism), a history of type 1 diabetes or other autoimmune disorders, and finally a family history of thyroid disorders. Based on these criteria, 413 women (25.6%) were considered to be 'high-risk'. By systematic screening, hypothyroidism was diagnosed in 40 women, with only 28 belonging to the high-risk group. Thus, 1/3 of pregnant hypothyroid women would have been missed by applying a targeted screening procedure (adapted from Vaidya et al., 2007).
* "L–D" TSH: low but still detectable serum TSH;
  "F–S" TSH: fully suppressed serum TSH.

6.7 Summary for Hypothyroidism

This summary was adapted from the recent Clinical Guidelines of the Endocrine Society for the management of thyroid disorders during pregnancy (Abalovich et al., 2007).

– Maternal and foetal hypothyroidism is known to have serious adverse effects on the foetus. Therefore, maternal hypothyroidism should be avoided. Targeted case finding (or universal screening?) should be recommended at 1st prenatal visit.
– If hypothyroidism has been diagnosed before pregnancy, adjustment of preconception thyroxine dosage is recommended to reach a TSH ≤2.5 µU/mL prior to pregnancy. The thyroxine dosage usually needs to be incremented by 4–6 weeks gestation and will require usually a 30% – 50% increase in dosage. For overt hypothyroidism diagnosed during pregnancy, thyroid function tests should be normalised as rapidly as possible and thyroxine dosage titrated to rapidly reach and thereafter maintain a serum TSH concentration ≤2.5 µU/mL in the 1st trimester (or ≤3 µU/mL in the 2nd and 3rd trimesters).
– Euthyroid women with thyroid autoimmunity in early gestation are at risk of developing hypothyroidism later on and should be monitored for elevation of TSH above the normal range. SCH (defined as a serum TSH concentration above the upper limit of the reference range with a normal free T_4) has been shown to be associated with adverse outcomes for both mother and offspring. Thyroxine treatment improves obstetrical outcome, but has not yet been proved to improve long-term neurological development in offspring. However, given that potential benefits outweigh potential risks, thyroxine administration is recommended in women with SCH.
– Finally, after delivery, most hypothyroid women need to decrease the thyroxine dosage they received during pregnancy.

Fig. 6.1 *Graph A:* Changes in microsomal antibodies (log scale on the ordinate) between 1st trimester and 2 months after delivery in 3 groups of women, according to maximal serum TSH level reached during postpartum (modified from Jansson et al., 1984). *Graph B:* Changes in TPO-Ab during gestation in women with AITD. Solid lines represent euthyroid pregnancies and dotted lines women with subclinical hypothyroidism in early gestation. The decrement in TPO-Ab was similar in both groups and independent of the initial TPO-Ab titres. The rate of TPO-Ab positivity declined from 74% in the 1st trimester to <40% near term (modified from Glinoer et al., 1994). *Graphs C:* Changes in TPO-Ab (right panel) and Tg-Ab (left panel) between early and late pregnancy in 4 groups of women who presented different types of thyroid dysfunction during postpartum (modified from Nøhr et al., 2000). *Graph D:* Changes in TPO-Ab titres in a large group of Chinese pregnant women. The ordinate is shown as a log scale; the 3 horizontal lines show the 95th (upper) percentile, the median, and the 5th (lower) percentile limits for TPO-Ab in non-pregnant controls. The prevalence of a positive antibody status declined from 47% to 39% and finally to 16%, respectively, in the 1st, 2nd, and 3rd trimesters of gestation (modified from Panesar et al., 2006).

Table 6.**4**   Serial changes in TBII and TSAb during pregnancy.

Type of assay	Stage of Pregnancy Early (< 13 weeks)	Middle (14–27 weeks)	Late (> 28 weeks)	Statistical difference Late *vs.* Early
TRAb$_1$ (%)[a]	24.2	21.1	17.4	$p < 0.01$
pTRAB$_2$ (%)[b]	46.1	40.0	35.3	$p < 0.01$
hTRAb$_2$ (IU/L)[c]	12.3	7.2	5.1	$p < 0.01$
pTRAb$_3$ (%)[d]	48.5	41.3	35.4	$p < 0.01$
TSAb (%)[e]	281.1	250.3	224.0	$p < 0.01$

[a]   TRAb$_1$: 1st generation assay (Cosmic Corporation, Tokyo, Japan): the cut-off value for normal serum yields binding inhibition of < 10%.
[b]   pTRAb$_2$: 2nd generation assay using purified porcine TSH receptor in a coated plate ELISA (Cosmic Corporation, Tokyo, Japan): the cut-off value for normal serum yields binding inhibition of < 20%.
[c]   hTRAb$_2$: 2nd generation assay using recombinant human TSH receptor in a coated tube radioassay (DYNO-test 'TRAb' human, Yamasa-Shou Ltd, Tokyo, Japan); the cut-off value for normal serum yields binding inhibition of < 1.0 IU/L.
[d]   pTRAb$_3$: 3rd generation assay measuring the binding inhibition of human monoclonal thyroid stimulating antibody M22 (biotin-labeled) to porcine TSH receptor coated ELISA plate wells: the cut-off value for normal serum yields binding inhibition of < 20%.
[e]   TSAb: thyroid stimulating antibody bioassay using PEG 22.5% assay & porcine thyroid cells (Yamasa-Shouyu Ltd, Tokyo, Japan) and measuring cAMP production compared with normal sera: the cut-off value for normal serum yields cAMP production < 180%. (Adapted with modifications from Kamijo, 2007.)

6.8   Graves' Disease during Pregnancy

Hyperthyroidism complicates approximately 0.1–0.4% of pregnancies, with 85% of the cases due to Graves' disease (GD). Patients with GD during pregnancy can present *de novo*, or as a recurrence after a prior treatment (and remission) with antithyroid drug therapy (ATD), or with clinical and/or biochemical exacerbation while still taking ATD in the case of women with an active disease, or (rarely) with signs of foetal hyperthyroidism despite the mother being euthyroid (or even hypothyroid) after prior radical cure of GD by radioiodine or surgical ablation (Chan et al., 2007). GD is an autoimmune disorder due to circulating TSH-receptor auto-antibodies (TSHR-Ab), capable of stimulating growth and function of both the maternal and (later on) the foetal thyroid gland. Different assays exist for the determination of TSHR-Ab. The most commonly used methodology is 'TBII' assays (TSH binding inhibitory immunoglobulin), radio-receptor assays in which the ligand (radiolabelled TSH) is displaced from the TSH receptor by specific antibodies present in maternal serum. Albeit highly sensitive and specific, these assays do not discriminate between stimulating antibodies (responsible for GD), neutral antibodies (shown to exist), and blocking-type antibodies (rarely found in women with Hashimoto's disease) (Morgenthaler et al., 1999; Akamizu, 2001). Currently available bioassays are 'TSAb' (thyroid stimulating immunoglobulin or TSI). These assays use

CHO cells expressing (by transfection) the human TSH receptor, and measure increased cAMP generation when incubated with sera from patients with GD. There is presently no strong evidence to indicate that one assay (i.e., TSAb) is more useful than the other (i.e., TBII) in the context of a pregnancy with the suspicion of GD although, in theory at least, there are arguments to favour the determination of TSAb (especially for women with long-term AITD in whom a suspicion of the potential presence of blocking antibodies may be raised).

In pregnant women with GD, the pattern of TSHR-Ab generally fluctuates and such fluctuation reflects broadly the clinical course of the disease. Although the number of studies that have evaluated systematically changes in TSHR-Ab during pregnancy is much smaller than for TG-Ab and TPO-Ab, most studies concur to conclude that the pattern of changes in TSHR-Ab parallels the marked decrease known to occur for TPO-Ab and TG-Ab. Most pregnant women with active GD have detectable TSHR-Ab and, although the diagnosis of GD during pregnancy is often clinical, measurements of TSHR-Ab are of great value to help distinguishing GD from GTT (gestational transient thyrotoxicosis) in the 1st trimester (Abalovich et al., 2007; Baloch et al., 2003). Since GD tends to undergo immunological remission after the late 2nd trimester, detection of TSHR-Ab may depend upon gestational age at measurement (Amino et al., 1982). Clinically, patients

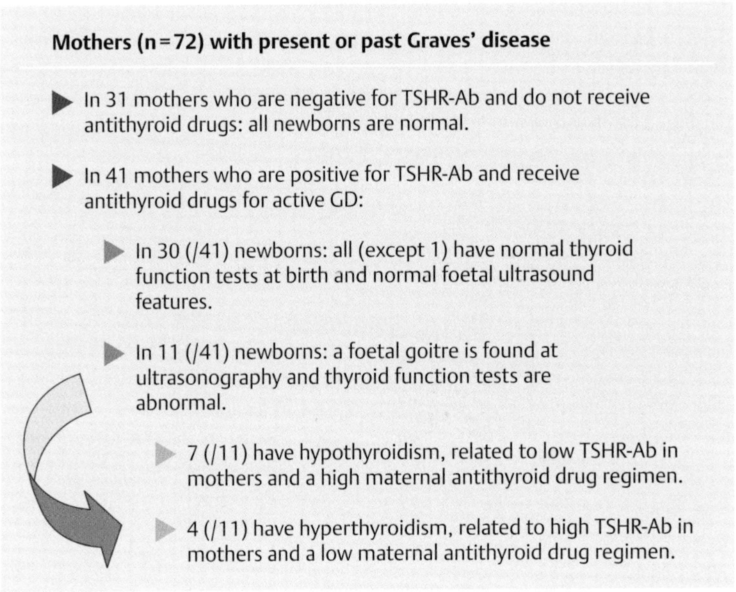

Mothers (n = 72) with present or past Graves' disease

▶ In 31 mothers who are negative for TSHR-Ab and do not receive antithyroid drugs: all newborns are normal.

▶ In 41 mothers who are positive for TSHR-Ab and receive antithyroid drugs for active GD:

▷ In 30 (/41) newborns: all (except 1) have normal thyroid function tests at birth and normal foetal ultrasound features.

▷ In 11 (/41) newborns: a foetal goitre is found at ultrasonography and thyroid function tests are abnormal.

▷ 7 (/11) have hypothyroidism, related to low TSHR-Ab in mothers and a high maternal antithyroid drug regimen.

▷ 4 (/11) have hyperthyroidism, related to high TSHR-Ab in mothers and a low maternal antithyroid drug regimen.

Fig. 6.**3** Main results of a French retrospective study on the risk of foetal-neonatal hyperthyroidism in the infants born to 72 mothers with past or present Graves' disease (adapted from Luton et al., 2005).

with GD can experience relapse or exacerbation in the 1st trimester. This is not surprising since women with GD are submitted to the combined stimulating actions of TSHR-Ab and peak hCG concentrations on maternal thyrocytes (Tagami et al., 2007). During the 2nd and 3rd trimesters, patients with GD often undergo apparent remission of hyperthyroidism, which has been attributed to the immunosuppressive effect of pregnancy on maternal stimulating TSHR-Ab. In a recent article, Kamijo (2007) investigated serially a group of pregnant women with active GD. By comparing five TSHR-Ab assays at various pregnancy stages, the author was able to confirm a significant decrease in TSHR-Ab titres, as gestation progressed. Table 6.**4** illustrates the TSHR-Ab values obtained between early and late gestation, showing a mean decrement of 32% (range: 20.3% to 58.5%), depending upon the type of assay used.

To explain the partial remission frequently observed during late gestation in women with GD, there has been a suggestion that a specificity change, from the stimulatory- to the blocking-type TSHR-Ab, might contribute to apparent remission of disease activity (Kung and Jones, 1998; Kung et al., 2001). Even though rare cases have been reported in the literature in favour of such a hypothesis (both during gestation and the postpartum period), the potential impact of such findings remains largely controversial (Yoshida et al., 1992; Hara et al., 1990; Amino et al., 2003).

6.8.1 Foetal Immunological Aspects Related to Maternal Graves' Disease

One to five percent of neonates born to mothers with GD have neonatal GD, due to the transplacental passage of stimulating TSHR-Ab (Weetman, 2000). Risk factors for neonatal thyroid dysfunction include history of a previously affected baby, prior ablative treatment with radioiodine, and elevated maternal TSHR-Ab at the time of delivery (Mitsuda et al., 1992; Laurberg et al., 1998). Foetal signs to suggest intra-uterine thyrotoxicosis include tachycardia, intra-uterine growth retardation, accelerated bone maturation, foetal cardiac failure and foetal goitre. However, foetal goitre associated with the maternal treatment of GD can be due to either foetal hypothyroidism (because of ATD administered to the mother) or foetal hyperthyroidism (due to stimulation of the foetal gland by maternal TSHR-Ab).

In a remarkable study carried out by Michel Polak and colleagues (Paris), a large group of women (n = 72) with past or present GD was investigated (Luton et al., 2005). The results provide a prospective view on how to handle this difficult clinical challenge (see Fig. 6.**3**). When mothers had a *history of past GD* (i.e., negative for TSHR-Ab and no ATD treatment), there was no risk of foetal-neonatal hyperthyroidism: thus, no particular screening or follow-up is required in those circumstances. Even in *mothers with active GD*, the risk remained negligible in ~ 70% of the cases and this reassuring information was provided by a normal foetal thyroid ultrasonography at 32 weeks. Finally, a *minority of foetuses* (11/72) presented a goitre (at ultrasonography) and in these circumstances, there was a risk for foetal hypo- or hyperthyroidism. Diagnosis of foetal hyperthyroidism was associated with high maternal TSHR-Ab titres and low doses of maternal ATD treatment. Conversely, diagnosis of foetal hypothyroidism was associated with low TSHR-Ab titres and high doses of maternal ATD treatment. The authors recommended therefore to measure TSHR-Ab in all women with current or past GD at the onset of pregnancy, and a close observation of pregnant women with elevated TSHR-Ab and/or ATD treatment, by performing foetal ultrasonography monthly after 20 weeks.

6.9   Summary for Hyperthyroidism

Summary was adapted from the recent Clinical Guidelines of the Endocrine Society for the management of thyroid disorders during pregnancy (Abalovich et al., 2007).
- The two most common causes of hyperthyroidism during pregnancy are GD and gestational transient thyrotoxicosis (GTT). Differentiation of GD from GTT rests on the presence of typical goitre and autoimmunity (specifically TSHR-Ab).
- For the management of active GD, antithyroid drug (ATD) therapy should be initiated with the aim to control maternal hyperthyroidism. Maternal serum free T_4 levels should be maintained in the upper non-pregnant free T_4 reference range.
- An important concept is that maternal and foetal outcomes are directly related to adequate control of thyrotoxicosis. Obstetric repercussions of poorly controlled thyrotoxicosis include the risk of miscarriage, gestational hypertension, foetal malformation, premature delivery and low birth weight.
- Maternal GD can affect the foetus in several ways. TSHR-Ab freely cross the placenta to stimulate the foetal thyroid. These antibodies should be measured before pregnancy or by the end of the 2nd trimester in mothers with current GD, a history of GD and prior curative treatment (with radioiodine or after thyroidectomy), or a previous neonate with GD at birth. Women with negative TSHR-Ab and those who

do not require ATD have a very low risk of foetal or neonatal thyroid dysfunction. In women with positive TSHR-Ab, foetal and neonatal thyrotoxicosis constitute a real risk when maternal TSHR-Ab titres have not substantially decreased during the 2nd part of gestation. In such women, foetal ultrasound should be performed to search for evidence of foetal thyroid dysfunction.

6.10   Conclusion

Pregnancy has profound effects on the regulation of thyroid function in healthy women and in patients with thyroid disorders. These effects need to be recognised, precisely assessed, clearly interpreted, and correctly managed in order to drastically reduce the detrimental effects of thyroid dysfunction on pregnancy outcome.

Acknowledgements

Daniel Glinoer acknowledges the support of *Ministère de la Communauté Française, Administration Générale de l'Enseignement & de la Recherche Scientifique* within the framework of *Actions de Recherche Concertées* (ARC: Convention N°04/09-314).

References

Aagaard-Tillery KM, Silver R, Dalton J. Immunology of normal pregnancy. Sem Fetal Neonatal Med 2006; 11: 279–95.

Abalovich M, Amino N, Barbour LA, Cobin RH, DeGroot LJ, Glinoer D, Mandel SJ, Stagnaro-Green A. Management of thyroid dysfunction during pregnancy and postpartum: an Endocrine Society clinical practice guideline. J Clin Endocrinol Metab 2007; 92: S1–S47.

Abalovich M, Guttierez S, Alcaraz G, Maccallini G, Garcia A, Levalle O. Overt and subclinical hypothyroidism complicating pregnancy. Thyroid 2002; 12: 63–8.

Akamizu T. Antithyrotropin receptor antibody: an update. Thyroid 2001; 11: 1123–34.

Allan WC, Haddow JE, Palomaki GE, Williams JR, Mitchell ML, Hermos RJ, Klein RZ. Maternal thyroid deficiency and pregnancy complications: implications for population screening. J Med Screen 2000; 7: 127–30.

Amino N, Izumi Y, Hidaka Y, Takeoka K, Nakata Y, Tatsumi KI, Nagata A, Takano T. No increase of blocking type anti-thyrotropin receptor antibodies during pregnancy in patients with Graves' disease. J Clin Endocrinol Metab 2003; 88: 5871–4.

Amino N, Tanizawa O, Mori H, Iwatani Y, Yamada T, Kurachi K, Kumahara Y, Miyai K. Aggravation of thyrotoxicosis in early pregnancy and after delivery in Graves' disease. J Clin Endocrinol Metab 1982; 55: 108–12.

Badenhoop K. Microchimerism and the model of postpartum thyroiditis. In: The Thyroid and Autoimmunity. Wiersinga WM, Drexhage HA, Weetman AP, Butz S, eds. Georg Thieme Verlag (Stuttgart, New York), 2007; 99–103.

Bagis T, Gokcel A, Saygili ES. Autoimmune thyroid disease in pregnancy and the postpartum period: relationship to spontaneous abortion. Thyroid 2001; 11: 1049–53.

Baloch Z, Carayon P, Conte-Devolx B, Demers LM, Feldt-Rasmussen U, Henry JF, LiVosli VA, Niccoli-Sire P, John R, Ruf J, Smyth PP, Spencer CA, Stockigt JR. Laboratory medicine practice guidelines. Laboratory support for the diagnosis and monitoring of thyroid disease. Thyroid 2003; 13: 3–126.

Casey BM, Dashe JS, Spong CY, McIntire DD, Leveno KJ, Cunningham GF. Perinatal significance of isolated maternal hypothyroxinemia identified in the first half of pregnancy. Obstet Gynecol 2007; 109: 1129–35.

Chan GW, Mandel SJ. Therapy insight: management of Graves' disease during pregnancy. Nature Clin Pract Endocrinol Metab 2007; 3: 470–8.

D'Armiento M, Salabe H, Vetrano G, Scucchia M, Pachi A. Decrease of thyroid antibodies pregnancy. J Endocrinol Invest 1980; 4: 437–8.

Dosiou C, Giudice L. Natural killer cells in pregnancy recurrent pregnancy loss: endocrine and immunologic perspectives. Endocrine Rev 2005; 26: 44–62.

Fukushi M, Honma K, Fujita K. Letter to the Editor. New Engl J Med 1999; 341: 2016.

Fung HY, Kologlu M, Collison K, John R, Richards CJ, Hall R, McGregor AM. Postpartum thyroid dysfunction in Mid Glamorgan. Brit Med J 1988; 296: 241–4.

Glinoer D. Management of hypo- and hyperthyroidism during pregnancy. Growth Hormone & IGF Research 2003; 13: S45–54.

Glinoer D. Regulation of thyroid function in pregnancy: Pathways of endocrine adaptation from physiology to pathology. Endocrine Rev 1997; 18: 404–33.

Glinoer D. The systematic screening and management of hypothyroidism and hyperthyroidism during pregnancy. Trends Endocrinol Metab 1998; 9: 403–11.

Glinoer D. The thyroid in pregnancy: a European perspective. Thyroid Today 1995; 18: 1–11.

Glinoer D, Fernandez Soto M, Bourdoux P, Lejeune B, Delange F, Lemone M, Kinthaert J, Robijn C, Grün JP, De Nayer P. Pregnancy in patients with mild thyroid abnormalities: maternal and neonatal repercussions. J Clin Endocrinol Metab 1991; 73: 421–7.

Glinoer D, Rihai M, Grün JP, Kinthaert J. Risk of subclinical hypothyroidism in pregnant women with asymptomatic autoimmune thyroid disorders. J Clin Endocrinol Metab 1994; 79: 197–204.

Haddow JE, Palomaki GE, Allan WC, Williams JR, Knight GJ, Gagnon J, O'Heir CE, Mitchell ML, Hermos RJ, Waisbren SE, Faix JD, Klein RZ. Maternal thyroid efficiency during pregnancy and subsequent neuropsychological development of the child. New Engl J Med 1999; 341: 549–55.

Hara T, Tamai H, Mukuta T, Fukata S, Kuma K, Sugawara M. Transient postpartum hypothyroidism caused by thyroid-stimulation-blocking antibody. Lancet 1990; 1: 946.

Hayslip CC, Fein HG, O'Donnell VM, Friedman DS, Klein TA, Smallridge RC. The value of serum antimicrosomal antibody testing in screening for symptomatic postpartum thyroid dysfunction. Am J Obstet Gynecol 1988; 159: 203–9.

Hunt JS. Stranger in a strange land. Immunol Rev 2006; 213: 36–47.

Iijima T, Tada H, Hidaka Y, Mitsuda N, Murata Y, Amino N. Effects of autoantibodies on the course of pregnancy and fetal growth. Obstet Gynecol 1997; 90: 364–9.

Jansson R, Bernander S, Karlsson A, Levin K, Nilsson G. Autoimmune thyroid dysfunction in the postpartum period. J Clin Endocrinol Metab 1984; 58: 681–7.

Kamijo K. TSH-receptor antibodies determined by the first, second and third generation assay and thyroid-stimulating antibody in pregnant patients with Graves' disease. Endocr J 2007; 54: 619–24.

Klein RZ, Haddow JE, Faix JD, Brown RS, Hermos RJ, Pulkkinen A, Mitchell ML. Prevalence of thyroid deficiency in pregnant women. Clin Endocrinol 1991; 36: 41–6.

Kung AWC, Jones BM. A change from stimulatory to blocking antibody activity in Graves' disease during pregnancy. J Clin Endocrinol Metab 1998; 83: 514–8.

Kung AWC, Lau KS, Kohn LD. Epitope mapping of TSH receptor-blocking antibodies in Graves' disease that appear during pregnancy. J Clin Endocrinol Metab 2001; 86: 3647–53.

Laurberg P, Nygaard B, Glinoer D, Grussendorf M, Orgiazzi J. Guidelines for TSH-receptor antibody measurements in pregnancy: results of an evidence-based symposium organized by the European Thyroid Association. Eur J Endocrinol 1998; 139: 564–8 l.

Leung AS, Millar LK, Koonings PP, Montoro M, Mestman JH. Perinatal outcome in hypothyroid pregnancies. Obstet Gynecol 1993; 81: 349 – 53.

Luton D, Le Gac I, Vuillard E, Castanet M, Guibourdenche J, Noel M, Toubert ME, Leger J, Boissinot C, Schlageter MH, Garel C, Tebeka B, Oury JF, Czernichow P, Polak M. Management of Graves' disease during pregnancy: the key role of fetal thyroid gland monitoring. J Clin Endocrinol Metab 2005; 90: 6093 – 8.

Mitchell ML, Klein RZ, Sargent JD, Meter RA, Haddow JE, Waisbren SE, Faix JD. Iodine sufficiency and measurements of thyroid function in maternal hypothyroidism. Clin Endocrinol 2003; 58: 612 – 6.

Mitsuda N, Tamaki H, Amino N, Hosono T, Miyai K, Tanizawa O. Risk factors for developmental disorders in infants born to women with Graves disease. Obstet Gynecol 1992; 80: 359 – 64.

Moffett A, Loke YW. The immunological paradox of pregnancy: a reappraisal. Placenta 2004; 25: 1 – 8.

Morgenthaler NG, Hodak K, Seissler J, et al. Direct binding of thyrotropin receptor autoantibody to *in vitro* translated thyrotropin receptor: a comparison of radioreceptor assay and thyroid stimulating assay. Thyroid 1999; 9: 467 – 75.

Negro R, Formoso G, Mangieri T, Pezzarossa A, Dazzi D, Hassan H. Levothyroxine treatment in euthyroid pregnant women with autoimmune thyroid disease: effects on obstetrical complications. J Clin Endocrinol Metab 2006; 91: 2587 – 91.

Nøhr SB, Jorgensen A, Pedersen KM, Laurberg P. Postpartum thyroid dysfunction in pregnant thyroid peroxidase antibody-positive women living in an area with mild to moderate iodine deficiency: is iodine supplementation safe? J Clin Endocrinol Metab 2000; 85: 3191 – 8.

Panesar NS, Chan KW, Li CY, Rogers MS. Status of antithyroid peroxidase during normal pregnancy and in patients with hyperemesis gravidarum. Thyroid 2006; 16: 481 – 4.

Pop VJ, de Vries E, van Baar AL, Waelkens JJ, de Rooy HA, Hosten M, Donkers MM, Komproe IH, van Son MM, Vader HL. Maternal thyroid peroxidase antibodies during pregnancy: a marker of impaired child development? J Clin Endocrinol Metab 1995; 80: 3561 – 6.

Pop VJ, Kuijpens JL, van Baar AL, Verkerk G, van Son MM, de Vijlder JJ, Vulsma T, Wiersinga WM, Drexhage HA, Vader HL. Low maternal free thyroxine concentrations during early pregnancy are associated with impaired psychomotor development in infancy. Clin Endocrinol 1999; 50: 149 – 55.

Poppe K, Glinoer D. Thyroid autoimmunity and hypothyroidism before and during pregnancy. Human Reprod Update 2003; 9: 149 – 61.

Premawardhana LD, Parkes AB, Ammari F, John R, Darke C, Adams H, Lazarus JH. Postpartum thyroiditis and long-term thyroid status: prognostic influence of thyroid peroxidase antibodies and ultrasound echogenicity. J Clin Endocrinol Metab 2000; 85: 71 – 5.

Sieiro Netto S, Medina Coeli M, Micmacher E, Mamede Da Costa S, Nazar L, Galvao D, Buescu A, Vaisman M. Influence of thyroid autoimmunity and maternal age on the risk of miscarriage. Am J Reprod Immunol 2004; 52: 312 – 6.

Smallridge RC. Postpartum thyroid disease: a model of immunologic dysfunction. Clin & Appl Immunol Rev 2000; 1: 89 – 103.

Smyth PP, Wijeyaratne CN, Kaluarachi WN, Smith DF, Premawardhana LD, Parkes AB, Jayasinghe A, de Silva DG, Lazarus JH. Sequential studies on thyroid antibodies during pregnancy. Thyroid 2005; 15: 474 – 7.

Stagnaro-Green A, Chen X, Bogden JD, Davies TF, Scholl TO. The thyroid and pregnancy: a novel risk factor for very preterm delivery. Thyroid 2005; 15: 351 – 7.

Stagnaro-Green A, Roman SH, Cobin RH, El-Harazy E, Alvarez-Marfani M, Davies TF. Detection of an at-risk pregnancy by means of highly sensitive assays for thyroid autoantibodies. JAMA 1990; 264: 1422 – 5.

Stagnaro-Green A, Roman SH, Cobin RH, El-Harazy E, Wallenstein S, Davies TF. A prospective study of lymphocyte-initiated immunosuppression in normal pregnancy: evidence of a T-cell etiology for postpartum thyroid dysfunction. J Clin Endocrinol Metab 1992; 74: 645 – 53.

Tagami T, Hagiwara H, Kimura T, Usui T, Shimatsu A, Naruse M. The incidence of gestational hyperthyroidism and postpartum thyroiditis in the treated patients with Graves' disease. Thyroid 2007; 17: 767 – 72.

Vaidya B, Anthony S, Bilous M, Shields B, Drury J, Hutchinson S, Bilous R. Detection of thyroid dysfunction in early pregnancy: universal screening or targeted high-risk case finding. J Clin Endocrinol Metab 2007; 92: 203 – 7.

Veenstra van Nieuwenhoven AL, Heinemann MJ, Faas MM. The immunology of successful pregnancy. Human Reprod Update 2003; 9: 347 – 57.

Walfish PG, Meyerson J, Provias JP, Vargas MT, Papsin FR. Prevalence and characteristics of post-partum thyroid dysfunction: results of a survey from Toronto, Canada. J Endocrinol Invest 1992; 15: 265 – 72.

Weetman AP. Graves' disease. N Engl J Med 2000; 343: 1236 – 48.

Yoshida S, Takamatsu J, Kuma K, Ohsawa N. Thyroid-stimulating antibodies and thyroid stimulation-blocking antibodies during the pregnancy and postpartum period: a case report. Thyroid 1992; 2: 27 – 30.

7 Thyroid Hormone Action on the Developing Placental Unit

E. Vasilopoulon[1], M. D. Kilby[2]*

[1] School of Clinical and Experimental Medicine, Institute of Biomedical Research, Medical School, University of Birmingham, Birmingham B15 2TT, U.K.
[2] School of Clinical and Experimental Medicine, Birmingham Women's Foundation Trust/ University of Birmingham, Edgbaston, Birmingham B15 2TG, U.K.

Abstract

The human placenta provides 'direct' contact between the maternal blood and the chorionic villi forming a haemochorial placenta. In human pregnancy, the haemochorial placenta is pivotal in providing nutrients and oxygen to the developing foetus. One of the important placental functions is that of transport, both from maternal to the foetal and foetal to maternal circulations. The placenta has classically been considered as being relatively impermeable to thyroid hormones of maternal origin, expressing enzymes, especially type 3 deiodinase that metabolises thyroxine (T_4). However, contemporaneous data have shown that maternal/foetal transfer of both T_4 and triiodothyronine (T_3) occurs, with these thyroid hormones (TH) being present in foetal tissues, such as the coelomic cavity (at 5–7 weeks) before endogenous foetal TH production occurs at 14 weeks. There is thus now evidence that maternal thyroid hormones (TH) can cross the human placenta throughout gestation and that optimal TH levels are important for foetal brain development. A well functioning placenta is essential in mediating the supply of maternal TH to the foetus. In addition, TH is thought to be important for placental development. The action of TH on the developing foetoplacental unit is dependent on the circulating concentrations of TH in maternal serum, the presence of plasma membrane TH transporters that facilitate transplacental passage of TH, the activity of deiodinase enzymes that convert TH to its active and inactive forms and the presence of nuclear TH receptors that bind to TH response elements (TREs) and regulate gene expression. Disruption of these mechanisms may lead to abnormal foetal brain development and can also affect placental development. Further research is needed in order to determine the mechanisms by which TH acts on placental development and to elucidate its potential role in pregnancy complications such as intrauterine growth restriction.

7.1 Introduction

The thyroid hormones (TH) are synthesised in the thyroid gland and released into the circulation. The majority of released TH is in the form of T_4, as total serum T_4 and is 40-fold higher than serum T_3. Only 0.03 % of the total serum T_4 and 0.3 % of total serum T_3 is free (unbound). The majority of released T_3 and T_4 are bound to carrier proteins such as thyroxine binding globulin, albumin and thyroid binding prealbumin. The free TH enters target cells, where it exerts its biological actions (Yen, 2001). TH is important for the growth and differentiation of many organs and is essential for normal foetal development (Chan and Kilby, 2000; Schwartz et al., 1983). It plays a critical role in the development of the foetal brain, as demonstrated by studies showing an association of maternal hypothyroidism with poorer neurophysiological outcome in the offspring (Haddow et al., 1999; Pop et al., 2003; Pop et al., 1999). Foetal TH production does not begin until the second trimester of pregnancy (Fig. 7.**1**). However, TH is present in human embryonic cavities at the first trimester of pregnancy, indicating that TH from the maternal circulation is supplied to the developing foetus (Calvo et al., 2002; Calvo et al., 1990; Cotempre et al., 1993; Thorpe-Beeston et al., 1991; Vulsma et al., 1989). There is an ongoing foetal demand for maternal TH throughout pregnancy with 30 % of TH present in the foetus at term originating from the maternal circulation (Chan et al., 2002). The human placenta provides

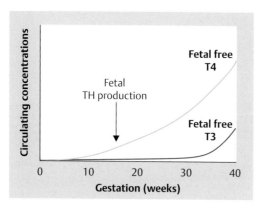

Fig. 7.1   Fetal TH production. Fetal production of thyroid hormone does not start until the second trimester of pregnancy. However, TH is present in human embryonic cavities since the first trimester of pregnancy indicating that transfer of TH occurs from the mother to the foetus. Circulating levels of foetal free T_3 and free T_4 increase with gestation.

'direct' contact between the maternal blood and the chorionic villi forming a haemochorial placenta. In human pregnancy, the haemochorial placenta is pivotal in providing nutrients and oxygen to the developing foetus. One of the important placental functions is that of transport, both from maternal to the foetal and from foetal to maternal circulations. The placenta has classically been considered as being relatively impermeable to thyroid hormones of maternal origin, expressing enzymes, especially type 3 deiodinase that metabolises thyroxine (T_4). However, contemporaneous data have shown that maternal/foetal transfer of both T_4 and triiodothyronine (T_3) occurs, with these thyroid hormones (TH) being present in foetal tissues, such as the coelomic cavity (at 5–7 weeks) before endogeneous foetal TH production occurs at 14 weeks. For maternal thyroid hormone to reach the foetal circulation it must pass through the various cell layers of the placenta. It is therefore essential that an efficient transport system is available for both uptake and export of TH into the cells through the plasma membrane (James et al., 2007). As well as facilitating the transport of maternal TH to the foetal circulation, the human placenta is thought to be sensitive to the action of TH for the regulation of its metabolism, differentiation and development (Kilby et al., 2005). *In vitro* experiments indicate that TH induces the differentiation of placental cells in early but not late pregnancy (Maruo et al.,

1991). It is also thought that TH acts in synergy with EGF to regulate the survival, proliferation and differentiation of placental cells (Barber et al., 2005; Canettieri et al., 2008; Maruo et al., 1995; Matsuo et al., 1993). Therefore, TH availability is postulated to play an important role in both foetal and placental development.

7.2   Mechanisms Regulating TH Action

Whilst circulating concentrations of THs are the major determinants of cellular supply of T_3, many other factors may modulate T_3 action at the tissue level. These include the expression of TH receptors in the target cells, the activity of deiodinase enzymes and the expression of TH transporters (Fig. 7.**2**). All these factors regulate the availability of T_3 to the placenta and the amounts of T_3 that are released to the foetal circulation.

7.2.1   Thyroid Hormone Receptors

T_3, the active TH ligand, exerts its biological function by binding to TH receptors (TRs). These are ligand-regulated transcription factors that belong to the nuclear hormone receptor superfamily (Yen, 2001). TRs are the product of two genes. The TRα (*c-erbAα*) gene is located on chromosome 17 and encodes the separate isoforms TRα1 and TRα2 (Weinberger et al., 1986). The TRβ (*c-erbAβ*) gene is found on chromosome 3 and encodes the isoforms TRβ1 and TRβ2. TRs form homo- and hetero-dimers that interact with T_3-response elements (TREs) in order to repress or activate gene expression. TRα1, TRβ1 and TRβ2 are known to bind T_3. In contrast, TRα2 does not bind T_3 and may therefore inhibit the function of the other TRs by competitive binding to the TRE site. TRα1 and TRβ1 are ubiquitously expressed. In contrast, TRβ2 is only found in specific tissues, namely in the anterior pituitary gland, in the hypothalamus and in the developing brain (Yen, 2001). Several studies have investigated the expression of TRs in the placenta. The presence of nuclear T_3 binding was first described in placental homogenates using radiolabelling techniques (Banovac et al., 1980; Banovac et al, 1986). These experiments were extended using trophoblast cells, which demonstrated that nuclear binding of radiolabelled T_3 was specific to this cell type (Ashitaka et al., 1988; Nishii et al., 1989). Our group investigated the expression of TRs in human placenta across gestation (Kilby et al., 1998). Using immunohisto-

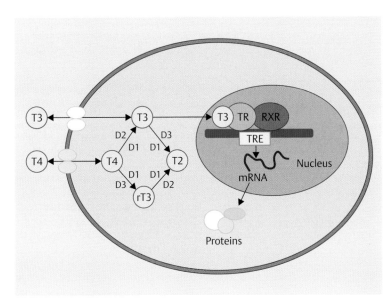

Fig. 7.**2** **Mechanisms regulating TH action.** The action of TH at the cellular level is dependent upon four factors. These include (1) the circulating levels of free T_3 and T_4, (2) the presence of TH plasma membrane transporters that facilitate entry of TH to the cells, (3) the activity of deiodinase enzymes that metabolise TH to its active (T_3) and inactive (T_4, rT_3, T_2) forms and (4) the presence of the nuclear thyroid hormone receptors (TRs). Binding of T_3 to TRs regulates the expression of TH responsive genes by interactions with thyroid hormone response elements (TREs) found on the DNA molecule.

chemistry we defined the expression of TRα1, TRα2 and TRβ1 in trophoblasts and stromal placental cells. The staining for all isoforms increased with increasing gestation. The expression levels of TRs were also assessed at the mRNA level by semi-quantitative RT-PCR. There was an increase in the mRNA levels of TRα1, TRα2 and TRβ1 with increasing gestation. The expression of TRs has also been studied in rat placenta (Leonard et al., 2001). Semi-quantitative RT-PCR showed no change in the expression levels of TRα1 and TRβ1 between the 16th and 21st day of gestation. However, the maximal T_3 binding capacity doubled over the same period, indicating that placental TR binding capacity is post-transcriptionally regulated in the rat.

7.2.2 Deiodinase Enzyme Activity

The biological activity of thyroid hormone is regulated locally by tissue specific regulation of the different deiodinase enzymes. The iodothyronine deiodinases are selenocysteine-containing enzymes that determine the availability of the active TH ligand, T_3, within the tissues. There are three deiodinase subtypes, type I (D1), type II (D2) and type III (D3) (St. Germain and Galton, 1997). They are responsible for the outer-ring deiodination (ORD) of T_4 to T_3 and for the inner-ring deiodination (IRD) of T_4 and T_3 to their inactive metabolites (rT_3, T_2). D1 catalyses the monodeiodination of T_4 to T_3 and is responsible for 80% of the circulating T_3 in humans. It is expressed predominantly in the liver, kidney and thyroid (Mandel et al., 1992). D2 is the primary activating enzyme in tissues and locally catalyses the monodeiodination of T_4 to T_3 (Salvatore et al., 1996). It is found in the brain, anterior pituitary, thyroid, brown fat, skeletal muscle, heart and is also present at low levels in the human placenta (Croteau et al., 1996; Kuiper et al., 2005). D3 is the deactivating enzyme. It catalyses the monodeiodination of T_4 to rT_3 and of T_3 to T_2 (Kohrle, 1999). It is present in the placenta, pregnant uterus, fetal tissues and in the brain (Chan et al., 2002; Kuiper et al., 2005; Chan et al., 2003; Kaplan and Yaskoski, 1981; Koopdonk-Kool et al., 1996). Our group has studied the mRNA expression and enzymatic activities of deiodinases in the placenta throughout gestation (Chan et al., 2003). The predominant deiodinase expressed in the placenta was D3. The mRNA levels and the activities of D2 and D3 were decreased with increasing gestation. *In vitro* experiments using primary cultures of term cytotrophoblasts and JEG-3 choriocarcinoma cells showed that treatment with T_3 causes an increase in the expression of D2 and/or D3.

7.3 Expression of TH Transporters

Transporter proteins are required to facilitate the passage of TH into and out of the cells. A variety of proteins that are capable of transporting TH have

Table 7.**1**   TH transporters present in the human placenta.

Transporter family	MCTs	LATs	OATPs
Subtypes in the placenta	MCT8; MCT10	LAT1; LAT2	OATP 1A2; OATP 4A1
Obligate heterodimer	Unknown	4F2hc	Unknown
Also transports	MCT8: unknown; MCT10: aromatic amino acids and derivatives	Amino acids	Amphipathic organic compounds (e.g., bile acids, steroid hormones, prostaglandins, penicillins)

been identified to date. They belong to different families including the monocarboxylate transporter family, L-type amino acid transporters and organic anion transporting polypeptides. The TH transporters expressed in the placenta are summarised in Table 7.1. They play an important role in regulating TH uptake by the placental cells and efflux of TH into the fetal circulation.

7.3.1   Monocarboxylate Transporters (MCT) 8 and 10

The MCT family consists of 14 members, of which four (MCT1–4) have been characterised as monocarboxylate transporters. Two members of the MCT family, MCT8 and MCT10, have been identified as TH transporters (Friesema et al., 2008; Friesema et al., 2003). The MCT8 gene (SLC16A2) is located on the X chromosome and encodes a 67 kDa protein containing 12 transmembrane putative domains (Lafreniere et al., 1994). MCT8 is highly expressed in the liver, kidney, brain, heart, lung and placenta. Studies in human placenta show increased expression of MCT8 with advancing gestation (Chan et al., 2006). MCT8 was demonstrated to be a potent transporter of T_4, T_3, rT_3 and T_2 with a Km value of $2-5\,\mu M$ (37). It does not transport monocarboxylates or aromatic amino acids and no other ligands for MCT8 have been found so far. MCT8 facilitates both influx and efflux of THs (Friesema et al., 2008). Mutations in the MCT8 gene have been associated with an X-linked psychomotor retardation syndrome. Mutations have been reported in several unrelated families (Schwartz et al., 2005; Maranduba et al., 2006; Holden et al., 2005; Friesema et al., 2004; Biebermann et al., 2005). The affected males have abnormal concentrations of circulating iodothyronines, namely elevated serum T_3 and free T_3 and decreased serum T_4 and free T_4. The levels of TSH are normal. The patients demonstrate neurological abnormalities including global developmental delay, central hypotonia, spastic quadraplegia, dystonic movements, rotary nystagmus and impaired gaze and hearing. Heterozygous females have a milder thyroid phenotype and no neurological defects.

The human MCT10, also known as T-type amino acid transporter-1 (TAT1), was characterised in 2002 (Kim et al., 2002). The MCT10 gene (SLC16A10) is localised on chromosome 6 and encodes a 55 kDa protein with 12 transmembrane putative domains. MCT10 is highly expressed in the human intestine, kidney, heart and placenta. MCT10 is responsible for the efflux of aromatic amino acids (Ramadan et al., 2006). Due to its high homology with MCT8, it was hypothesised that MCT10 can also transport iodothyronines. In order to investigate this hypothesis COS1 cells were transfected with human MCT10. Transfection with MCT10 caused a marked stimulation of cellular T_3 and particularly T_4 uptake. Co-transfection with hCRYM, a cytosolic protein with high affinity for iodothyronines, demonstrated that MCT10 also facilitates efflux of T_3 and T_4. T_3 uptake by MCT10-transfected COS1 cells was inhibited in the presence of the aromatic amino acids phenylalanine, tyrosine and tryptophan. However, T_3 efflux was not affected (Friesema et al., 2008).

7.3.2   L-Type Amino Acid Transporters (LAT) 1 and 2

L-Type amino acid transporters (system L) are members of the heterodimeric amino acid transporter (HAT) family. They consist of a heavy chain (4F2/CD98) and a light chain (LAT1 or LAT2) linked together by a disulphide bridge. System L is responsible for the transport of neutral amino acids (Verrey, 2003). LAT2 is primarily expressed in the human kidney and intestine (Rossier et al., 1999). LAT1 mRNA is expressed widely including human liver, bone marrow, brain, intestine, testis and adipose tissue (Yanagida et al., 2001). LAT1, LAT2 and 4F2hc are expressed in the human placenta. Expression studies in the human placenta showed that mRNA levels of both LAT1 and 4F2hc were increased at full term compared to mid-trimester (Okamoto et al., 2002). Furthermore, LAT1 expression was localised at the syncytiotrophoblast layer on the apical (maternal blood-facing) side (Okamoto et al., 2002; Ritchie et al., 2001). The ability of the system L to facilitate transport of iodothyronines as well as of amino acids was investigated using X. laevis oocytes, which have negligible expression of system L, and the choriocarcinoma cell line BeWo, which has high endogeneous expression of system L, as models (Ritchie et al., 2001; Friesema et al., 2001; Ritchie et al., 2003). These experiments demonstrated that system L facilitates the transport of amino acids, such as phenylalanine, tyrosine, tryptophan and leucine and of iodothyronines, namely T_3, rT_3 and T_4. They also demonstrated that this is an Na^+-independent transport mechanism.

7.3.3 Organic Anion Transporting Polypeptides (OATP) 1A2 and 4A1

The OATP family includes eleven different OATPs in humans, which are expressed in various tissues including the liver, kidney, brain, lung, intestine and placenta. They mediate Na^+-independent transport of a variety of amphipathic organic compounds, such as bile acids, steroid hormones and their conjugates, linear and cyclic peptides, prostaglandins and thyroid hormones (Hagenbuch, 2007). OATP1A2 and OATP4A1 are expressed in the human placenta (Sato et al., 2003; Patel et al., 2003; Briz et al., 2003). Immunohistochemistry studies in human placental samples showed that OATP4A1 is predominantly expressed at the apical surface of syncytiotrophoblasts in the human placenta (Sato et al., 2003). Transfection studies using Xenopus oocytes demonstrated the ability of OATP4A1 to transport T_3, T_4 and rT_3 (Fujiwara et al., 2001). In a similar study it was shown that OATP1A2 facilitates the transport of T_3 and T_4 in X. laevis oocytes (Kullak-Ublick et al., 2001). These transporters could therefore be important for maternal thyroid hormone transport to the developing fetus.

7.4 Effect of TH on Foetal Development

The critical role of thyroid hormones in growth and differentiation of many organs and thus overall development in man is well recognised (Cahn and Kliby, 2000; Schwartz et al., 1983). This is of particular significance in the central nervous system (CNS) where thyroid hormone deficiency is known to be associated with neurodevelopment morbidity. It appears that in many species thyroid hormones, via influence on thyroid-responsive genes, synchronise neuronal differentiation, polarity, synaptogenesis, cytoplasmic outgrowths and myelin formation (Bernal, 2005; Bernal and Nunez, 1995; Guadano-Ferraz et al., 1999). The thyroid status of neonates and children has a significant long-term impact on their behaviour, locomotor ability, speech, hearing and cognition (Legrand, 1986). Development of different areas of the CNS has been associated with the timing and duration of TH deficiency, suggesting that there are critical periods during which various parts of the brain are sensitive to TH supply (Rovet et al., 1992).

The placenta has been considered as being impermeable to thyroid hormones of maternal origin, partly as a result of it expressing enzymes, especially type III deiodinase, that metabolise T_4. However, there is now evidence that transfer of T_3 and T_4 occurs from the mother to the foetus. Thyroid hormones are present in human embryonic cavities during the first trimester of pregnancy, before the onset of foetal TH production, which does not occur until the second trimester (Comtempre et al., 1993; Thorpe-Beeston et al., 1991). Between 6 and 11 weeks of pregnancy T_4 concentration increases with gestational age and with rising maternal serum T_4 (Contempre et al., 1993). These data suggest that maternal T_4 can cross the placental barrier as early as the second month of pregnancy. More recent studies have confirmed that foetal tissues are exposed to biologically relevant free T_4 concentrations during early pregnancy (Calvo et al., 2002). Studies in infants with severe congenital hypothyroidism have shown that substantial amounts of T_4 are transferred from mother to foetus during late gestation (Vulsma et al., 1989). A similar study using a rat model of congenital hypothyroidism demonstrated that infusion of T_4 into the mothers caused an increase in T_4 and particularly T_3 in the foetal brain (Calvo et al., 2002).

The association of maternal hypothyroidism with poorer neuropsychological outcome in the offspring demonstrates the critical role of TH in foetal brain development (Haddow et al., 1999; Pop et al., 2003; Pop et al., 1999). Children of women with free T_4 levels below the fifth and tenth percentiles at 12 weeks of gestation had significantly lower scores on the Bayley psychomotor developmental index (PDI) scale at ten months of age, compared to children of mothers with higher free T_4 levels (Pop et al., 1999). Furthermore, there was a positive correlation between maternal free T_4 levels and PDI scores. In a three-year follow-up study, children of women with hypothyroxinaemia at 12 weeks of gestation had delayed mental and motor functions compared to matched controls (Pop et al., 2003). These data suggest that low maternal plasma free T_4 concentrations during early pregnancy are an important risk factor for impaired infant development. A study investigating the effects of maternal hypothyroxinaemia in a rat model showed that maternal hypothyroxinaemia during early pregnancy alters fetal brain histogenesis and cytoarchitecture (Lavado-Autric et al., 2003).

The sensitivity of the developing brain to TH is indicated by the presence of molecules involved in TH supply, action and metabolism in the fetal brain. Nuclear binding sites for T_3 have been identified in the human fetal brain from week 10 of gestation and they were shown to increase with gestational age (Bernal et al., 1984). In a more recent study the expression of thyroid hormone receptors in the first trimester foetal brain was investigated by semi-quantitative PCR (Iskaros et al., 2000). The expression of TRα1, TRα2 and TRβ1 was detected as early as week 8. The expression of TRα1 and TRα2 increased with gestation, while there was a nadir in the expression of TRβ1 between weeks 8 and 12. Our own group has studied the mRNA and protein expression of TRs in the human foetal brain (Kilby et al., 2000). TRα1, TRα2, TRβ1 and TRβ2 mRNAs were present in the foetal brain from week 10 of human pregnancy. The presence of TRs at the protein level was determined by immunohistochemistry. TRα1 and TRα2 proteins were present in the foetal brain from gestation week 11 and their expression increased with gestational age. The expression of these proteins was confined to the pyramidal neurons of the cerebral cortex and the Purkinje cells of the cerebellum, indicating that these cell types are probably the targets of TH action.

The expression and activity levels of the deiodinase enzymes in the developing brain have also been investigated. Our group has studied the mRNA expression and the activity of the deiodinases in human foetal cerebral cortex during the first and second trimesters of pregnancy (Chan et al., 2002). The expression of D1 was variable across gestation and D1 activity was undetectable. D2 mRNA and activity were present from 7–8 weeks of gestation and they peaked at 15–16 weeks. D3 mRNA expression and enzymatic activity were detected from early first trimester. The D3 activity levels detected in the human foetal cortex were higher than those in the adult, indicating the importance of this mechanism to protect the developing foetal brain from excessive T_3 supply. In a similar study D1, D2 and D3 activities were assessed in the human foetal brain (Kester et al., 2004). D1 activity was undetectable. There was considerable D2 activity in foetal cortex, which correlated positively with T_4 levels. D3 activity was found in the cerebellum, midbrain, basal ganglia, brain stem, spinal cord and hippocampus and it decreased after midgestation. T_3 levels in these tissues were low until midgestation, when D3 activity started decreasing. These results suggest that D2 and D3 play important roles in regulating the local availability of T_3 in the human foetal brain. Their spatial and temporal expression is essential in protecting brain regions from excessive T_3 until differentiation is required. Experiments in hypothyroid rat brain showed an increase in D2 mRNA expression in relay nuclei and cortical targets of the primary somatosensory and auditory pathways during postnatal development. These results indicate that T_3 has a role in the development of these structures (Guadano-Ferraz et al., 1999).

The expression of TH transporters is also critical for the supply of TH to the developing brain. Members of the OATP, LAT and MCT families that are known to transport thyroid hormones are expressed in the brain (Frieseam et al., 2003; Lafreniere et al., 1994; Yanagida et al, 2001; Hagenbuch, 2007; Heuer, 2007; Taylor and Ritchie, 2007). These include LAT1, OATP1C1 and MCT8. OATP1C1 is expressed in the blood-brain barrier and is thought to play an important role in the delivery of thyroid hormones, mainly T_4, to the brain. The blood-brain barrier is the route by which thyroid hormone is preferentially distributed throughout the brain and this transporter could facilitate uptake of T_4 by the astrocytes (Hagenbuch, 2007; Bernal, 2005; Pizzagalli et al., 2002). MCT8 expression was studied in the murine CNS (Heuer et al., 2005). High levels of MCT8 mRNA were detected in the choroid plexus and in neo- and allocortical regions including the olfactory bulb, cerebral cortex, hippocampus and amygdala. Moderate levels of MCT8 mRNA were found in the striatum and cerebellum and low levels in a few neuroendocrine nuclei. According to this study, MCT8 is predominantly expressed by neurons. It is therefore postulated that OATPs are responsible for the transport of T_4 through the blood-brain barrier. T_4 is then converted to T_3 in the astrocytes by the action of D2. The uptake of T_3 by the neighbouring neurons, where T_3 acts upon cell differentiation and migration, is facilitated by MCT8. The importance of MCT8 in CNS development is demonstrated by the psychomotor retardation that has been reported in males affected by MCT8 mutations (Schwartz et al., 2005; Maranduba et al., 2006; Holden et al., 2005; Friesema et al., 2004; Dumitrescu et al., 2004; Biebermann et al., 2005).

7.5 Effect of TH on Placental Development

A well functioning placenta is necessary to mediate the transport of nutrients from the maternal to the foetal circulation. The development of the human placenta involves a complex process of tightly regulated proliferation, invasion into the uterine decidua and differentiation into a multinucleated syncytiotrophoblast layer. Early human placentation involves proliferation of cytotrophoblast cells from the tips of anchoring chorionic villi to form cytotrophoblast columns. Cytotrophoblast cells differentiate into extravillous trophoblasts (EVTs), which invade the maternal endometrium and transform the maternal spiral arteries resulting in dilated, low-capacitance vessels, thus facilitating the blood flow from the maternal circulation to the placenta (Craven et al., 2000; Naneev et al., 2000; Pijnenborg et al., 1983). Furthermore, cytotrophobast cells in floating villi fuse together to form a multinucleated syncytiotrophoblast (ST) layer, which forms a physical barrier between the maternal and fetal cells and is responsible for gas and nutrient exchange between the maternal circulation and the developing fetus (Jurisicova et al., 2005). The syncytiotrophoblast layer is continuously renewed as aged syncytiotrophoblast nuclei are packed into syncytial knots and released into the maternal circulation and new cytotrophoblasts continuously fuse with the syncytiotrophoblast layer (Jurisico-

va et al., 2005; Huppertz et al., 2006). The formation of the syncytium is linked to the initiator stages of the apoptotic cascade, while the formation of syncytial knots is the results of the final "execution" stages of the apoptotic cascade (Huppertz et al., 2006).

It has been postulated that the human placenta is sensitive to the actions of thyroid hormone for the regulation of its metabolism, differentiation and development. It has been shown that placental tissue has a high nuclear binding capacity for T_3 (Banovac et al., 1980; Banovac et al., 1986; Ashitaka et al., 1988; Nishii et al., 1989). Our own study has demonstrated the expression of TRα1, TRα2 and TRβ1 within the nuclei of trophoblasts and stromal placental cells throughout gestation (Kilby et al., 1998). TRα1, TRα2 and TRβ1 are also found in EVTs, as demonstrated by immunohistochemistry in 1st and 2nd trimester placental bed biopsies and in expression studies in primary cultures of 1st trimester EVTs (Barber et al., 2005; Laoag-Fernandez et al., 2004). These data indicate that the placenta is a target organ for TH action. A study by Maruo et al. (1991) investigated the effect of TH on trophoblast differentiation. Explants from early and term placentae were treated with T_3 or T_4. TH treatment caused an increase in the secretion of progesterone, 17β-oestradiol, hCGα, hCGβ and hPL by early placenta explants. In contrast, term placenta explants did not respond to TH treatment with increased endocrine activity, indicating that TH is important for the differentiation of placental cells in early but not late pregnancy. The effect of TH on placental apoptosis in EVTs isolated from 1st trimester placentae was investigated in another study (Laoag-Fernandez et al., 2004). T_3 treatment reduced apoptosis by down-regulating the expression of Fas and Fas ligand. Therefore, TH might promote EVT invasion of the endometrium by suppressing apoptosis in early pregnancy.

It has also been suggested that TH acts in synergy with epidermal growth factor (EGF) to regulate placental growth and function. Indeed, treatment of first trimester placental explants with T_3 resulted in increased EGF secretion (Maruo et al., 1995; Matsuo et al., 1993). EGF has been shown to increase cytotrophoblast proliferation in placental explants isolated at 4–5 weeks of pregnancy. In contrast, EGF did not affect proliferation in 6–12 week placental expants, however it resulted in increased secretion of hCG and hPL (Maruo et al., 1995). A study performed by our group also investigated the effects of EGF and T_3 on trophoblast function (Barber et al., 2005). EGF enhanced the survival of primary term cytotrophoblasts. Furthermore, it enhanced the invasion of fibrin gels by EVT-like SGHPL-4 cells; an effect that was attenuated by co-treatment with T_3. Co-treatment with T3 and EGF had an anti-proliferative effect on SGHPL-4 cells, while it enhanced their motility. In contrast treatment with T_3 and EGF stimulated proliferation of JEG-3 cells. Interestingly, a study performed in JEG-3 choriocarcinoma cells showed that EGF modulates the transcription of human type II deiodinase (Canettieri et al., 2008). EGF was shown to induce a short-lived D2 mRNA expression and enzymatic activity. The authors propose that this indicates that EGF transcriptionally regulates the activation of TH. These results indicate that EGF and TH are important in both the proliferation and differentiation of placental cells in early pregnancy and may act in synergy to regulate placental development.

A series of studies have also been performed using hypothyroid animal models in order to investigate the importance of TH in placental development, however, their findings have not always been consistent. One study investigated the effect of maternal TH on rat placental TH content (Morreale de Escobar et al., 1985). It was shown that T_3 and T_4 were undetectable in the rat placenta before the onset of foetal thyroid function. Measurements in 21-day old placentae revealed that T_3 and T_4 were still markedly reduced after the onset of foetal thyroid function. In another study investigating the foetal and neonatal development of the rat, it was shown that maternal hypothyroidism results in impaired reproduction and intrauterine growth restriction (IUGR) (Kumar and Chaudhuri, 1989). In contrast similar studies suggested that maternal hypothyroxinaemia did not consistently affect rat placental development (Pickard et al., 1993; Pickard et al., 1999). They showed that placental weight was normal in hypothyroxinaemic pregnancies, however, cytosolic and total placental protein concentrations were reduced at 15 and 19 weeks of gestation, respectively.

7.6   TH and Pregnancy Complications – Intrauterine Growth Restriction

Intrauterine growth restriction (IUGR) is a pregnancy complication that is characterised by reduced birth weight and increased risk of foetal

and neonatal death. The ultrasound features of IUGR are increased head/abdomen circumference ratio, oligohydramnios, vasodilation of the foetal middle cerebral artery circulation and increased impedence to blood flow in the umbilical arteries (Chang et al., 1993). This pathological process may cause significant long-term morbidity, with 10% of very low birthweight babies having some physical handicap (Gaffney et al., 1994) and a further 5% demonstrating neurodevelopmental delay at the age of 9 years (Kok et al., 1998). Thyroid status is one of several factors that have been postulated to play a critical role in the pathogenesis of such morbidity, especially with respect to the growth and development of the CNS (Fisher, 1986).

The serum concentrations of free T_4 and free T_3 are lower in foetuses affected by IUGR compared to matched controls, while there is no difference in serum TSH levels (Kilby et al., 1998). Assessment of the endocrine profile of children (2–10 years old) with IUGR revealed no differences in TH levels compared to the control group (Fattal-Valevski et al., 2005). In contrast, a study performed in lambs showed that placental restriction and small size at birth correlates with reduced plasma total T_4 and increased plasma total T_3 postnatally (De Blasio et al., 2006). Furthermore, soft tissue growth was increased in placental restriction compared with control lambs at the same circulating TH concentrations. These results suggest that placental restriction and small size at birth may increase activation of T_4 to T_3 and sensitivity of soft tissues to TH in the lamb, which may contribute to catch-up growth following IUGR. However, interactions between thyroid hormone levels and growth often differ in man from animal studies (Laron, 2003).

Another important consideration concerning the implications of thyroid status in IUGR is the expression patterns of TRs, deiodinases and TH transporters in pregnancies complicated by IUGR. Our group has studied the changes in the expression of TRs in human placenta and foetal CNS with IUGR. In the placenta, there was no significant difference in the mRNA levels of TRα1, TRα2 and TRβ1, but the protein levels of these molecules were increased with IUGR (Kilby et al., 1998). In contrast, the protein expression of TRα1, TRα2 and TRβ1 was lower in the cerebral cortex and cerebellum of IUGR foetuses compared to matched controls (Kilby et al., 2000). Therefore, thyroid status is potentially important in influencing CNS development and long-term foetal outcome in IUGR pregnancies. Comparisons of the mRNA expression and activity of the deiodinase enzymes D2 and D3 in human placentae from pregnancies complicated by IUGR compared to normal placentae of similar gestational ages revealed no significant differences, indicating that placental deiodinases are not responsible for the low TH concentrations observed in IUGR foetuses (Chan et al., 2003).

7.7 Conclusions

There is increasing evidence that transplacental passage of maternal T_4 and T_3 is important for the development of the human central nervous system. TH deficiency or excess alters cell differentiation, migration and gene expression in the developing brain and can have a long-term impact on psychomotor functions. Furthermore, TH seems to be important for placental development. A well functioning placenta is essential for normal foetal development. IUGR is often associated with malplacentation and is a significant contributor to perinatal mortality and morbidity. It is postulated that the changes observed in the expression of TRs with IUGR may contribute to the development of this pathology. The availability of maternal TH to the developing foetoplacental unit is also an important consideration. It is now known that plasma membrane transporter proteins are necessary for the passage of TH in and out of the cells. Further research is needed in order to identify the transporter proteins that are responsible for influx and efflux of TH from the different placental layers. Different molecules may be involved in the uptake of maternal TH by the placenta, and the release of TH to the foetal circulation. Further research would elucidate whether changes in these transporters are contributing to the lower TH concentrations found in growth restricted foetuses.

Acknowledgements

EV is supported by a PhD studentship funded by the MRC (UK). Her work is also part funded by grants from Acton Medical Research and Well-being of Women.

References

Ashitaka Y, Maruo M, Takeuchi Y, Nakayama H, Mochizuki M. 3, 5, 3′-triiodo-L-thyronine binding sites in nuclei of human trophoblastic cells. Endocrinol Jpn 1988; 35: 197–206.

Banovac K, Bzik L, Tislaric D, Sekso M. Conversion of thyroxine to triiodothyronine and reverse triiodothyronine in human placenta and fetal membranes. Horm Res 1980; 12: 253–9.

Banovac K, Ryan EA, O'Sullivan MJ. Triiodothyronine (T_3) nuclear binding sites in human placenta and decidua. Placenta 1986; 7: 543–9.

Barber KJ, Franklyn JA, McCabe CJ, Khanim FL, Bulmer JN, Whitley GS et al. The *in vitro* effects of triiodothyronine on epidermal growth factor-induced trophoblast function. J Clin Endocrinol Metab 2005; 90: 1655–61.

Bernal J, Nunez J. Thyroid hormones and brain development. Eur J Endocrinol 1995; 133: 390–8.

Bernal J, Pekonen F. Ontogenesis of the nuclear 3, 5, 3′-triiodothyronine receptor in the human fetal brain. Endocrinology 1984; 114: 677–9.

Bernal J. Thyroid hormones and brain development. Vitam Horm 2005; 71: 95–122.

Biebermann H, Ambrugger P, Tarnow P, von Moers A, Schweizer U, Grueters A. Extended clinical phenotype, endocrine investigations and functional studies of a loss-of-function mutation A150V in the thyroid hormone specific transporter MCT8. Eur J Endocrinol 2005; 153: 359–66.

Briz O, Serrano MA, Maclas RI, Gonzalez-Gallego J, Marin JJ. Role of organic anion-transporting polypeptides, OATP-A, OATP-C and OATP-8, in the human placenta-maternal liver tandem excretory pathway for foetal bilirubin. Biochem J 2003; 371: 897–905.

Calvo MR, Jauniaux E, Gulbis B, Asuncion M, Gervy C, Contempre B et al. Fetal tissues are exposed to biologically relevant free thyroxine concentrations during early phases of development. J Clin Endocrinol Metab 2002; 87: 1768–77.

Calvo R, Obregón MJ, Ruiz de Oña C, Escobar del Rey F, Morreale de Escobar G. Congenital hypothyroidism, as studied in rats. Crucial role of maternal thyroxine but not of 3, 5, 3′-triiodothyronine in the protection of the fetal brain. J Clin Invest 1990; 86: 889–99.

Canettieri G, Franchi A, Guardia MD, Morantte I, Santaguida MG, Harney JW et al. Activation of thyroid hormone is transcriptionally regulated by epidermal growth factor in human placenta-derived JEG3 cells. Endocrinology 2008; 149: 695–702.

Chan S, Kachilele S, Hobbs E, Bulmer JN, Boelaert K, McCabe CJ et al. Placental iodothyronine deiodinase expression in normal and growth-restricted human pregnancies. J Clin Endocrinol Metab 2003; 88: 4488–95.

Chan S, Kachilele S, McCabe CJ, Tannahill LA, Boelaert K, Gittoes NJ et al. Early expression of thyroid hormone deiodinases and receptors in human fetal cerebral cortex. Brain Res Dev Brain Res 2002; 138: 109–16.

Chan S, Kilby MD. Thyroid hormone and central nervous system development. J Endocrinol 2000; 165: 1–8.

Chan SY, Franklyn JA, Pemberton HN, Bulmer JN, Visser TJ, McCabe CJ et al. Monocarboxylate transporter 8 expression in the human placenta: the effects of severe intrauterine growth restriction. J Endocrinol 2006; 189: 465–71.

Chang TC, Robson SC, Spencer JA, Gallivan S. Identification of fetal growth retardation: comparison of Doppler waveform indices and serial ultrasound measurements of abdominal circumference and fetal weight. Obstet Gynaecol 1993; 82: 230–6.

Contempre B, Jauniaux E, Morreale de Escobar G, Calvo R, Jurkovic D, Campbell S et al. Detection of thyroid hormones in human embronic cavities during the first trimester of pregnancy. J Clin Endocrinol Metab 1993; 77: 1719–22.

Craven CM, Zhao L, Ward K. Lateral placental growth occurs by trophoblast cell invasion of decidual veins. Placenta 2000; 21: 160–9.

Croteau W, Davey JC, Galton VA, St Germain DL. Cloning of the mammalian type II iodothyronine deiodinase. A selenoprotein differentially expressed and regulated in human and rat brain and other tissues. J Clin Invest 1996; 98: 405–17.

De Blasio MJ, Gatford KL, Robinson JS, Owens JA. Placental restriction alters circulating thyroid hormone in the young lamb postnatally. Am J Physiol Regul Integr Comp Physiol 2006; 291: 1016–24.

Dumitrescu AM, Liao XH, Best TB, Brockmann K, Refetoff S. A novel syndrome combining thyroid and neurological abnormalities is associated with mutations in a monocarboxylate transporter gene. Am J Hum Genet 2004; 74: 168–75.

Fattal-Valevski A, Toledano-Alhadef H, Golander A, Leitner Y, Harel S. Endocrine profile of children with intrauterine growth retardation. J Pediatr Endocrinol Metab 2005; 18: 671–6.

Fisher D. The unique endocrine milieu of the fetus. J Clin Invest 1986; 78: 603–11.

Friesema EC, Docter R, Moerings EP, Verrey F, Krenning EP, Hennemann G et al. Thyroid hormone transport by the heterodimeric human system L amino acid transporter. Endocrinology 2001; 142: 4339–48.

Friesema EC, Ganguly S, Abdalla A, Manning Fox JE, Halestrap AP, Visser TJ. Identification of monocarboxylate transporter 8 as a specific thyroid hormone transporter. J Biol Chem 2003; 278: 40128–35.

Friesema EC, Grueters A, Biebermann H, Krude H, von Moers A, Reeser M et al. Association between mutations in a thyroid hormone transporter and severe X-linked psychomotor retardation. Lancet 2004; 364 (9443): 1435–7.

Friesema EC, Jansen J, Jachtenberg JW, Visser WE, Kester MH, Visser TJ. Effective cellular uptake and efflux of thyroid hormone by human monocarboxylate transporter 10 (MCT10). Mol Endocrinol 2008; 22: 1357–69.

Fujiwara K, Adachi H, Nishio T, Unno M, Tokui T, Okabe M et al. Identification of thyroid hormone transporters in humans: different molecules are involved in a tissue-specific manner. Endocrinology 2001; 142: 2005–12.

Gaffney G, Squier MV, Johnson A, Flavell V, Sellers S. Clinical associations of prenatal ischaemic white matter injury. Arch Dis Childhood 1994; 70 (Suppl. 2): F101–6.

Guadano-Ferraz A, Escamez MJ, Rausell E, Bernal J. Expression of type 2 iodothyronine deiodinase in hypothyroid rat brain indicates an important role of thyroid hormone in the development of specific primary sensory systems. J Neurosci 1999; 19: 3430–9.

Haddow JE, Palomaki GE, Allan WC, Williams JR, Knight GJ, Gagnon J et al. Maternal thyroid deficiency during pregnancy and subsequent neuropsychological development of the child. N Engl J Med 1999; 341: 549–55.

Hagenbuch B. Cellular entry of thyroid hormones by organic anion transporting polypeptides. Best Pract Res Clin Endocrinol Metab 2007; 21: 209–21.

Heuer H, Maier MK, Iden S, Mittag J, Friesema EC, Visser TJ et al. The monocarboxylate transporter 8 linked to human psychomotor retardation is highly expressed in thyroid hormone-sensitive neuron populations. Endocrinology 2005; 146: 1701–6.

Heuer H. The importance of thyroid hormone transporters for brain development and function. Best Pract Res Clin Endocrinol Metab 2007; 21: 265–76.

Holden KR, Zuniga OF, May MM, Su H, Molinero MR, Rogers RC et al. X-linked MCT8 gene mutations: characterization of the pediatric neurologic phenotype. J Child Neurol 2005; 20: 852–7.

Huppertz B, Kadyrov M, Kingdom JC. Apoptosis and its role in the trophoblast. Am J Obstet Gynecol 2006; 195: 29–39.

Iskaros J, Pickard MR, Evans IM, Sinha AK, Hardiman P, Ekins RP. Thyroid hormone receptor gene expression in first trimester human fetal brain. J Clin Endocrinol Metab 2000; 85: 2620–3.

James SR, Franklyn JA, Kilby MD. Placental transport of thyroid hormone. Best Pract Res Clin Endocrinol Metab 2007; 21: 253 – 64.

Jurisicova A, Detmar J, Caniggia I. Molecular mechanisms of trophoblast survival: from implantation to birth. Birth Defects Res C Embryo Today 2005; 75: 262 – 80.

Kaplan MM, Yaskoski KA. Maturational patterns of iodothyronine phenolic and tyrosyl ring deiodinase activities in rat cerebrum, cerebellum, and hypothalamus. J Clin Invest 1981; 67: 1208 – 14.

Kester MH, Martinez de Mena R, Obregon MJ, Marinkovic D, Howatson A, Visser TJ et al. Iodothyronine levels in the human developing brain: major regulatory roles of iodothyronine deiodinases in different areas. J Clin Endocrinol Metab 2004; 89: 3117 – 28.

Kilby MD, Barber K, Hobbs E, Franklyn JA. Thyroid hormone action in the placenta. Placenta 2005; 26: 105 – 13.

Kilby MD, Gittoes N, McCabe C, Verhaeg J, Franklyn JA. Expression of thyroid receptor isoforms in the human fetal central nervous system and the effects of intrauterine growth restriction. Clin Endocrinol (Oxf) 2000; 53: 469 – 77.

Kilby MD, Verhaeg J, Gittoes N, Somerset DA, Clark PM, Franklyn JA. Circulating thyroid hormone concentrations and placental thyroid hormone receptor expression in normal human pregnancy and pregnancy complicated by intrauterine growth restriction (IUGR). J Clin Endocrinol Metab 1998; 83: 2964 – 71.

Kim DK, Kanai Y, Matsuo H, Kim JY, Chairoungdua A, Kobayashi Y et al. The human T-type amino acid transporter-1: characterization, gene organization, and chromosomal location. Genomics 2002; 79: 95 – 103.

Kohrle J. Local activation and inactivation of thyroid hormones: the deiodinase family. Mol Cell Endocrinol 1999; 151: 103 – 19.

Kok JH, Den Ouden AL, Verloove-Vanhorick SP, Brand R. Outcome of very preterm small for gestational age infants: the first nine years of life. Br J Obstetr Gynaecol 1998; 105: 162 – 6.

Koopdonk-Kool JM, de Vijlder JJ, Veenboer GJ, Ris-Stalpers C, Kok JH, Vulsma T, et al. Type II and type III deiodinase activity in human placenta as a function of gestational age. J Clin Endocrinol Metab 1996; 81: 2154 – 8.

Kuiper GG, Kester MH, Peeters RP, Visser TJ. Biochemical mechanisms of thyroid hormone deiodination. Thyroid 2005; 15: 787 – 98.

Kullak-Ublick GA, Ismair MG, Stieger B, Landmann L, Huber R, Pizzagalli F et al. Organic anion-transporting polypeptide B (OATP-B) and its functional comparison with three other OATPs of human liver. Gastroenterology 2001; 120: 525 – 33.

Kumar R, Chaudhuri BN. Altered maternal thyroid function: fetal and neonatal development of rat. Indian J Physiol Pharmacol 1989; 33: 233 – 8.

Lafreniere RG, Carrel L, Willard HF. A novel transmembrane transporter encoded by the XPCT gene in Xq13.2. Hum Mol Genet 1994; 3: 1133 – 9.

Laoag-Fernandez JB, Matsuo H, Murakoshi H, Hamada AL, Tsang BK, Maruo T. 3, 5, 3′-Triiodothyronine down-regulates Fas and Fas ligand expression and suppresses caspase-3 and poly (adenosine 5′-diphosphate-ribose) polymerase cleavage and apoptosis in early placental extravillous trophoblasts *in vitro*. J Clin Endocrinol Metab 2004; 89: 4069 – 77.

Laron Z. Interactions between the thyroid hormones and the hormones of the growth hormone axis. Pediatr Endocrinol Rev 2003; Suppl 2: 244 – 9.

Lavado-Autric R, Ausó E, V. G-VJ, del Carmen Arufe M, Escobar del Rey F, Berbel P et al. Early maternal hypothyroxinemia alters histogenesis and cerebral cortex cytoarchitecture of the progeny. J Clin Invest 2003; 111: 1073 – 82.

Legrand J. Thyroid hormone effects on growth and development. Thyroid Horm Metab 1986: 503 – 34.

Leonard AJ, Evans IM, Pickard MR, Bandopadhyay R, Sinha AK, Ekins RP. Thyroid hormone receptor expression in rat placenta. Placenta 2001; 22: 353 – 9.

Mandel SJ, Berry MJ, Kieffer JD, Harney JW, Warne RL, Larsen PR. Cloning and *in vitro* expression of the human selenoprotein, type I iodothyronine deiodinase. J Clin Endocrinol Metab 1992; 75: 1133 – 9.

Maranduba CM, Friesema EC, Kok F, Kester MH, Jansen J, Sertie AL et al. Decreased cellular uptake and metabolism in Allan-Herndon-Dudley syndrome (AHDS) due to a novel mutation in the MCT8 thyroid hormone transporter. J Med Genet 2006; 43: 457 – 60.

Maruo T, Matsuo H, Mochizuki M. Thyroid hormone as a biological amplifier of differentiated trophoblast function in early pregnancy. Acta Endocrinol (Copenh) 1991; 125: 58 – 66.

Maruo T, Matsuo H, Otani T, Mochizuki M. Role of epidermal growth factor (EGF) and its receptor in the development of the human placenta. Reprod Fertil Dev 1995; 7: 1465 – 70.

Matsuo H, Maruo T, Murata K, Mochizuki M. Human early placental trophoblasts produce an epidermal growth factor-like substance in synergy with thyroid hormone. Acta Endocrinol (Copenh) 1993; 128: 225 – 9.

Morreale de Escobar G, Pastor R, Obregon MJ, Escobar del Rey F. Effects of maternal hypothyroidism on the weight and thyroid hormone content of rat embryonic tissues, before and after onset of fetal thyroid function. Endocrinology 1985; 117: 1890 – 900.

Nanaev AK, Kosanke G, Reister F, Kemp B, Frank HG, Kaufmann P. Pregnancy-induced de-differentiation of media smooth muscle cells in uteroplacental arteries of the guinea pig is reversible after delivery. Placenta 2000; 21: 306–12.

Nishii H, Ashitaka Y, Maruo M, Mochizuki M. Studies on the nuclear 3, 5, 3′-triiodo-L-thyronine binding sites in cytotrophoblast. Endocrinol Jpn 1989; 36: 891–8.

Okamoto Y, Sakata M, Ogura K, Yamamoto T, Yamaguchi M, Tasaka K et al. Expression and regulation of 4F2hc and hLAT1 in human trophoblasts. Am J Physiol Cell Physiol. 2002; 282: C196–204.

Patel P, Weerasekera N, Hitchins M, Boyd CA, Johnston DG, Williamson C. Semi quantitative expression analysis of MDR3, FIC1, BSEP, OATP-A, OATP-C, OATP-D, OATP-E and NTCP gene transcripts in 1st and 3rd trimester human placenta. Placenta 2003; 24: 39–44.

Pickard MR, Sinha AK, Ogilvie L, Ekins RP. The influence of the maternal thyroid hormone environment during pregnancy on the ontogenesis of brain and placental ornithine decarboxylase activity in the rat. J Endocrinol 1993; 139: 205–12.

Pickard MR, Sinha AK, Ogilvie LM, Leonard AJ, Edwards PR, Ekins RP. Maternal hypothyroxinemia influences glucose transporter expression in fetal brain and placenta. J Endocrinol 1999; 163: 385–94.

Pijnenborg R, Bland JM, Robertson WB, Brosens I. Uteroplacental arterial changes related to interstitial trophoblast migration in early human pregnancy. Placenta 1983; 4: 397–413.

Pizzagalli F, Hagenbuch B, Stieger B, Klenk U, Folkers G, Meier PJ. Identification of a novel human organic anion transporting polypeptide as a high affinity thyroxine transporter. Mol Endocrinol 2002; 16: 2283–96.

Pop VJ, Brouwers EP, Vader HL, Vulsma T, van Baar AL, de Vijlder JJ. Maternal hypothyroxinaemia during early pregnancy and subsequent child development: a 3-year follow-up study. Clin Endocrinol (Oxf) 2003; 59: 282–8.

Pop VJ, Kuijpens JL, van Baar AL, Verkerk G, van Son MM, de Vijlder JJ et al. Low maternal free thyroxine concentrations during early pregnancy are associated with impaired psychomotor development in infancy. Clin Endocrinol (Oxf) 1999; 50: 149–55.

Ramadan T, Camargo SM, Summa V, Hunziker P, Chesnov S, Pos KM et al. Basolateral aromatic amino acid transporter TAT1 (Slc16a10) functions as an efflux pathway. J Cell Physiol 2006; 206: 771–9.

Ritchie JW, Shi YB, Hayashi Y, Baird FE, Muchekehu RW, Christie GR et al. A role for thyroid hormone transporters in transcriptional regulation by thyroid hormone receptors. Mol Endocrinol 2003; 17: 653–61.

Ritchie JW, Taylor PM. Role of the system L permease LAT1 in amino acid and iodothyronine transport in placenta. Biochem J 2001; 356: 719–25.

Rossier G, Meier C, Bauch C, Summa V, Sordat B, Verrey F et al. LAT2, a new basolateral 4F2hc/CD98-associated amino acid transporter of kidney and intestine. J Biol Chem 1999; 274: 34948–54.

Rovet JF, Ehrlich RM, Sorbara DL. Neurodevelopment in infants and preschool children with congenital hypothroidism: etiological and treatment factors affecting outcome. J Pediat Psychol 1992; 17: 187–213.

Salvatore D, Bartha T, Harney JW, Larsen PR. Molecular biological and biochemical characterization of the human type 2 selenodeiodinase. Endocrinology 1996; 137: 3308–15.

Sato K, Sugawara J, Sato T, Mizutamari H, Suzuki T, Ito A et al. Expression of organic anion transporting polypeptide E (OATP-E) in human placenta. Placenta 2003; 24: 144–8.

Schwartz CE, May MM, Carpenter NJ, Rogers RC, Martin J, Bialer MG et al. Allan-Herndon-Dudley syndrome and the monocarboxylate transporter 8 (MCT8) gene. Am J Hum Genet 2005; 77: 41–53.

Schwartz HL, Trence D, Oppenheimer JH, Jiang NS, Jump DB. Distribution and metabolism of L- and D-triiodothyronine (T$_3$) in the rat: preferential accumulation of L–T$_3$ by hepatic and cardiac nuclei as a probable explanation of the differential biological potency of T$_3$ enantiomers. Endocrinology 1983; 113: 1236–43.

St Germain DL, Galton VA. The deiodinase family of selenoproteins. Thyroid 1997; 7: 655–68.

Taylor PM, Ritchie JW. Tissue uptake of thyroid hormone by amino acid transporters. Best Pract Res Clin Endocrinol Metab 2007; 21: 237–51.

Thorpe-Beeston JG, Nicolaides KH, Felton CV, Butler J, McGregor AM. Maturation of the secretion of thyroid hormone and thyroid-stimulating hormone in the fetus. N Engl J Med 1991; 324: 559–61.

Verrey F. System L: heteromeric exchangers of large, neutral amino acids involved in directional transport. Pflugers Arch 2003; 445: 529–33.

Vulsma T, Gons MH, de Vijlder JJ. Maternal-fetal transfer of thyroxine in congenital hypothyroidism due to a total organification defect or thyroid agenesis. N Engl J Med 1989; 321: 13–6.

Weinberger C, Thompson CC, Ong ES, Lebo R, Gruol DJ, Evans RM. The c-erb-A gene encodes a thyroid hormone receptor. Nature 1986; 324 (6098): 641–6.

Yanagida O, Kanai Y, Chairoungdua A, Kim DK, Segawa H, Nii T et al. Human L-type amino acid transporter 1 (LAT1): characterization of function and expression in tumor cell lines. Biochim Biophys Acta 2001; 1514: 291–302.

Yen PM. Physiological and molecular basis of thyroid hormone action. Physiol Rev 2001; 81: 1097–142.

8 Thyroid Function and Fertility

G. E. Krassas*, A. Kaprara

Department of Endocrinology, Diabetes and Metabolism, Panagia General Hospital, N. Plastira 22, 551 32 Thessaloniki, Greece

Abstract

Thyroid dysfunction in the context of hyper- and hypothyroidism has an adverse effect on female reproduction. Steroid and gonadotropin alterations as well as abnormal menstruation have been reported. In particular, menstrual irregularities in hyperthyroid women are at the level of about 20%, while in hypothyroid patients they are at the level of about 25%, mainly oligomenorrhoea. Fertility is also reduced. Women with menstrual disturbances or conception difficulties should be investigated for thyroid dysfunction and, if the latter is confirmed, then appropriate treatment should be considered. Regarding thyroid autoimmunity all available studies have found an increased prevalence of thyroid autoimmunity in women attending infertility clinics, although many of the studies are uncontrolled and include heterogeneous groups of patients with different types of infertility.

8.1 Introduction

Infertility or the absence of pregnancy after one year of unprotected intercourse occurs in 10–15% of couples (Mosher and Pratt, 1991). The causes of infertility among couples can be subdivided into 4 categories: a) male infertility (30%), b) female infertility (35%), c) the combination of both (20%) and finally d) unexplained or idiopathic infertility (15%) (Evers, 2002; Thonneau et al., 1991; Healy et al., 1994).

Female causes of infertility comprise endometriosis, tubal damage and ovulatory dysfunction. In the presence of a normal spermiogram and the absence of female infertility, the diagnosis of idiopathic infertility is established.

Thyroid autoimmunity (TAI) is the most common autoimmune disorder in women and a common feature in the reproductive age, with a prevalence varying between 5 and 15% according to the area investigated. It is 5 to 10 times more common in women than in men and can be present without thyroid dysfunction and thus remains undiagnosed (Wang and Crapo, 1997; Bjoro et al., 2000; Hollowell et al., 2002). This female predominance may potentially be explained by the effects of oestrogens in promoting autoimmunity, by genetic factors and, perhaps, maternal microchimerism.

8.2 Hyper- and Hypothyroidism and Fertility

Thyroid dysfunction affects the reproductive system in women more than in men. Clinicians have long recognised that hyper- and hypothyroidism are often associated in premenopausal women with menstrual abnormalities and infertility (Krassas, 2000). Moreover, in the last decade many reports have linked thyroid autoimmunity with infertility in euthyroid individuals (Krassas et al., 2008). Although many of the studies are uncontrolled and include heterogeneous groups of patients with different types of infertility, the final conclusion of all the studies is in favour of an increased prevalence of thyroid autoimmunity in women attending infertility clinics.

Thyrotoxicosis occurring in prepubertal girls may result in a slightly delayed menarche. In adult women, the effects of thyrotoxicosis on the reproductive system are present at the hypothalamic pituitary level with alterations in gonadotrophin (Gns) release and in the circulating levels of sex hormone binding globulin (SHBG), which result in alterations in the metabolism of sex steroids or their biological activity (Krassas, 2005). Specifically, SHBG is increased, and plasma levels of 17β-oestradiol (E_2) may be two- or three-fold higher in hyperthyroid than in normal women during all phases of the menstrual cycle (Akande

Table 8.1   Steroid and gonadotropin alterations in female hyperthyroid patients.

Parameter	Change
SHBG	Increased
E_2	Increased
Metabolic clearance rate of E_2	Decreased
Testosterone	Increased
Androstenedione	Increased
Production rate of T and A	Increased
Conversion ratio of A to oestrone	Increased
Conversion ratio of T to E_2	Increased
LH, FSH	Increased or unchanged
Pulsatile secretion of LH, FSH	No change
Gns response to GnRH	Increased

Table 8.2   Steroid and gonadotropin alterations in female hypothyroid patients.

Parameter	Change
Total testosterone	Decreased
Total oestrogens	Decreased
Free testosterone	Increased
Free oestrogens	Increased
Activity of SHBG	Decreased
FSH, LH levels	Normal
Gns response to GnRH	Blunted
PRL	Increased

and Hockaday, 1972a). The metabolic clearance rate of E_2 is decreased in hyperthyroidism and is thought to be largely due to increased binding of E_2 to SHBG (Ridgeway et al., 1975). Mean plasma levels of testosterone (T) and androstenedione (A) increase (Southren et al., 1974). The production rates of T and A are significantly elevated in hyperthyroid women in comparison with normal females. The conversion ratio of A to estrone, as well as that of T to E_2, is increased in hyperthyroid women (Burrow, 1986). Akande and Hockaday (1972b) found that the mean luteinising hormone (LH) levels in both the follicular and luteal phases of the menstrual cycle are significantly higher in hyperthyroid women than in normal women. LH secretion is increased (Zahringer et al., 2000), while the pulsatile secretion characteristics of LH and follicle-stimulating hormone (FSH) secretion (frequency, peak and shape) do not differ in patients when compared with controls (Zahringer et al., 2000). Serum LH levels decrease to normal after a few weeks of treatment with antithyroid drugs (Akande, 1974). There is discrepancy regarding FSH levels in hyperthyroid patients. Some reports claim that they are normal, while others state that they are elevated (Zahringer et al., 2000; Tanaka et al., 1981; Distiller et al., 1975). Tanaka et al. (1981) reported that hyperthyroxinaemia results in an augmented Gns response to gonadotrophin-releasing hormone (GnRH). Others have been unable to confirm this finding. All the above data are presented in Table 8.1.

The variable clinical symptoms seen in women with thyrotoxicosis are the consequence of these alterations. Menstrual disturbances have also been described in thyrotoxic females since the second half of the last century. The frequency of menstrual abnormalities in more recent studies is not the same as that in earlier series. Older studies estimated that menstrual irregularities are at the level of about 60% (Goldsmith et al., 1952; Joshi et al., 1993), while a more recent study found irregular cycles in only 20% of thyrotoxic patients (Krassas et al., 1994). This is mainly the result of earlier diagnosis of thyroid disturbances, when the symptoms are still mild. It was also found that smoking aggravates the development of menstrual disturbances in thyrotoxicosis and also that the latter group had higher total thyroxine levels (Krassas et al., 1994). Thyrotoxicosis in women has been linked with reduced fertility, although most thyrotoxic women remain ovulatory according to the results of endometrial biopsies. It is estimated that approximately 6% of thyrotoxic women have primary or secondary infertility (Joshi et al., 1993).

Hypothyroidism affects the female reproductive system in a number of ways. Women with hypothyroidism have decreased plasma levels of both TH and oestrogens, but their unbound fractions are increased. The binding activity of SHBG in plasma is decreased. Gns levels are usually normal. However, a blunted or delayed LH response to GnRH has been reported in some female patients with hypothyroidism. Serum prolactin (PRL) concentrations may be increased (Krassas, 2005) (Table 8.2). Galactorrhoea may occur. These disturbances usually disappear when the euthyroid state is restored (Stoffer et al., 1981).

In women of fertile age, hypothyroidism results in changes in cycle length and amount of bleeding (i.e., oligomenorrhoea and amenorrhoea, polymenorrhoea, and menorrhagia). The latter is probably due to oestrogen breakthrough bleeding secondary to anovulation (Krassas et al., 1999). Older studies found that menstrual disturbances in such patients were at the level of about 60–80% (Goldsmith et al., 1952 3; Scott and Mussey, 1964; Benson and Dailey, 1955), while a more recent study estimated that only 25% of hypothyroid women have irregular cycles, mainly oligomenorrhoea (Krassas et al., 1999). Moreover, it was found, as expected, that patients with more severe hypothyroidism had higher thyrotropin (TSH) levels and the latter group had more menstrual disturbances (Krassas et al., 1999).

In women, severe hypothyroidism is commonly associated with diminished libido and failure of ovulation. Hypothyroid women who become pregnant have a higher probability for miscarriage (Kaprara and Krassas, 2008). Gestational hypertension often occurs in pregnant women with untreated hypothyroidism. Moreover, it has been suggested that subclinical hypothyroidism may be of greater clinical importance in infertile women with menstrual disorders, especially when the luteal phase is inadequate, than is usually thought. This was also confirmed in a recent study reporting that mean serum TSH levels and antithyroid peroxidase antibodies were higher among women with infertility compared with controls (Glinoer et al., 1994). Finally, it has been reported that in a group of infertile women, those with elevated TSH levels had a higher incidence of out-of-phase biopsies than women with normal serum TSH concentrations (Gerhard et al., 1991).

The conclusion from the above studies is that women with menstrual disturbances or conception difficulties should be investigated for hypothyroidism and, if the latter is confirmed, then thyroxine treatment should be considered (Krassas et al., 2008).

8.3   Thyroid Autoimmunity and Fertility

Several studies have evaluated the relationship between TAI and infertility in euthyroid individuals. Most series document a significant association between the presence of thyroid antibodies, infertility and a higher risk of miscarriage. It is of interest that patients with higher titres of thyroid antibodies do not have a higher rate of miscarriage compared with patients with only modest elevations of thyroid peroxidase (TPO) antibody titres (Stagnaro-Green et al., 1990 M Iijima et al., 1997). Although many of the studies are uncontrolled and include heterogeneous groups of patients with different types of infertility, the final conclusion of all the studies is in favour of an increased prevalence of TAI in women attending infertility clinics (Krassas et al., 2008).

Specifically, Roussev et al. (1996) published the first controlled study on this topic. The aim was to determine the frequency of abnormal immunological tests in women with reproductive failure. They investigated 108 patients (45 with a diagnosis of unexplained infertility), with a variety of immunological assessments, including thyroglobulin (TG) and microsomal (TPO) antibodies. Comparisons were made with 15 normal controls. Seventy out of 108 (65%) women experiencing reproductive failure had at least one positive test, compared to 1 of 15 (7%) controls (p = 0.0001).

Geva et al. (1997) reported a high incidence of thyroid antibodies in women with unexplained and mechanical infertility, compared to healthy controls.

Kutteh et al. (1999), investigated the prevalence of TG and TPO antibodies in women undergoing assisted reproduction technology (ART). 688 women undergoing ART and 200 healthy controls were investigated. 29 out of 200 (14.5%) controls and 132 of 688 (19.2%) of women undergoing ART had positive thyroid antibodies. No significant difference was found between the two groups. This study, which is the sole outlier in Table 8.**3** merits further comment. Close examination of the control data in Figures 1 and 2 of this paper reveals that control women under 30 years of age provided most of the positive thyroid antibody tests. The more appropriate control group, women over 30 years of age, had significantly less thyroid autoimmunity that the ART patients as well as the younger groups of controls. This permits us to accept that the control individuals were not properly recruited. The same year Kaider et al. (1999) investigated 122 patients undergoing *in vitro* fertilization (IVF) (97 with unexplained infertility) and 100 controls. Of the unexplained infertility group, 81% had at least one abnormal immunological test including TPO and TG antibodies compared to 10% of the normal fertile controls. These differences were statistically significant.

Reimand et al. (2001) investigated 108 females with different pathologies leading to the sterility,

Table 8.3   Published studies indicating the percentage of thyroid antibody-positive patients in a cohort of female women with infertility as compared with controls.

A/A	First author	Year of publication	Number of individuals investigated	Results	Statistical analysis
1	Roussev et al.	1996	108 p + 15 c	65% vs. 7%	p = 0.0001
2	Geva et al.	1997	40 p + 40 c	20% vs. 5%	p < 0.05
3	Kutteh et al.	1999	688 p (IVF) + 200 c	19.2% vs. 14.5%	n.s.
4	Kaider et al.	1999	122 p (IVF) + 100 c	81% vs. 10%	p < 0.0004
5	Reimand et al.	2001	108 p + 392 c	40.7% vs. 14.8%	p < 0.001
6	Poppe et al.	2002	438 p + 100 c	18% vs. 8%	p < 0.05
7	Janssen et al.	2004	175 p + 168 c	26.9 vs. 8.3%	p < 0.001

From Krassas et al. (2008); p = patients, c = controls; ns = not significant.

including unexplained infertility, and 392 normal fertile controls. Common antibodies were assessed by indirect immunofluorescence, including TPO and TG antibodies. The results showed that 40.7% of patients' sera contained one or more common antibodies, compared to 14.8% of controls.

Poppe et al. (2002) investigated 438 couples presenting for the first time to their infertility clinic and 100 fertile controls, matched for age. In couples where the infertility was thought to be of female origin, there was an increased risk (RR = 2.25; CI: 1.02 – 1.52; p = 0.024) of associated TAI in the female partner, compared with the control population. The risk was further increased in the presence of endometriosis (RR = 3.57; CI: 1.09 – 11.8; p = 0.016). The prevalence of thyroid dysfunction in the study group was comparable with that in the control population but, overall, the median TSH was significantly higher in patients with infertility compared to controls [1.3 (0.9) vs. 1.1 (0.8) mU/L].

In a further prospective case-control study Poppe et al. (2003) investigated the outcome of pregnancy in euthyroid infertile women, who required ART in the context of their TAI status. Two hundred and thirty-four infertile women presenting for their first ART cycle were included. Pregnancy rates after ART were comparable in the two study groups (with/without TAI; 53% vs. 43%).

Finally, Janssen et al. (2004) investigated the prevalence of TAI in patients with polycystic ovary syndrome (PCOS). They evaluated thyroid function and morphology in 175 patients with PCOS and 168 age-matched women without PCOS. Thyroid function and thyroid-specific antibody tests revealed elevated TPO and TG antibodies in 14 of 168 controls (8.3%) and 47 of 175 patients with PCOS (26.9%, p < 0.001). On thyroid ultrasound, 42.3% of PCOS patients showed hypoechoic areas typical of TAI, compared to 6.5% of the controls (p < 0.001); while thyroid hormone levels were normal in all subjects, PCOS patients had a higher mean TSH level (p < 0.001) and a higher incidence of TSH levels above the upper limit of normal than controls (PCOS 10.9%, controls 1.8%; p < 0.001). The study concluded that the prevalence of TAI in patients with PCOS is three times greater when compared with controls. Table 8.3 presents a summary of all the above studies.

Pooling all the published studies together, the overall conclusion favours a significantly increased incidence of TAI in women presenting with infertility. The underlying pathogenetic mechanisms regarding TAI and infertility remain speculative since the existence of animal data, as well as *in vitro* data, are scarce. However, it must be emphasised that adequate levels of circulating thyroid hormones are of primary importance for normal reproductive function and any impairment of the available triidothyronine in glanulose and stromal cells, as could be the case in thyroid autoimmunity, may disrupt normal female reproductive functions (Wakim et al., 1993; Maruo et al., 1991).

8.4   Conclusion

Thyroid dysfunction in the context of hyper- and hypothyroidism has an adverse effect on female reproduction. Steroid and gonadotropin alterations as well as abnormal menstruation have been reported. Fertility is also reduced. Regarding TAI, all available studies have found an increased prevalence of TAI in women attending infertility clinics, although many of the studies are uncontrolled and include heterogeneous groups of patients with different types of infertility.

References

Akande EO. The effect of oestrogen on plasma levels of luteinizing hormone in euthyroid and thyrotoxic postmenopausal women. J Obstet Gynecol 1974; 81: 795–801.

Akande EO, Hockaday TD. Plasma oestrogen and luteinizing hormone concentrations in thyrotoxic menstrual disturbance. Proc R Soc Med 1972a; 65: 789–90.

Akande EO, Hockaday TD. Plasma luteinizing hormone levels in women with thyrotoxicosis. J Endocrinol 1972b; 53: 173–4.

Benson RC, Dailey ME. Menstrual pattern in hyperthyroidism and subsequent post-therapy hypothyroidism. Surg Gynaecol Obstet 1955; 100: 19–26.

Bjoro T, Holmen J, Krüger O et al. Prevalence of thyroid disease, thyroid dysfunction and thyroid peroxidase antibodies in a large, unselected population. The Health Study of Nord-Trondelag (HUNT). Eur J Endocrinol 2000; 143: 639–47.

Burrow GN. The thyroid gland and reproduction. In: Reproductive Endocrinology. Yen SSC, Jaffe RB, eds., Philadelphia: WB Saunders, 1986: 424–40

Distiller LA, Sagel J, Morley JE. Assessment of pituitary gonadotropin reserve using luteinizing hormone–releasing hormone (LRH) in states of altered thyroid function. J Clin Endocrinol Metab 1975; 40: 512–5.

Evers JL. Female subfertility. Lancet 2002; 360: 151–9.

Gerhard I, Becker T, Eggert-Kruse W et al. Thyroid and ovarian function in infertile women. Hum Reprod 1991; 6: 338–45.

Geva E, Lessing JB, Lerner-Geva L, Azem F, Yovel I, Amit A. The presence of antithyroid antibodies in euthyroid patients with unexplained infertility and tubal obstruction. Am J Reprod Immunol 1997; 37: 184–6.

Glinoer D, Riahi M, Grün JP, Kinthaert J. Risk of subclinical hypothyroidism in pregnant women with asymptomatic autoimmune thyroid disorders. J Clin Endocrinol Metab 1994; 79: 197–204.

Goldsmith RE, Sturgis SH, Lerman J et al. The menstrual pattern in thyroid disease. J Clin Endocrinol Metab 1952; 12: 846–55.

Healy DL, Trounson AO, Andersen AN. Female infertility: causes and treatment. Lancet 1994; 343: 1539–44.

Hollowell JG, Staehling NW, Flanders WD et al. Serum TSH, T(4), and thyroid antibodies in the United States population (1988 to 1994): National Health and Nutrition Examination Survey (NHANES III). J Clin Endocrinol Metab 2002; 87: 489–99.

Iijima T, Tada H, Hidaka Y, Mitsuda N, Murata Y, Amino N. Effects of autoantibodies on the course of pregnancy and fetal growth. Obstet Gynecol 1997; 9: 364–9.

Janssen OE, Mehlmauer N, Hahn S, Offner AH, Gärtner R. High prevalence of autoimmune thyroiditis in patients with polycystic ovary syndrome. Eur J Endocrinol 2004; 150: 363–9.

Joshi JV, Bhandakar SD, Chadha M et al. Menstrual irregularities and lactation failure may precede thyroid dysfunction or goitre. J Postgad Med 1993; 39: 137–41.

Kaider AS, Kaider BD, Janowicz PB, Roussev RG. Immunodiagnostic evaluation in women with reproductive failure. Am J Reprod Immunol 1999; 42: 335–46.

Kaprara A, Krassas GE. Thyroid autoimmunity and miscarriage. Hormones (Athens) 2008; 7: 294–302.

Krassas GE. The male and female reproductive system in hypothyroidism. In: Werner's and Ingbar: The Thyroid. A fundamental and clinical text. 9th edn., Braverman L, Utiger R, eds., Philadelphia: Lippincott, 2005: 824–29.

Krassas GE. The male and female reproductive system in thyrotoxicosis. In: Werner's and Ingbar: The Thyroid. A fundamental and clinical text. 9th edn., Braverman L, Utiger R, eds., Philadelphia: Lippincott, 2005: 621–29.

Krassas GE. Thyroid disease and female reproduction. Fertil Steril 2000; 74: 1063–70.

Krassas GE, Perros P, Kaprara A. Thyroid autoimmunity, infertility and miscarriage. Expert Rev Endocrinol Metab 2008; 3: 127–36.

Krassas GE, Pontikides N, Kaltsas T et al. Disturbances of menstruation in hypothyroidism. Clin Endocrinol (Oxf) 1999; 50: 655–9.

Krassas GE, Pontikides N, Kaltsas T, Papadopoulou P, Batrinos M. Menstrual disturbances in thyrotoxicosis. Clin Endocrinol (Oxf) 1994; 40: 641–4.

Kutteh WH, Yetman DL, Carr AC, Beck LA, Scott RT Jr. Increased prevalence of antithyroid antibodies identified in women with recurrent pregnancy loss but not in women undergoing assisted reproduction. Fertil Steril 1999; 71: 843–8.

Maruo T, Matsuo H, Mochizuki M. Thyroid hormone as a biological amplifier of differentiated trophoblast function in early pregnancy. Acta Endocrinol (Copenh) 1991; 125: 58–66.

Mosher WD, Pratt WF. Fecundity and infertility in the United States: incidence and trends. Fertil Steril 1991; 56: 192–3.

Poppe K, Glinoer D, Tournaye H et al. Assisted reproduction and thyroid autoimmunity: an unfortunate combination? J Clin Endocrinol Metab 2003; 88: 4149–52.

Poppe K, Glinoer D, Van Steirteghem A et al. Thyroid dysfunction and autoimmunity in infertile women. Thyroid 2002; 12: 997–1001.

Reimand K, Talja I, Metsküla K, Kadastik U, Matt K, Uibo R. Autoantibody studies of female patients with reproductive failure. J Reprod Immunol 2001; 51: 167–176.

Ridgway EC, Longcope C, Maloof F. Metabolic clearance and blood production rates of estradiol in hyperthyroidism. J Clin Endocrinol Metab 1975; 4: 491–7.

Roussev RG, Kaider BD, Pride DE, Coulam CB. Laboratory evaluation of women experiencing reproductive failure. Am J Reprod Immunol 1996; 35: 415–20.

Scott JC, Mussey E. Menstrual patterns in myxedema. Am J Obstet Gynecol 1964; 90: 161–5.

Southren AL, Olivo J, Gordon GG et al. The conversion of androgens to estrogens in hyperthyroidism. J Clin Endocrinol Metab 1974; 38: 207–14.

Stagnaro-Green A, Roman SH, Cobin RH, el-Harazy E, Alvarez-Marfany M, Davies TF. Detection of at-risk pregnancy by means of highly sensitive assays for thyroid autoantibodies. JAMA 1990; 264: 1422–5.

Stoffer SS, McKeel DW Jr, Randall RV et al. Pituitary prolactin cell hyperplasia with autonomous prolactin secretion and primary hypothyroidism. Fertil Steril 1981; 36: 682–5.

Tanaka T, Tamai H, Kuma K et al. Gonadotropin response to luteinizing hormone releasing hormone in hyperthyroid patients with menstrual disturbances. Metabolism 1981; 30: 323–6.

Thonneau P, Marchand S, Tallec A et al. Incidence and main causes of infertility in a resident population (1,850,000) of three French regions (1988–1989). Hum Reprod 1991; 6: 811–6.

Wakim AN, Polizotto SL, Buffo MJ, Marrero MA, Burholt DR. Thyroid hormones in human follicular fluid and thyroid hormone receptors in human granulosa cells. Fertil Steril 1993; 59: 1187–90.

Wang C, Crapo LM. The epidemiology of thyroid disease and implications for screening. Endocrinol Metab Clin North Am 1997; 26: 189–218.

Zahringer S, Tomova A, von Werder K et al. The influence of hyperthyroidism on the hypothalamic-pituitary-gonadal axis. Exp Clin Endocrinol Diabetes 2000; 108: 282–9.

Session III

Management of Thyroid Disorders in Pregnancy

Chairperson: D. Glinoer (Brussels)

9 Which Thyroid Function Tests Should We Be Measuring during Gestation?

U. Feldt-Rasmussen

Department of Medical Endocrinology, Rigshospitalet, National University Hospital, Copenhagen University, Blegdamsvej 9, DK-2100 Copenhagen, Denmark

Abstract

It is important to know about a number of physiological changes in thyroid function variables in relation to the measurement and interpretation of thyroid function tests during gestation. The circulating binding protein TBG increases due to the high oestrogen concentration, there is an increased need for iodine supply to the thyroid, the synthesis of thyroid hormones is increased, changed deiodinase activity and, furthermore, in the first trimester there is an increase of HCG, which has a TSH-like effect on the TSH receptor. Finally, thyroid autoimmune activity is usually decreasing due to a general immune suppressive action from the pregnancy. The measurement of serum TSH is the first-line screening variable for thyroid dysfunction, also in pregnancy, with the caveats of early gestationally suppressed TSH (by HCG in approx. 18%). However, serum TSH measurement cannot be used to control the treatment of maternal thyroid dysfunction. If using serum TSH, the mother is likely to be undertreated with levothyroxine and overtreated with antithyroid drugs, both of which infer an increased risk for foetal brain development. Measurement of the peripheral thyroid hormones is hampered by the fact that many clinical biochemical laboratories do not have appropriate reference intervals, in general, and none during pregnancy, in particular, despite recommendations in the field. Even with appropriate reference intervals, the methods for the measurement of all the hormones are highly different among laboratories, despite calibration against the same calibrators. More important, however, is probably that the intra-individual variability of the thyroid hormone measurements (reflecting an individual genetic set-point) is much narrower than the inter-individual variation (reflecting the reference interval). Due to the high TBG concentration, the best laboratory assessment of thyroid function is a free thyroid hormone estimate – in hypothyroidism free T_4 combined with TSH, and in hyperthyroidism free T_4 and T_3 combined with TSH. These free thyroid hormone measurements do not always correct completely for the binding protein abnormalities. Thus, if in doubt, samples should be measured in another laboratory or combined with total hormone measurement and a T_3 uptake test. Measurement of anti-TPO and/or TSH receptor antibodies may give additional information in some cases. There is a need for normative gestational age-related reference ranges for TSH and T_4. Measurement of TPO antibodies predicts the risk of hypothyroidism and in pregnant women with low TSH hyperthyroidism will be predicted by TSH receptor antibodies in 60–70%.

9.1   Introduction

Diagnosing maternal thyroid dysfunction during pregnancy is very important for the outcome for both mother and foetus at all stages of pregnancy (Glinoer, 1997; Casey and Leveno, 2006). Women with hypothyroidism treated insufficiently with levothyroxine [high serum concentration of thyrotropin (TSH) or serum free thyroxine (T_4) in the low normal range] deliver babies with significantly lower IQ and/or other inhibited neuropsychological development (Haddow et al., 1999; Pop et al., 1999). Such offspring outcome has even been demonstrated in women with a serum concentration of T_4 in the low normal range during pregnancy (Morreale de Escobar et al., 2000).

As a natural consequence of these findings much focus has been given to diagnosing both overt and subclinical (or mild) thyroid dysfunction as early as possible in pregnant women, and in as many women as possible worldwide, recently resulting in international consensus guidelines (Endocrine Society Clinical Practice Guideline). Apart from general global problems in accomplishing this type of care due to financial and/or infrastructure restrictions, there are also many other reasons why these efforts have limited success. One of them is associated with the biochemical measurements of thyroid function undergoing many complicated changes during pregnancy, and the corresponding issue of educating these important matters to the physicians who are caretakers of pregnant women. The question of whether detection and treatment of thyroid insufficiency in pregnancy are feasible, is still unanswered but recent progress and better insights into physiological changes, trimester-specific reference ranges, and inter- versus intraindividual variability on the assessment of thyroid function in the single pregnant woman should give a better background for the future (Mandel et al., 2005). The present review will focus on the choice of tests for assessment of biochemical thyroid function together with their strengths and limitations. Information from two recent guidelines have been used in part as reference (Endocrine Society Clinical Practice Guideline; National Academy of Clinical Biochemistry Guidelines for Laboratory Practice).

9.2   Physiological Changes during Pregnancy and Consequences for Thyroid Function Assessment

Normal pregnancy entails complicated and substantial changes in thyroid function. The circulating thyroid hormone binding globulin (TBG) increases due to an oestrogen-induced increase in its production and at the same time the serum iodine decreases, the synthesis of thyroid hormones is increased, there are changes in the deiodinase activity, and towards the end of the first trimester, when chorionic gonadotropin (hCG) levels are highest, a significant fraction of the thyroid-stimulating activity is from HCG. Furthermore, thyroid autoimmune activity is usually decreasing due to a general immune suppressive action from the pregnancy, and finally there is an approximately 50% expansion in plasma volume. Serum concentrations of total T_4 and T_3 increase due to the increase of TBG. Serum concentrations of free thyroid hormones and TSH physiologically should be normal, except in the short period of time when TSH is suppressed due to the HCG effect. But it must be emphasised that normal reference ranges from a non-pregnant population are not "normal" in pregnancy. All the above-mentioned physiological changes, including the high TBG concentration, influence the laboratory measurements even of the free thyroid hormones. There is therefore a huge risk of false interpretation of thyroid function tests in pregnancy.

9.3   Biochemical Diagnosis of Thyroid Dysfunction in Pregnancy

9.3.1   Measurement of Serum TSH

The most sensitive method for screening for thyroid dysfunction in a healthy, non-pregnant population is the measurement of TSH serum concentration due to the log-linear relationship between TSH and free T_4. Even small changes in T_4 concentrations will provoke very large changes in serum TSH. However, in pregnant women thyroid and pituitary functions are not stable and, therefore, measuring TSH is not sufficient and often inappropriate for the assessment of thyroid function during gestation. If serum TSH measurement is used alone, the mother is likely to be insufficiently treated with levothyroxine for hypothyroidism or overtreated with antithyroid drugs for thyrotoxicosis, both of which may result in maternal hypothyroidism which, in turn, seriously affects the foetal brain development.

A typical example of such biochemical misdiagnosis during follow-up of antithyroid drug-treated Graves' disease is demonstrated in a case from our tertiary referral department. A 32-years-old 24-weeks pregnant woman was referred from a local hospital due to the finding of a large foetal goitre by routine scan. It was her second pregnancy, and she had been treated with antithyroid drugs for Graves' disease for 9 years. This included treatment during a previous pregnancy 5 years before, which resulted in a male baby with severely reduced cerebral capacity. Upon referral she was being treated with 20 mg thiamazole daily. At the local hospital she had been considered sufficiently euthyroid based on a normal TSH of 2.9 mU/L (population-based reference range: 0.4–4.0 mU/L), total T_4 97 nmol/L (60–140 nmol/L), and free T_4 7.8 pmol/L (7–20 pmol/L). She had a high level of TSH receptor antibodies at 24 U/L (< 1.5 U/L). A more elaborate foetal ultrasound showed a male foetus with polyhydramnios, and an enlarged thyroid gland with dimensions of $1.4 \times 3.5 \times 3.5$ cm, which was predominantly intrathoracic. Cord blood TSH was highly elevated at 34.5 mU/L, and free T_4 was reduced to 13.8 pmol/L. The misdiagnosis of the thyroid function had been based primarily on the normal maternal levels particularly of TSH but also of total and free T_4, which were, however, reflecting a delayed pituitary reaction to the lowered thyroid hormone levels. It is mandatory for doctors taking care of pregnant women with thyroid diseases to have a thorough knowledge of the evolution of the normal thyroid function during pregnancy as well as during treatment of thyroid dysfunction in order to avoid such unfortunate and unnecessary cases.

9.3.2 Measurement of Total or Free Thyroid Hormones?

Also the measurement of the peripheral thyroid hormones themselves is complicated by a number of problems, the most important of which is the relationship to the gestation-induced elevation of the serum concentration of TBG. Since mostly immunoassays are used, biased values can derive from thyroid hormone antibodies in a woman with autoimmune thyroid disease, or heterophilic antibodies interfering in either the assays for TSH or thyroid hormones (Sapin et al., 2004). The elevated total hormone concentrations during gestation can display diverse reactions in the free thyroid hormone assays, either correcting completely or in some situations either overcorrecting or correcting insufficiently. Consequently, results of free thyroid hormone measurements may very likely be either over- or underestimated. A more reliable free thyroid hormone estimate is provided by measurement of total hormone concentrations (T_3 and T_4) and correction for the increased binding proteins by either direct measurement of TBG (to provide T_4/TBG or T_3/TBG ratios) or by a T_3 or T_4 uptake test to provide free thyroid hormone indices. The availability of these measurements depends on the clinical biochemical laboratory.

From a clinical biochemical point of view total hormone measurements and creation of free thyroid hormone measurements are strictly the most reliable tests with the highest precision and accuracy. Very recently free thyroid hormones have been measured by tandem mass spectrometry, which provides accurate, precise, fast and simple measurements (Soukhova et al., 2004; Soldin et al., 2004; Kahric-Janicic et al., 2007). Such methods are, however, not generally available yet, and most laboratories use immunoassays. Overall, the results of thyroid function testing during pregnancy are still difficult, and often impossible to interpret.

Do trimester dependent reference ranges solve the problem of assessing thyroid dysfunction in pregnancy?

Another problem in thyroid function tests are the population-based reference ranges, because they depend not only on the composition of the population and the iodine intake, but also highly on the laboratory methods used. Therefore, there is a strong need of laboratory-dependent reference ranges, in order not to rely only on the reference range provided by the assay manufacturer. Because the progression of pregnancy and foetal, neonatal and child health are dependent on adequate thyroid hormone supplementation throughout pregnancy, trimester-specific reference intervals for thyroid functions can be crucial for both maternal and foetal health. The physiological changes associated with pregnancy require an increased availability of thyroid hormones by 40% to 100% to meet the needs of mother and foetus. Trimester-specific population-based reference ranges in order to correct for the physiological changes with increasing total hormone concentration and de- or increasing free hormones and suppressed TSH have been published from many sources in recent years (Soldin et al., 2004; Kahric-Janicic et al., 2007; Dashe et al., 2005; Soldin, 2006; Stricker et al., 2007; Cotzias et al., 2008; Marwaha et al., 2008; La'ulu and Roberts, 2007; Gilbert etal., 2008; Dhatt et al., 2006; Price et al., 2001; Ong and Hoffman, 2008; Soldin et al., 2007; Pearce et al., 2008). Even though this approach will reduce the global variability of thyroid hormone assessment, it is important to stress that laboratory- and population-specific ranges are crucial, since measurements by different methods in different populations do provide very different ranges (examples shown in Table 9.**1**). This table is not extensive but just includes examples of the most recent publications. When producing trimester-specific reference ranges it is important that seemingly normal women with thyroperoxidase antibodies should not be included in the population (Pearce et al., 2008).

9.4   The Problem of Population-Based Reference Ranges

Another, probably even more important problem complicating the use of population-based reference ranges is that each individual has his/her own genetic set-point, as has been shown by Feldt-Rasmussen et al. (1980) and more recently by Andersen et al. (2002) in a non-pregnant population. In the initial studies when the methods for measurement of thyroid function had a lower sensitivity and higher imprecision the intra-individual coefficient of variation (CV%) was between 6 and 17% (Feldt-Rasmussen et al., 1980), also confirmed in a recent publication using more modern methods (Ankrah-Tetteh et al., 2008), while the inter-individual CV was 11 to 25%. A more relevant way of evaluating this is through an individuality assessment which was in these studies below 0.5, indicating that the thyroid function cannot be meaningfully assessed by the population-based reference range (Feldt-Rasmussen et al., 1980; Andersen et al., 2002; Ankrah-Tetteh et al., 2008; Biersack et al., 2004). Boas et al. (2007) found a similar magnitude of variability in healthy pregnant women with an inter-individual variability of 13–20% for both total and free T_3 and T_4, independent of gestational week, and an intra-individual variability of the same variables of 8–10%.

It is therefore very possible that also during pregnancy changes within the same women are more important than the specific single measurement in relation to a specific reference range. In this case it applies also when using gestation-specific reference ranges, although the latter has to be considered also as a reduction of the total variability of the thyroid hormone function tests. The mentioned gestation-specific reference ranges should, however, be assessed in a given population with the given assays used in the laboratory, and should not solely be based on information from the kit manufacturer or from the literature.

9.5   Conclusions

In conclusion, in clinical practice doctors should use all available thyroid functions tests relevant for the diagnosis in question (see Table 9.**2**) to avoid the risk of false interpretations and the resulting potentially irreversible damage to the foetal brain. Both total and free thyroid hormones are liable to false results during pregnancy, and the biochemical panel of measurements performed when there is a suspicion of hypo- and hyperthyroidism should therefore be supplemented with anti-thyroperoxidase antibodies, and TSH receptor antibodies, respectively. TSH is insufficient as a sole and first line diagnostic variable due to the thyroid-pituitary instability during pregnancy and to suppression during the high peak of HCG at the end of first trimester. Only women without thyroperoxidase antibodies should be included when producing trimester-specific reference ranges. The finding of low intra-individual variation of the thyroid hormones in serum would speak in favour of using the woman's own evolution of the thyroid hormones when diagnosing hypo- or hyperfunction. Since this is for obvious reasons not always possible, the use of trimester-specific references may at least serve to reduce the variability and improve diagnostics.

Due to the high TBG concentration, the best laboratory assessment of thyroid function is a free thyroid hormone estimate – in hypothyroidism free T_4 combined with TSH, and in hyperthyroidism free T_4 and T_3 combined with TSH. These free thyroid hormone measurements do not always correct completely for the binding protein abnormalities. Thus, if in doubt, samples should be measured in another laboratory or combined with total hormone measurement and a T_3-uptake test. Measurement of anti-TPO and/or TSH receptor antibodies may give additional information in some cases. Thus, presence of TPO antibodies very often predicts the risk of hypothyroidism and in pregnant women with low TSH,

Table 9.1 Trimester-specific reference ranges in various studies. Only a sample of studies is shown in order to exemplify the variety of values obtained in different populations of pregnant women and by different methods. Free thyroid hormone values are given – in some of the studies also total hormones have been measured together with T_3 uptake to perform a free T_4 index/estimate. Not all studies excluded pregnant women with thyroid autoantibodies.

Authors	Trimester	Method	TSH 1st trim.	TSH 2nd trim.	TSH 3rd trim.	Free T_4 1st trim.	Free T_4 2nd trim.	Free T_4 3rd trim.	Free T_3 1st trim.	Free T_3 2nd trim.	Free T_3 3rd trim.
Pearce et al.	1st trim., cross sectional		0.04–3.6	ND	ND	ND	ND	ND	ND	ND	ND
Cotzias et al.	All trim., cross sectional	Advia Centaur System	0–5.5	0.5–3.5	0.5–4.0	10–16	9–15.5	8–14.5	3–7	3–5.5	2.5–5.5
Marwaha et al.	All trim., cross sectional	Roche Modular Elecsys	0.6–5.0	0.4–5.8	0.7–5.7	12–19.5	9.5–19.6	11.3–17.7	1.9–5.9	3.2–5.7	3.3–5.2
La'ulu et al.	2nd trim., cross sectional	Abbott Architect i2000SR	ND	0.1–3.3	ND	ND	9.1–15.4	ND	ND	3.8–6.0	ND
Soldin et al.	All trim., longitudinal	Tandem mass spectrometry	0.2–2.99	0.5–3.0	0.4–2.8	3.7–23.4	7.4–18.9	8.3–15.6	ND	ND	ND
Gilbert et al.	1st trim	Abbott Architect	0.02–2.2	ND	ND	10–17.8	ND	ND	3.3–5.7	ND	ND
Dhatt et al.	All trim./Arabs, cross sectional	Abbott Architect	0.06–8.3	0.17–5.9	0.2–6.9	8.9–24.6	8.4–19.3	8.0–18.0	ND	ND	ND
Dhatt et al.	All trim./Asians, cross sectional	Abbott Architect	0.12–7.4	0.3–5.5	0.3–4.9	11.3–21.9	9.7–18.5	8.9–16.6	ND	ND	ND
Price et al.	1st and 2nd trim./Asians, cross sectional	Bayer Diagnostics ACS:180	0.6–1.3	1.0–1.8	ND	11.8–13.4	10.9–12.1	ND	ND	ND	ND
Price et al.	1st and 2nd trim./Caucasian, cross sectional	Bayer Diagnostics ACS:180	0.7–1.1	1.2–1.5	ND	12.0–12.8	11.2–11.8	ND	ND	ND	ND
Gong and Hoffman	All trim., cross sectional	Roche Modular Elecsys	ND	ND	ND	11–19	9.7–17.5	8.1–15.3	ND	ND	ND

TSH was measured in mU/L, free T_4 in pmol/L and free T_3 in pmol/L. ND = not done

Table 9.**2**   What to do in clinical practice concerning thyroid function tests in pregnancy, when diagnosing hypo- or hyperthyroidism, respectively?

State	Test	Problem
Hypothyroidism	Serum TSH, evaluation respecting the gestation induced suppression	Direct measurement with difficulty of interpretation
	Measurement of anti-TPO	Measurement of total T_4 and T_3-uptake test – more reliable
	Free T_4 estimate	Measurement of total T_4 and correcting by 50% increase for pregnancy/TBG effect
Hyperthyroidism	Serum TSH, evaluation respecting the gestation induced suppression	Direct measurement with difficulty of interpretation
	Measurement of TSH receptor antibodies	
	Free T_4 estimate/free T_3 estimate	Measurement of total T_4/T_3 and T_3-uptake test – more reliable

JCEM 2007; 92, Suppl 1: 1–47

hyperthyroidism will be predicted by TSH receptor antibodies in 60–70%.

References

Andersen S, Pedersen KM, Bruun NH, Laurberg P. Narrow individual variations in serum T(4) and T(3) in normal subjects: a clue to the understanding of subclinical thyroid disease. J Clin Endocrinol Metab 2002; 87: 1068–1072.

Ankrah-Tetteh T, Wijeratne S, Swaminathan R. Intra-individual variation in serum thyroid hormones, parathyroid hormone and insulin-like growth factor-1. Ann Clin Biochem 2008; 45: 167–169.

Biersack H-J, Hartmann F, Rödel R, Reinhardt M. Long term changes in serum T_4, T_3 and TSH in benign thyroid disease. Proof of a narrower individual variation. Nuklearmedizin 2004; 43: 158–160.

Boas M, Juul A, Feldt-Rasmussen U, Skakkebaek NE, Chellakooty M, Larsen T, Falck Larsen J, Main KM. Thyroid hormones in pregnancy: Intraindividual variation and correlation to foetal growth. Hot Thyroidology. ETA Abstract Book 2007: 203.

Casey BM, Leveno KJ. Thyroid disease in pregnancy. Obstet Gynecol 2006; 108: 1283–1292.

Cotzias C, Wong S-J, Taylor E, Seed P, Girling J. A study to establish gestation-specific reference intervals for thyroid function testings in normal singleton pregnancy. Eur J Obst Gynaecol 2008; 137: 61–66.

Dashe JS, Casey BM, Wells CE, McIntire DD, Byrd EW, Leveno KJ, Cunningham FG. Thyroid stimulating hormone in singleton and twin pregnancy: importance of gestational age-specific reference ranges. Obstet Gynecol 2005; 106: 753–757.

Dhatt GS, Jayasundaram R, Wareth LA, Nagelkerke N, Jayasundaram K, Darwish EA, Lewis A. Thyrotropin and free thyroxine trimester-specific reference intervals in a mixed ethnic pregnant population in the United Arab Emirates. Clin Chim Acta 2006; 370: 147–151.

Endocrine Society Clinical Practice guideline: Management of thyroid dysfunction during pregnancy and postpartum. www.endo-society/thyroidand-pregnancy; www.jcem

Feldt-Rasmussen U, Hyltoft Petersen P, Blaabjerg O, Hørder M. Long-term variability in serum thyroglobulin and thyroid related hormones in healthy subjects. Acta Endocrinol (Copenh) 1980; 95: 328–334.

Gilbert RM, Hadlow NC, Walsch JP, Fletcher SJ, Brown SJ, Stuckey BG, Lim EM. Assessment of thyroid function during pregnancy. The Medical Journal of Australia. 2008; 189: 250–253.

Glinoer D. The regulation of thyroid function in pregnancy: pathways of endocrine adaptation from physiology to pathology. Endocr Rev 1997; 18: 404–433.

Gong Y, Hoffman BR. Free thyroxine reference interval in each trimester of pregnancy determined with the Roche Modular E-170 electrochemiluminescent immunoassay. Clin Biochem 2008; 41: 902–906.

Haddow JE, Palomaki GE, Allan WC, Williams JR, Knight GJ, Gagnon J, O'Heir CE, Mitchell ML, Hermos RJ, Waisbren SE, Faix JD, Klein RZ. Maternal thyroid deficiency during pregnancy and subsequent neuropsychological development of the child. N Engl J Med 1999; 341: 549–555.

Kahric-Janicic N, Soldin SJ, Soldin OP, West T, Gu J, Jonklaas J. Tandem mass spectrometry improves the accuracy of free thyroxine measurements during pregnancy. Thyroid 2007; 17: 303–311.

La'ulu SL, Roberts W. Second-Trimester reference intervals for thyroid tests: The role of ethnicity. Clin Chem 2007; 1658–1664.

Mandel SJ, Spencer CA, Hollowell JG. Are detection and treatment of thyroid insufficiency in pregnancy feasible? Thyroid 2005; 15: 44–53.

Marwaha RK, Chopra S, Gopalakrishnan S, Sharma B, Kanwar RS, Sastry A, Singh S. Establishment of reference range for thyroid hormones in normal pregnant Indian women. Br J Obstet Gynaecol 2008; 115: 602–606.

Morreale de Escobar G, Obregon MJ, Escobar del Rey F. Is neuropsychological development related to maternal hypothyroidism or to maternal hypothyroxinaemia? J Clin Endocrinol Metab 2000; 85: 3975–3987

National Academy of Clinical Biochemistry Guidelines for Laboratory Practice. www.nacb.org

Pearce EN, Oken E, Gillman MW, Lee SL, Magnani B, Platek D, Braverman LE. Association of first-trimester thyroid function test values with thyroperoxidase antibody status, smoking, and multivitamin use. Endocr Pract 2008; 14: 33–39.

Pop VJ, Kuijpens JL, van Baar AL, Verkerk G, van Son MM, de Vijlder JJ, Vulsma T, Wiersinga WM, Drexhage HA, Vader HL. Low maternal free thyroxine concentrations during early pregnancy are associated with impaired psychomotor development in infancy. Clin Endocrinol 1999; 50: 149–155.

Price A, Obel O, Cresswell J, Catch I, Rutter S, Barik S, Heller SR, Weetman AP. Comparison of thyroid function in pregnant and non-pregnant Asian and western Caucasian women. Clin Chim Acta 2001; 308: 91–98.

Sapin R, D'Herbomez M, Schlienger JL. Free thyroxine measured with equilibrium dialysis and nine immunoassays decreases in late pregnancy. Clin Lab 2004; 50: 581–584.

Soldin OP. Thyroid function testing in pregnancy and thyroid disease. Trimester-specific reference intervals. Ther Drug Monit 2006; 28: 8–11.

Soldin OP, Soldin D, Sastoque M. Gestation-specific thyroxine and thyroid stimulating hormone levels in the United States and worldwide. Ther Drug Monit 2007; 29: 553–559.

Soldin OP, Tractenberg RE, Hollowell JG, Jonklaas J, Janicic N, Soldin SJ. Trimester-specific changes in maternal thyroid hormone, thyrotropin, and thyroglobulin concentrations during gestation: Trends and associations across trimesters and iodine sufficiency. Thyroid 2004; 14: 1084–1090.

Soukhova N, Soldin OP, Soldin SJ. Isotope dilution tandem mass spectrometric method for T_4/T_3. Clin Chim Acta 2004; 343: 185–190.

Stricker R, Echenard M, Eberhart R, Chevailler MC, Perez V, Quinn FA, Stricker R. Evaluation of maternal thyroid function during pregnancy: The importance of using gestational age-specific reference intervals. Eur J Endocrinol 2007; 157: 509–514.

10 Significance and Management of Low TSH in Pregnancy

R. Negro

Department of Endocrinology, "V. Fazzi" Hospital, Piazza F. Muratore, 73100 Lecce, Italy

Abstract

Normal pregnancy is characterised by major changes in thyroid economy, thyroid function tests and iodine metabolism, so that normal reference ranges usually valid for the non-pregnant state should not be applied during gestation. In fact, the stimulatory action exerted by human chorionic gonadotropin (hCG) on the thyroid gland, with a consequent reduction of thyroid-stimulating hormone (TSH) concentration, must always be taken into account when evaluating thyroid function tests, especially during the first trimester of pregnancy. This concept is valid either for the upper or for the lower TSH reference range. Furthermore, the employment of third-generation TSH assays has really improved the accuracy of detection of TSH concentration, allowing us to distinguish between low and suppressed values. The right interpretation of TSH, in conjunction with free thyroxine (FT_4) and TSH-receptor antibodies (TRAb), is of pivotal importance to distinguish not dangerous situations (gestational transient thyrotoxicosis – GTT) from health-threatening ones (Graves' disease). Graves' hyperthyroidism is associated with an increased risk of maternal and foetal complications, and an appropriate treatment with anti-thyroid drugs is able to abolish these adverse effects; on the contrary, GTT does not require a specific treatment and alterations of thyroid function tests usually recover during the second and the third trimesters of gestation. Then, of pivotal importance are a) the right recognition of low TSH aetiology and, b) an adequate knowledge in the management of pregnant women with low TSH values.

10.1 Introduction

Normal pregnancy is characterised by significant changes in thyroid economy, thyroid function tests and iodine metabolism (Glinoer, 1997; Casey and Leveno, 2006). Particularly concerning thyroid-stimulating hormone (TSH), its regulation is influenced by the rise of human chorionic gonadotropin (hCG), whose concentration increases during the first trimester. As hCG and TSH share a common α subunit, the former exerts a stimulatory action on the thyroid gland; the rising in maternal hCG concentration during gestation results in a reciprocal reduction in TSH (Glinoer et al., 1990; Glinoer, 1993) (Fig. 10.1). Then, hCG represents a physiological regulator of thyroid function, as it displays a TSH-like activity; it has been estimated that an hCG increase of 10 000 UI/L results in a corresponding TSH reduction of 0.1 mIU/L. Given the thyroid stimulating action exerted by hCG and the increased levels of TBG, the first trimester of pregnancy is characterised by increased concentrations of thyroxine (T_4) (Glinoer, 1997). These and many others modifications mean that the normal reference ranges which are valid for the non-pregnant state, are not fully applicable, in particular during the first trimester of gestation. The inverse logarithmic relationship between TSH and free T_4 (FT_4) is not always respected, and the laboratory evaluation of thyroid function is further complicated by interfering factors which may alter the accuracy of FT_4 dosage (Mandel et al., 2005). Even today, normal reference ranges to be universally applied for the pregnancy state are still lacking. The elaboration of such reference ranges should be trimester-specific and requires that the population sample has to be characterised by a sufficient iodine intake, be free from thyroid disease, and be without thyroid antibodies.

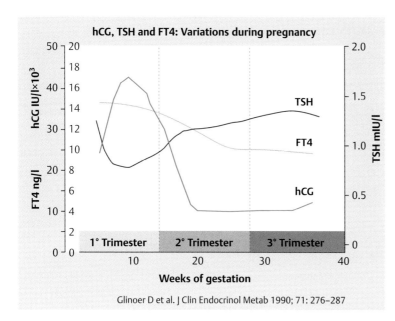

Fig. 10.**1** Serum TSH, hCG, and FT$_4$ as a function of gestational age in healthy pregnant women. From Glinoer et al. (1990).

Glinoer D et al. J Clin Endocrinol Metab 1990; 71: 276–287

10.2   Aetiology of Low TSH Values in Pregnancy

Hyperthyroidism during pregnancy is relatively uncommon, with a prevalence estimated to range between 0.1% and 1% (Becks and Burrow, 1991; Wang and Crapo, 1997; LeBeau and Mandel, 2006; Hollowell et al., 2002). Causes of low TSH during pregnancy are listed in Table 10.**1**. Aetiologies such as single toxic adenoma, multinodular toxic goitre, subacute or silent thyroiditis, iodide-induced thyrotoxicosis, or thyrotoxicosis factitia are quite uncommon during pregnancy. Molar disease should always be considered, even if an uncomplicated hydatidiform mole is easily diagnosed and rarely leads to severe thyrotoxicosis (Hersghman, 1997; Narasimhan et al., 2002). Other extremely rare causes of hyperthyroidism include hyperplacentosis and struma ovarii (Coughlin and Haddad, 2000; Ginsberg et al., 2001). In women in the childbearing age, a frequent cause of hyperthyroidism is Graves' disease, but the most frequent cause of low TSH is represented by high hCG levels encountered during the first trimester; this condition may be associated with high thyroid hormones concentration, which is usually transient (gestational transient thyrotoxicosis – GTT) (LeBeau and Mandel, 2008; Yoshimura and Hershman, 1995; Glinoer, 1998; Goodwin et al., 1992). Women develop GTT when they have an abnormally elevated peak of hCG, and

Table 10.**1**   Causes of low TSH during pregnancy.

Causes of low TSH during pregnancy
High hCG, Gestational transient thyrotoxicosis
Hyperplacentosis, struma ovarii
Molar pregnancy
Graves' hyperthyroidism
Subacute thyroiditis
Uni-multinodular toxic goitre
Factitious

when high hCG values are sustained during an unusually prolonged period (Grün et al., 1997). Twin pregnancy, for example, is a clinical condition associated with sustained and high hCG concentrations. In women with a twin pregnancy, hCG values are significantly higher and of a much longer duration than in a singleton one. In fact, twin pregnancy is associated with a more profound and more frequent suppression of TSH values. Also, while serum FT$_4$ levels are comprised within the normal range in a singleton pregnancy, they often rise above normal in a twin pregnancy.

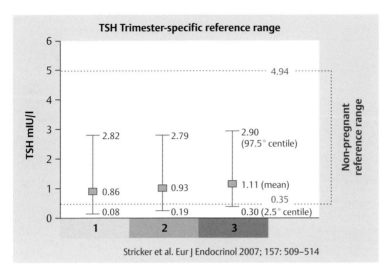

Fig. 10.**2** Serum TSH values during gestation in a population of pregnant women (free from thyroid disease and with a sufficient daily iodine intake), compared with non-pregnant normal reference range. From Stricker et al. (2007).

Stricker et al. Eur J Endocrinol 2007; 157: 509–514

10.3   Normal TSH Reference Ranges in Pregnancy

Serum TSH values are influenced by the thyrotropic action of hCG, above all near the end of the first trimester, so that about 20% of healthy pregnant women show transiently low TSH values at this time of gestation (Burrow, 1993: Pekonen et al., 1988; Guillaume et al., 1985; Weeke et al., 1982; Chan and Swaminathan, 1988; Yamamoto et al., 1979). Thus, above all during the first trimester, by using the classical non-pregnant reference range for serum TSH (0.4–4.0 mIU/L), a normal pregnant woman may be misdiagnosed as having subclinical hyperthyroidism. During the second and the third trimester, serum TSH progressively increases, but is still within the normal range. Several authors measured TSH values during pregnancy to derive normal reference ranges to be applied in physiological pregnancy. These studies are sometimes very different one from another, because of differences in the population examined. In fact, ethnicity, iodine intake, and antibody status, profoundly influence thyroid function tests during pregnancy. Anyway, also taking into account all the above-mentioned differences among the studies published, the 2.5 percentile in the first trimester resulted to be around 0.03 mIU/L, 0.1 mIU/L in the second trimester, and 0.2 mIU/L in the third trimester; the 97.5 percentile in the first trimester resulted at around 2.5 mIU/L, and 3.0 mIU/L in the second and the third trimesters; mean TSH values resulted to be around 0.8 mIU/L in the first trimester,

and comprised between 1.0–1.3 mIU/L in the second and the third trimesters (Panesar et al., 2001: Haddow et al., 2004; Stricker et al., 2007; Spencer et al., 2005; Walker etal., 2005) (Fig. 10.2). A recent study by Pearce et al. (2008) evaluated thyroid function tests during the first trimester in pregnant women with and without thyroid antibodies. Results showed, as expected, that the median TSH value (range containing 95% of the data points) in antibody-negative women was 1.1 mIU/L (0.04–3.6), a significantly lower value than in antibody-positive women [(1.8 mIU/L (0.3–6.4)]. Then, the study outlined that TPOAb status should be considered in pregnant women when constructing trimester-specific reference ranges, because elevated serum TPOAb levels are associated with higher TSH (and lower T_4) values. Given the changes occurring to thyroid function during pregnancy, it is becoming clearer and clearer that trimester-specific reference ranges are needed to correctly identify either hypo- or hyperthyroid patients. The importance of gestational age reference ranges is shown in a study conducted by Dashe et al. (2005), where if a non-pregnant reference (0.4–4.0 mU/L) had been used, 28% of 342 singletons with TSH greater than 2 standard deviations above the mean would not have been identified. In conclusion, the concrete risk in applying non-pregnant reference ranges in pregnant women is represented by an underestimation of diagnosis of hypothyroidism and an overestimation of hyperthyroidism.

10.4   Prevalence of Low TSH in Pregnancy

The employment of third-generation TSH assays has allowed a greater accuracy in the detection of low TSH values. From studies which examined the thyroid function during pregnancy the incidence of low and/or suppressed TSH values may be derived. In a study involving Asian pregnant women examined between the 8th and 14th weeks of gestation, 1.1% of the population were found to be affected by Graves' disease, while suppressed TSH was observed in 33%, and 11% were diagnosed as having GTT (using a TSH lower limit of 0.36 mIU/L and an FT_4 higher limit of 9.1 pmol/L (Yeo et al., 2001). In the Japanese study by Kurioka et al. (2005) during the first trimester, 21.8% of the pregnant women examined had TSH values lower than the normal range of healthy non-pregnant controls; this percentage progressively decreased to 4.5% in the second trimester and to 0.74% in the third trimester; FT_4 was found to be higher than the normal reference range in 6.7% during the first trimester, while none of the pregnant women showed high FT_4 levels during the second and the third trimesters. In the same study, trimester-specific reference ranges for thyroid function were proposed, with a TSH lower limit corresponding to 0.04 mIU/L for the first trimester (Kurioka et al, 2005). Vaidya et al. (2007) examining 1560 women screened mostly between the 9th and 12th weeks of gestation, found 7.8% with low and 1.9% with suppressed TSH values. Currently, a randomised study by Lazarus and Premawardhana (2005) (Controlled Antenatal Thyroid Screening Study – CATS) is being undertaken where pregnant women provide a blood sample before 16 weeks of gestation. The samples are randomised to a screen group (with immediate estimation of FT_4 and TSH) and a control group with estimation of these parameters occurring after delivery. Levothyroxine treatment is given to those in the screen group whose FT_4 is in the lowest 2.5th percentile or whose TSH is above the 97.5th percentile. This study design will produce two groups of children whose neurodevelopment will subsequently be tested at 3 years of age; that is, those from treated hypothyroid mothers and those from untreated mothers (undiagnosed during gestation). Aim of the study is to assess if LT_4 supplementation may prevent neurointellectual deficits in children born from mothers with thyroid impairment. Thanks to data collected from this pivotal study, the authors have taken the chance to assess the prevalence of low TSH in a large number of patients between the 9th and 15th weeks of gestation. Of 1497 samples, a TSH lower than 0.02 mIU/L was found in 1.47% of patients, while 0.17% had also elevated FT_4 (Kaköamanou et al., 2006). To evaluate pregnancy outcomes in women with suppressed TSH and normal FT_4 levels, Casey et al. (2006) screened 25 765 women, and found that 2.0% had low TSH values, with 1.7% having subclinical hyperthyroidism. In this study, suppressed TSH values were considered as values at or below the 2.5th percentile for gestational age and normal FT_4 values as less than 1.75 ng/dL (Casey et al., 2006). In conclusion, during the first trimester of pregnancy, TSH values lower than the non-pregnant reference range are a common finding. If a trimester-specific reference range is applied, the number of pregnant women with low TSH values decreases, but it still represents a very significant percentage that needs to be followed and sometimes treated.

10.5   Complications in Conditions of Low TSH in Pregnancy

Well known are the complications of Graves' hyperthyroidism during pregnancy and an important clinical concept is that the risk of complications for the mother and the newborn is directly related to the duration and the control of maternal hyperthyroidism. The most common complication is gestational hypertension, with a risk of preeclampsia that is ~5-fold greater in women with uncontrolled hyperthyroidism. Other obstetrical complications include miscarriage, foetal malformation, placenta abruptio, preterm delivery and low birth weight (LeBeau and Mandel, 2006; Mestman, 2004; Amino et al., 1982; Millar et al., 1994; Davis et al., 1989; Phoojaroenchanachal et al., 2001). Women with untreated Graves' disease often experience multiple abortions consistent with severe foetal hyperthyroidism. Several studies suggest foetal death rates up to 20% (Chopra, 1992). Congestive heart failure may rarely occur in thyrotoxic women, especially in the presence of gestational hypertension or in case of Caesarean delivery (Sheffield and Cunningham, 2004). In a study from Australia, the outcome of pregnancy was evaluated in women with unrecognised maternal Graves' disease (Smith et al., 2001). The results showed increased risk of severe prematurity (mean gestational age of 30 weeks at delivery) associated with very low birth weight (<2 kg) and neonatal hyperthyroidism requiring treatment with ATD. In contrast, for those patients in whom the diagnosis was made early and the treatment started promptly, the outcome was excellent. In fact, in another study from Japan, involving 230 pregnant women with Graves' disease, no adverse impact on the outcome of pregnancy was found in patients with adequately treated Graves' disease (Mitsuda et al., 1992). An important issue concerning Graves' disease is that it has profound effects on the foetus and the newborn. Maternal autoimmune thyroid disorders may affect foetal and neonatal thyroid function through placental transfer of anti-TSH-receptor antibodies (TRAb). These antibodies, mainly of the IgG class, usually elicit thyroid-stimulating activity but in rare cases may have an inhibitory action. Thus, maternal TRAb may have stimulatory or inhibiting effects on the foetal thyroid gland causing foetal and neonatal hyper- or hypothyroidism, respectively (Rapoport et al., 1998; Matsuura et al., 1997; Radetti et al., 1999; Peleg et al., 2002). One to 5% of neonates of mothers with Graves' disease have hyperthyroidism due to the trans-placental passage of stimulating maternal TRAb (McKenzie and Zakarjia, 1992). The overall incidence is low probably because of the state of immune tolerance, the balance between stimulatory and inhibitory antibodies, and also thanks to the use of antithyroid drug (ATD) in the mothers (Laurberg et al., 1998). The incidence of neonatal Graves' disease is not directly related to maternal thyroid hormones concentrations, but to TRAb titres (Mitsuda et al., 1992). Foetal dysfunction may be suspected on the base of detection of foetal goitre. The presence of foetal hyperthyroidism is associated with high TRAb titres, low ATD dosages, accelerated foetal bone maturation, high foetal heart beat rate (> 160/min), and growth retardation (Mestman, 2004; Polak et al., 2004). Conversely, foetal hypothyroidism is associated with low TRAb titres, high ATD dosages, and delayed foetal bone maturation. The employment of colour Doppler thyroid ultrasound may help in making the differential diagnosis. In particular, a Doppler signal throughout the gland is a typical feature of hyperthyroidism, while a Doppler signal confined to the periphery of the gland is a feature of hypothyroidism (Luton et al., 2005). Foetal blood sampling is indicated for cases in which the diagnosis of foetal dysfunction is uncertain and/or intra-amniotic thyroxine injection is required. In fact, as thyroid hormones play a crucial role in the foetal growth and foetal brain development, foetal hypothyroidism can cause permanent impairment in neurointellectual performance. In these cases, intra-amniotic thyroxine injection and ATD dosage reduction are effective in restoring normal foetal thyroid function (Volumenie et al., 2000). Finally, a condition of subclinical hyperthyroidism can be seen in maternal Graves' disease, but is more often found in association with GTT. In the above-mentioned study by Casey et al. (2006) the condition of subclinical hyperthyroidism was not associated with an increased risk of adverse pregnancy outcomes, either for the mother or for the newborn, the results of the paper leading to the conclusions that identification and treatment of subclinical hyperthyroidism is not warranted.

10.6 Interpretation of Low TSH in Pregnancy

Given the above-mentioned complications which may take place in conditions characterised by low TSH levels, it is of pivotal importance to correctly interpret thyroid function tests, to establish the diagnosis, and to initiate (or not) the treatment. Clinical signs and symptoms (in conjunction with maternal thyroid ultrasound) must always be considered when evaluating a pregnant woman. Even though the historical clues and physical findings are the same in pregnant and non-pregnant patients, the clinical diagnosis of thyrotoxicosis may be difficult to make during pregnancy. Non-specific symptoms such as fatigue, anxiety, tachycardia, heat intolerance, warm moist skin, tremor and systolic murmur may be present in a normal pregnancy as well. Alternatively, the presence of a goitre, ophthalmopathy or pretibial myxoedema obviously points to the suspicion of Graves' disease. A useful symptom of hyperthyroidism is that, instead of the expected weight gain associated with pregnancy, patients may report weight loss or, even more frequently, absence of weight gain despite an increased appetite (unless there is also excessive vomiting). Nausea (morning sickness) occurs frequently during normal pregnancy. However, the occurrence of hyperemesis gravidarum accompanied by weight loss must always raise the suspicion of hCG-induced hyperthyroidism. Patients suspected of having hyperthyroidism require measurement of serum TSH, FT_4, and TRAb. The presence of TRAb in the first trimester is highly useful in helping make the differential diagnosis between Graves' disease and other causes of gestational hyperthyroidism. Since TRAb production tends to undergo immunological remission during the second half of pregnancy, TRAb concentrations may depend upon gestational age (Amino et al., 1982; Davis and Weiss, 1981; Sridama et al., 1982; Kamijo, 2007). Graves' disease is an autoimmune disease and it is therefore important to consider that the production of TRAb may vary during pregnancy and, in turn, influence the clinical course of the disease. Usually, Graves' disease during pregnancy is characterised by an exacerbation of hyperthyroidism during the first trimester, followed by an improvement in the second half of gestation. Furthermore, it has to be remembered that maternal production of TRAb may be present, even after a previous thyroidectomy or thyroid ablation by radioiodine, or in a state of apparent remission of the disease thanks to ATD therapy given before pregnancy. For a euthyroid pregnant woman (with or without thyroid hormone replacement therapy) who has previously been treated with radioiodine or undergone thyroid surgery for Graves' disease, the risk of foetal/neonatal thyrotoxicosis derives from the level of TRAb produced by the mother. As a result, TRAb should be measured in early pregnancy and in each trimester to evaluate this risk. If TRAb titres have not substantially decreased during the second trimester, the chance of foetal thyrotoxicosis should be considered (Lauerberg et al., 1998; Burro et al., 1994). Maternal transfer of TRAb to the foetus in a hyperthyroid pregnant woman with active Graves' disease causes a marked increase in the foetal/maternal TRAb ratio (Radetti et al., 1999). Thus, the foetal-placental unit gradually concentrates proportionally larger fractions of thyroid stimulating antibodies from maternal blood, particularly during the second half of gestation, hence underlining the importance to systematically search for foetal thyroid dysfunction in all clinical conditions where the mother may produce large amounts of TRAb (Peleg et al., 2002). As mentioned above, hyperthyroidism due to Graves' disease usually tends to improve gradually during gestation, although exacerbations can be observed in the first weeks. Several reasons have been claimed to explain this spontaneous improvement: a) the partial immunosuppressive state characteristic of pregnancy, with a progressive decrease in TRAb production (Geva et al., 1997); b) the marked rise in maternal serum TBG levels that tends to reduce the free fractions of T_3 and T_4 (Soldin et al., 2004); c) the physiological iodine loss occurring during pregnancy that

may, paradoxically, constitute an advantage for women with Graves' disease (Smyth, 1999); d) changes in cytokine production between normal and Graves' disease pregnant women may also help explain the transient remission of the disease (Jones et al., 2000); and e) finally, two studies suggested that the balance between TRAb's blocking and stimulating activities may be modified in favour of blocking antibodies (Kung and Jones, 2001; Kung et al., 2001). This latter finding has been denied by Amino et al. (2003) who demonstrated that amelioration of Graves' disease during pregnancy is induced by a decrease of stimulating TRAb but not by the appearance of blocking ones. It is necessary to bear in mind that TRAb contain either a stimulating or an inhibiting class of antibodies and the commonly available kits for measuring TRAb cannot distinguish between these two types of antibodies. Anyway, in the great majority of cases, TRAb are mostly constituted by antibodies with a stimulatory action. Antibodies that stimulate the receptor can be measured by their ability to increase cAMP production in a preparation of cell membranes containing the TSH receptor, but this assay is not generally available in hospital or commercial laboratories. Some antibodies bind to the TSH receptor and inhibit the stimulating activity of TSH. Such antibodies may be clinically significant since they can cause hypothyroidism (including in the foetus), but they are usually measured only in a research setting (Gola et al., 2006). Patients with Graves' disease may have positive thyroid antibodies (TgAb and TPOAb) and, therefore, the presence of antibodies should alert the clinician that autoimmune thyroid disease is the cause of symptoms inducing hyperthyroidism. In the CATS study, 20.8% of hyperthyroid pregnant women were positive for TPOAb, with 70% of these sera testing positive for TRAb; 5.2% of women with subclinical hyperthyroidism were TPOAb positive, and about 50% of these sera tested positive for TRAb (Kaklamanou et al., 2006). Hence the determination of positive TPOAb in sera found to have low TSH in the first trimester is a moderate predictor of Graves' disease.

The complex picture represented by thyroid function in pregnancy is further complicated by serum FT_4 concentration. The state of pregnancy implies modifications due to the altered sensitivity of the hormone-protein binding (TBG and albumin) and each of the currently used kits has a certain variability compared with the gold standard, which is the equilibrium dialysis method (Roti et al., 1991; Soldin, 2006). At the end of gestation, the dosage of FT_4 concentrations when measured with different immunoassays, reveals a reduction that varies from −17% to −34% in respect to the normal reference ranges; the use of equilibrium dialysis further confirmed that during pregnancy FT_4 values are significantly reduced, as FT_4 decreases by about 40% (Sapin et al., 2004). The recent employment by Kahric-Janicic et al. (2007) of tandem mass spectrometry in the dosage of FT_4 has been demonstrated to be accurate as equilibrium dialysis; in the same study, the authors showed that FT_4 values in the second trimester are significantly lower than the first and that FT_4 values in the third trimester are lower than those of the first and the second trimesters, confirming that the FT_4 variations during pregnancy are not just a laboratory artefact.

10.7   Therapeutic Management of Low TSH Values

There are no available data to exactly determine if patients with GTT require a specific treatment. In most cases, no specific treatment is necessary and maternal symptoms due to thyrotoxicosis can be alleviated by the administration of beta-adrenergic blocking agents (propranolol) for a short period, while waiting for spontaneous recovery of elevated thyroid hormones to occur. In patients with a severe clinical presentation, some authors suggest treatment with ATD, usually for a few weeks only, and therapy is often discontinued by midgestation. It should be noted that treatment of subclinical hyperthyroidism does not improve pregnancy outcome and may risk unnecessary exposure of the foetus to ATD (Casey et al., 2006). Another point of discussion about the opportunity to treat or not to treat women with GTT, may derive from two particular cases of thyrotoxicosis, without production of TRAb. The first case is seen in women with genetic resistance to thyroid hormone: these patients show a significantly increased miscarriage rate in respect to controls, possibly due to foetal exposure to high thyroid hormones concentrations (Anselmo et al., 2004). The second case is where there are mutations of TSH receptor resulting in increased sensitivity of the receptor to normal concentrations of hCG (Rodien et al., 1998; Rodien et al., 2004). Also this latter condition is characterised by thyrotoxicosis and is complicated by an increased risk of miscarriage. The above-mentioned cases, being ex-

tremely rare, represent conditions of above normal FT_4 concentrations, similar to the ones encountered in GTT, although GTT is characterised by an amelioration of thyrotoxicosis during the second and the third trimesters of pregnancy.

Antithyroid drugs (ATD) are the main treatment for Graves' disease during pregnancy. The overall goal of therapy is to control maternal disease by maintaining the patient at high normal FT_4 values, while minimising the risk of fetal hyperthyroidism or hypothyroidism by using the smallest possible dose of ATD (LeBeau et al., 2006; Mestman, 2004; Mandel and Cooper, 2001; Cooper, 2005).

Propylthiouracil (PTU), methimazole (MMI) and *carbimazole (CMI)* are currently used during gestation. Pregnancy itself does not appear to alter significantly the pharmacokinetics of ATD and both PTU and MMI (or CMI) appear equally effective (Wing et al., 1994). The ATD dosage should be maintained at a minimum and drugs discontinued, when possible. Combined administration to the mother of ATD and thyroxine is not advised, since the transplacental passage of ATD is high, while it is negligible for thyroid hormones, and hence will not protect the foetus from ATD-induced hypothyroidism (Roti et al., 1981). All ATD cross the placenta and may thus inhibit foetal thyroid function. PTU is more water soluble and more extensively bound to albumin at physiological pH than MMI. Theoretically therefore, treatment with MMI may result in an increased transplacental passage relative to PTU. These facts have led authors to recommend preferentially the use of PTU both during pregnancy and lactation, based on the concept that the foetus might be at a higher risk of developing hypothyroidism when women receive MMI. From all the available information taken together, however, the placental transfer of PTU and MMI appears not to be so different, and the increased risk of foetal hypothyroidism associated with MMI compared with PTU is considered negligible (Mandel et al., 1994; Marchant et al., 1977; Skellern et al., 1980; Gardner et al., 1986; Cheron et al., 1981; Mortimer et al., 1997; Momotani et al., 1997). Then, either for MMI or PTU, the principle of therapy is to administer the lowest ATD dose needed for controlling clinical symptoms. Mild degrees of hyperthyroidism are acceptable as long as the patient tolerates this condition and pregnancy progresses satisfactorily. Patients should be followed closely, with careful monitoring of the patient.

10.8 Teratogenicity of Maternal Treatment with ATD

Both thyrotoxicosis by itself and the administration of ATD to pregnant women may raise concerns with regard to potential teratogenicity of the disease and/or the medications. To date, it remains unclear whether untreated Graves' disease is associated with a higher frequency of congenital abnormalities (Mandel and Cooper, 2001). There have been reports of two distinct teratogenic patterns associated with MMI administration, namely aplasia cutis congenita and choanal/oesophageal atresia, but data supporting these associations remain controversial (Frieden, 1986; Clementi et al., 1999; Johnsson et al., 1997; Bournard and Orgiazzi, 2003; Iwayama et al., 2007; Diav-Citrin and Ornoy, 2002; Valdez et al., 2007). Aplasia cutis has, so far, not been reported in mothers who received PTU. The prevalence of these malformations is extremely rare: 2/241 MMI-exposed infants (Di Gianantonio et al., 2001). In view of the potential danger – both for mother and offspring – of not treating active Graves' disease in pregnancy, it is clear that ATD administration is in any case mandatory and withholding ATD is not justified. However, due to a possible association between the use of MMI during pregnancy and above-mentioned foetal abnormalities, MMI may be less desirable as first-line treatment for Graves' disease in pregnancy than PTU. MMI should be considered a viable second choice if the patient is intolerant to PTU, has an allergic reaction to PTU, or fails to become euthyroid while receiving PTU (Chattaway and Klepser, 2007).

10.8.1 Beta-Adrenergic Blocking Agents

Propranolol may be used transiently to control symptoms of acute hyperthyroid disease and for pre-operative preparation. There are no significant teratogenic effects of propranolol reported in humans or in animals. If a patient requires long-term propranolol administration, careful monitoring of the foetus is recommended, because of a possible association with intrauterine growth restriction and impaired response to anoxic stress together with postnatal bradycardia and hypoglycaemia (Redmond, 1982).

10.8.2 Iodides

Chronic use of iodide during pregnancy has been associated with neonatal goitre and hypothyroidism, sometimes resulting in asphyxiation because of tracheal obstruction (Mandel et al., 1994). Because the experience with iodides is limited, iodide should not be used as a first-line therapy for Graves' disease during pregnancy, but can be used temporarily, when needed, in preparation for a thyroidectomy (Momotani et al., 1992).

10.8.3 Radioactive Iodine

Administration of radioactive iodine is contraindicated during pregnancy. In cases of inadvertent radioiodine administration, the foetus is exposed to radiation from mother's blood. Since foetal thyroid uptake of radioiodine begins after twelve weeks, exposure to maternal radioiodine prior to this time is not associated with foetal thyroid dysfunction (Zanzonico, 1997). However, treatment with radioiodine after twelve weeks, either for Graves' disease or for remnant ablation, leads to significant radiation to the foetal thyroid. Several incidents of inadvertent exposure to radioiodine have been reported, causing foetal thyroid destruction and congenital hypothyroidism (Berg et al., 1998; Lowe, 2004; Berg et al., 2008). Even if a routine pregnancy test is mandatory to confirm or exclude a suspected pregnancy, given the progressively reduced half-life and decreased degree of sialinisation of β-hCG, its detection may be missed from the 18th week onwards.

10.8.4 Surgery

Thyroidectomy for Graves' disease during pregnancy should be reserved as a second line of treatment in the following situations: 1) patients who have side effects to ATD (allergy, intolerance, etc.); 2) constantly high doses of ATD required to control maternal hyperthyroidism; 3) upper respiratory compressive symptoms due to goitre size. Thyrotoxic pregnant women should be prepared for surgery by using beta-blocking agents and super-saturated potassium iodide solution in order to reduce vascularity of the thyroid gland. Anaesthesia for non-obstetric surgery, whenever possible, should be deferred to the 2nd trimester (Kuczkowski, 2004; Van De Velde and De Buck, 2007).

10.9   Conclusions

Low TSH values during pregnancy are a quite common finding if non-pregnant reference ranges are used, involving up to 20% of women. This percentage lowers to 1.5–2.0% if trimester-specific reference ranges are applied. Thus, to help the clinician in the correct interpretation of thyroid function tests during pregnancy, there is a need for normative gestational age-related reference ranges that would avoid misdiagnosing a euthyroid pregnant woman with subclinical hyperthyroidism. Among women with real low TSH values, just a portion require treatment with anti-thyroid drugs. In fact, hyperthyroidism, above all during the first trimester, may represent a challenge for the endocrinologist who has to discriminate between Graves' disease and GTT. In this context, the concentration of TRAb is of pivotal importance. The differential diagnosis and the relative treatment are critical because, even if uncommon, hyperthyroidism due to Graves' disease is characterised by dangerous adverse effects for the mother and the foetus. Given the very low prevalence of Graves' disease during pregnancy, a screening programme for this specific condition would not be justified; but, as thyroid function tests are widely applied (even if screening is still not recommended), an adequate knowledge in the management of pregnant women with low TSH values is necessary to avoid unjustified alarms and inappropriate treatments, limiting the use of anti-thyroid drugs to targeted cases with health-threatening problems.

References

Amino N, Izumi Y, Hidaka Y et al. No increase of blocking type anti-thyrotropin receptor antibodies during pregnancy in patients with Graves' disease. J Clin Endocrinol Metab 2003; 88: 5871–4.

Amino N, Tanizawa O, Mori H et al: Aggravation of thyrotoxicosis in early pregnancy and after delivery in Graves' disease. J Clin Endocrinol Metab 1982; 55: 108–12.

Anselmo J, Cao D, Karrison T et al. Fetal loss associated with excess of thyroid hormone exposure. JAMA 2004; 292: 691–5.

Becks GP, Burrow GN. Thyroid disease and pregnancy. Med Clin N Amer 1991; 75: 121–50.

Berg G, Jacobsson L, Nystrom E et al. Consequences of inadvertent radioiodine treatment of Graves' disease and thyroid cancer in undiagnosed pregnancy. Can we rely on routine pregnancy testing? Acta Oncologica 2008; 47: 145–149.

Berg GE, Nystrom EH, Jacobsson L et al. Radioiodine treatment of hyperthyroidism in a pregnant woman. J Nucl Med 1998; 39: 357–61.

Bournaud C, Orgiazzi J. Embryopathies et anti-thyroïdiens. Ann Endocrinol (Paris) 2003; 64: 366–9.

Burrow GN. Thyroid function and hyperfunction during gestation. Endocr Rev 1993; 14: 194–202.

Burrow GN, Fisher DA, Larsen PR. Mechanisms of disease: Maternal and fetal thyroid function. N Engl J Med 1994; 331: 1072–8.

Casey BM, Dashe JS, Wells CE, McIntire DD, Leveno KJ, Cunningham FG. Subclinical hyperthyroidism and pregnancy outcomes. Obstet Gynecol 2006; 107: 337–41.

Casey MB, Leveno KJ. Thyroid disease in pregnancy. Obstet Gynecol 2006; 108: 1283–1292.

Chan BY, Swaminathan R. Serum thyrotropin concentration measured by sensitive assays in normal pregnancy. Br J Obstet Gynaecol 1988; 95: 1332–4.

Chattaway JM, Klepser TB. Propylthiouracil versus methimazole in treatment of Graves' disease during pregnancy. Ann Pharmacother 2007; 41: 1018–22.

Cheron RG, Kaplan MM, Larsen PR et al. Neonatal thyroid function after propylthiouracil therapy for maternal Graves' disease. N Engl J Med 1981; 304: 525–8.

Chopra IJ. Fetal and neonatal hyperthyroidism. Thyroid 1992; 2: 161–3.

Clementi M, Di Gianantonio E, Pelo E, et al. Methimazole embryopathy: delineation of the phenotype. Am J Med Genet 1999; 83: 43–6.

Cooper DS. Antithyroid drugs. N Engl J Med 2005; 352: 905–17.

Coughlin L, Haddad NG. Struma ovarii presenting as hyperemesis gravidarum in pregnancy. J Obstet Gynecol 2000; 20: 310.

Dashe JS, Casey BM, Wells CE, McIntire DD, Byrd EW, Leveno KJ, Cunningham FG. Thyroid stimulating hormone in singleton and twin pregnancy: importance of gestational age-specific reference ranges. Obstet Gynecol 2005; 106: 753–7.

Davies TF, Weiss I. Autoimmune thyroid disease and pregnancy. Am J Report Immunol 1981; 1187–92.

Davis LE, Lucas MJ, Hankins GD et al. Thyrotoxicosis complicating pregnancy. Am J Obstet Gynecol 1989; 160: 63–70.

Di Gianantonio E, Schaefer C, Mastroiacovo PP et al. Adverse effects of prenatal methimazole exposure. Teratology 2001; 64: 262–6.

Diav-Citrin O, Ornoy A. Teratogen update: antithyroid drugs-methimazole, carbimazole, and propylthiouracil. Teratology 2002; 65: 38–44.

Frieden IJ. Aplasia cutis congenita: a clinical review and proposal for classification. Acta Dermatol 1986; 14: 646–60.

Gardner DF, Cruikshank DP, Hays PM et al. Pharmacology of propylthiouracil (PTU) in pregnant hyperthyroid women: Correlation of maternal PTU concentration with cord serum thyroid function tests. J Clin Endocrinol Metab 1986; 62: 217–20

Geva E, Amit A, Lerner-Geva L, Lessing JB. Autoimmunity and reproduction. Fertil Steril 1997; 67: 599–611.

Ginsberg J, Lewanczuk RZ, Honore LH. Hyperplacentosis: a novel cause of hyperthyroidism. Thyroid 2001; 11: 393–6.

Glinoer D. The regulation of thyroid function in pregnancy: pathways of endocrine adaptation from physiology to pathology. Endocr Rev 1997; 18: 404–433.

Glinoer D. Thyroid hyperfunction during pregnancy. Thyroid 1998; 8: 859–64.

Glinoer D, De Nayer P, Bourdoux P et al. Regulation of maternal thyroid during pregnancy. J Clin Endocrinol Metab 1990; 71: 276–287.

Glinoer D, De Nayer P, Robyn C, et al: Serum levels of intact human chorionic gonadotropin (hCG) and its free alpha and beta subunits, in relation to maternal thyroid stimulation during normal pregnancy. J Endocrinol Invest 1993; 16: 881–8.

Gola S, Doga M, Mazziotti G et al. Development of Graves' hyperthyroidism during the early phase of pregnancy in a patient with pre-existing and long-standing Hashimoto's hypothyroidism. J Endocrinol Invest 2006; 29: 288–90.

Goodwin TM, Montoro M, Mestman JH. The role of chorionic gonadotropin in transient hyperthyroidism of hyperemesis gravidarum. J Clin Endocrinol Metab 1992; 75: 1333–7.

Grün JP, Meuris S, De Nayer P, Glinoer D. The thyrotropic role of human chorionic gonadotropin (hCG) in the early stages of twin (versus single) pregnancy. Clin Endocrinol 1997; 46: 719–25.

Guillaume J, Schussler GC, Goldman J. Components of the total serum thyroid hormone concentrations during pregnancy: high free thyroxine and blunted thyrotropin (TSH) response to TSH-releasing hormone in the first trimester. J Clin Endocrinol Metab 1985; 60: 678–84.

Haddow JE, Knight GJ, Palomaki GE et al. The reference range and within-person variability of thyroid stimulating hormone during the first and second trimesters of pregnancy. J Med Screen 2004; 11: 170–4.

Hershman JM. Hyperthyroidism induced by trophoblastic thyrotropin. Mayo Clin Proc 1997; 47: 913–8.

Hollowell JG, Staehling NW, Flanders WD et al. Serum TSH, T_4, and thyroid antibodies in the United States population (1988 to 1994): National Health and Nutrition Examination Survey (NHANES III). J Clin Endocrinol Metab 2002; 87: 489–99.

Iwayama H, Hosono H, Yamamoto H et al. Aplasia cutis congenita with skull defect in a monozygotic twin after exposure to methimazole in utero. Birth Defects Res A Clin Mol Teratol 2007; 79: 680–4.

Johnsson E, Larsson G, Ljunggren M. Severe malformations in infant born to hyperthyroid woman on methimazole. Lancet 1997; 350: 1520.

Jones BM, Kwok JSY, Kung AWC. Changes in cytokine production during pregnancy in patients with Graves' disease. Thyroid 2000; 10: 701–7.

Kahric-Janicic N, Soldin SJ, Soldin OP et al. Tandem mass spectrometry improves the accuracy of free thyroxine measurements during pregnancy. Thyroid 2007; 17: 303–11.

Kaklamanou M, Parkes AB, Taylor IL, Lazarus JH. Evaluation of low TSH in early gestation [abstract]. 77th Annual Meeting of the American Thyroid Association. Phoenix; 2006.

Kamijo K. TSH-receptor antibodies determined by the first, the second and the third generation assays and thyroid-stimulating antibody in pregnant patients with Graves' disease. Endocrine J 2007; 54: 619–24.

Kuczkowski KM. Nonobstetric surgery during pregnancy: what are the risks of anesthesia? Obstet Gynecol Surv. 2004; 59: 52–6.

Kung AWC, Jones BM. A change from stimulatory to blocking antibody activity in Graves' disease during pregnancy. J Clin Endocrinol Metab 1998; 83: 514–8.

Kung AWC, Lau KS, Kohn LD. Epitope mapping of TSH receptor-blocking antibodies in Graves' disease that appear during pregnancy. J Clin Endocrinol Metab 2001; 86: 3647–53.

Kurioka H, Takahashi K, Miyazaki K. Maternal thyroid function during pregnancy and puerperal period. Endocr J 2005; 52: 587–91.

Laurberg P, Nygaard B, Glinoer D et al. Guidelines for TSH-receptor antibody measurements in pregnancy: Results of an evidence-based symposium organized by the European Thyroid Association. Eur J Endocrinol 1998; 139: 584–6.

Lazarus JH, Premawardhana LD. Screening for thyroid disease in pregnancy. J Clin Pathol. 2005; 58: 449–52.

LeBeau SO, Mandel SJ. Thyroid disorders during pregnancy. Endocrinol Metab Clin N Am 2006; 35: 117–36.

Lowe SA. Diagnostic radiography in pregnancy: risks and reality. Aust NZ J Obstet Gynaecol 2004; 44: 191–6.

Luton D, Le Gac I, Vuillard E et al. Management of Graves' disease during pregnancy: the key role of fetal thyroid gland monitoring. J Clin Endocrionol Metab 2005; 90: 6093–8.

Mandel SJ, Brent GA, Larsen PR. Review of antithyroid drug use during pregnancy and report of a case of aplasia cutis. Thyroid 1994; 4: 129–33.

Mandel SJ, Cooper DS. The use of antithyroid drugs in pregnancy and lactation. J Clin Endocrinol Metab 2001; 86: 2354–9.

Mandel SJ, Spencer CA, Hollowell JG. Are detection and treatment of thyroid insufficiency in pregnancy feasible? Thyroid 2005; 15: 44–53.

Marchant B, Brownlie BEW, Hart DM et al. The placental transfer of propylthiouracil, methimazole and carbimazole. J Clin Endocrinol Metab 1977; 45: 1187–93.

Matsuura N, Harada S, Ohyama Y et al. The mechanisms of transient hypothyroxinemia in infants born to mothers with Graves' disease. Ped Res 1997; 42: 214–8.

McKenzie JM, Zakarjia M. Fetal and neonatal hyperthyroidism and hypothyroidism due to maternal TSH receptor antibodies. Thyroid 1992; 2: 155–9.

Mestman JH. Hyperthyroidism in pregnancy. Best Pract Res Clin Endocrinol Metab. 2004; 18: 267–88.

Millar LK, Wing DA, Leung AS, et al. Low birth weight and preeclampsia in pregnancies complicated by hyperthyroidism. Obstet Gynecol 1994; 84: 946–9.

Mitsuda N, Tamaki H, Amino N et al. Risk factors for developmental disorders in infants born to women with Graves' disease. Obstet Gynecol 1992; 80: 359–64.

Momotani N, Hisaoka T, Noh J et al. Effects of iodine on thyroid status of fetus versus mother in treatment of Graves' disease complicated by pregnancy. J Clin Endocrinol Metab 1992; 75: 738–44.

Momotani N, Noh JY, Ishikawa N et al. Effects of propylthiouracil (PTU) and methimazole (MMI) on fetal thyroid status in mothers with Graves' hyperthyroidism. J Clin Endocrinol Metab 1997; 82: 3633–6.

Mortimer R, Cannell GR, Addison R et al. Methimazole and propylthiouracil equally cross the perfused human term placental lobule. J Clin Endocrinol Metab 1997; 82: 3099–102.

Narasimhan KL, Ghobrial MW, Ruby EB. Hyperthyroidism in the setting of gestational trophoblastic disease. Amer J Med Sci 2002; 323: 285–7.

Panesar NS, Li CY, Rogers MS. Reference intervals of thyroid hormones in pregnant Chinese women. Ann Clin Biochem 2001; 38: 329–32.

Pearce EN, Oken E, Gillman MW, Lee SL, Magnani B, Platek D, Braverman LE. Association of first-trimester thyroid function test values with thyreoperoxidase antibody status, smoking, and multivitamin use. Endocr Pract 2008; 14: 33–39.

Pekonen F, Alfthan H, Stenman UH, Ylikorkala O. Human chorionic gonadotropin (hCG) and thyroid function in early pregnancy: Circadian variation and evidence for intrinsic thyrotropic activity of hCG. J Clin Endocrinol Metab 1988; 66: 853–6.

Peleg D, Cada S, Ben-Ami M. The relationship between maternal serum thyroid-stimulating immunoglobulins and fetal and neonatal thyrotoxicosis. Obstet Gynecol 2002; 99: 1040–3.

Phoojaroenchanachai M, Sriussadaporn S, Peerapatdit T et al. Effect of maternal hyperthyroidism during late pregnancy on the risk of neonatal low birth weight. Clin Endocrinol 2001; 54: 365–70.

Polak M, Le Gac I, Vuillard E et al. Fetal and neonatal thyroid function in relation to maternal Graves' disease. Best Pract Res Clin Endocrinol Metab 2004; 18: 289–302.

Radetti G, Persani L, Moroder W et al. Transplacental passage of anti-thyroid auto-antibodies in a pregnant woman with auto-immune thyroid disease. Prenatal Diagnosis 1999; 19: 468–71.

Rapoport B, Chazenbalk GD, Jaume JC, McLachlan SM. The thyrotropin (TSH)-releasing hormone receptor: interaction with TSH and autoantibodies. Endocrine Rev 1998; 19: 673–716.

Redmond GP. Propranolol and fetal growth retardation. Semin Perinatol 1982; 6: 142–7

Rodien P, Brémont C, Raffin Sanson M-L et al. Familial gestational hyperthyroidism caused by a mutant thyrotropin receptor hypersensitive to human chorionic gonadotropin. New Engl J Med 1998; 339: 1823–6.

Rodien P, Jordan N, Lefèvre A, et al. Abnormal stimulation of the thyrotrophin receptor during gestation. Hum Reprod Update 2004; 10: 95–105.

Roti E, Fang SL, Green K et al. Human placenta is an active site of thyroxine and 3, 3′,5-triiodothyronine tyrosyl ring deiodination. J Clin Endocrinol Metab 1981; 53: 498–501.

Roti E, Gardini E, Minelli R et al. Thyroid function evaluation by different commercially available free thyroid hormone measurement kits in term pregnant women and their newborns. J Endocrinol Invest 1991; 14: 1–9.

Sapin R, D'Herbomez M, Schlienger JL. Free thyroxine measured with equilibrium dialysis and nine immunoassays decreases in late pregnancy. Clin Lab 2004; 50: 581–4.

Sheffield JS, Cunningham FG. Thyrotoxicosis and heart failure that complicate pregnancy. Am J Obstet Gynecol 2004; 190: 211–7.

Skellern CG, Knight BI, Otter M. The pharmacokinetics of methimazole in pregnant patients after oral administration of carbimazole. Brit J Clin Pharmacol 1980; 9: 145–7.

Smith C, Thomsett, Choong C et al. Congenital thyrotoxicosis in premature infants. Clin Endocrinol 2001; 54: 371–6.

Smyth PP. Variation in iodine handling during normal pregnancy. Thyroid 1999; 9: 637–42.

Soldin OP. Thyroid function testing in pregnancy and thyroid disease. Trimester-specific reference intervals. Ther Drug Monit 2006; 28: 8–11.

Soldin OP, Tractenberg RE, Hollowell JG et al. Trimester-specific changes in maternal thyroid hormone, thyrotropin, and thyroglobulin concentrations during gestation: trends and associations across trimesters in iodine sufficiency. Thyroid 2004; 14: 1084–90.

Spencer C, Lee R, Kazarosyan M et al. Thyroid reference ranges in pregnancy: studies on a iodine sufficient cohort. Thyroid 2005; 15: 1–16.

Sridama V, Pacini F, Yang SL et al. Decreased levels of helper T cells. Possible cause of immunodeficiency in pregnancy. N Engl J Med 1982; 307: 352–6.

Stricker Rt, Echenard M, Eberhart R, Chevailler MC, Perez V, Quinn FA, Stricker RN. Evaluation of maternal thyroid function during pregnancy: the importance of using gestational age-specific reference intervals. Eur J Endocrinol 2007; 157: 509–514.

Vaidya B, Anthony S, Bilous M, Shields B, Drury J, Hutchison S, Bilous R. Detection of thyroid dysfunction in early pregnancy: Universal screening or targeted high-risk case finding? J Clin Endocrinol Metab 2007; 92: 203–7.

Valdez RM, Barbero PM, Liascovich RC et al. Methimazole embryopathy: a contribution to defining the phenotype. Reprod Toxicol 2007; 23: 253–5.

Van De Velde M, De Buck F. Anesthesia for non-obstetric surgery in the pregnant patient. Minerva Anestesiol 2007; 73: 235–40.

Volumenie JL, Polak M, Guibourdenche J et al. Management of fetal thyroid goitres: a report of 11 cases in a single perinatal unit. Prenatal Diagnosis 2000; 20: 799–806.

Walker JA, Illions EH, Huddleston JF, Smallridge RC. Racial comparisons of thyroid function and autoimmunity during pregnancy and the postpartum period. Obstet Gynecol 2005; 106: 1365–71.

Wang C, Crapo LM. The epidemiology of thyroid disease and implications for screening. Endocrinol Clin N Amer 1997; 26: 189–218.

Weeke J, Dykbjaer L, Granlie K, et al. A longitudinal study of serum TSH, and total and free iodothyronines during normal pregnancy. Acta Endocrinol 1982; 101: 531–7.

Wing DA, Millar LK, Koonings PP et al. A comparison of propylthiouracil versus methimazole in the treatment of hyperthyroidism in pregnancy. Am J Obstet Gynecol 1994; 170: 90–5.

Yamamoto T, Amino N, Tanizawa O et al. Longitudinal study of serum thyroid hormones, chorionic gonadotrophin during and after normal pregnancy. Clin Endocrinol 1979; 10: 459–68.

Yeo CP, Khoo DH, Eng PH et al. Prevalence of gestational thyrotoxicosis in Asian women evaluated in the 8th to 14th weeks of pregnancy: correlations with total and free beta human chorionic gonadotrophin. Clin Endocrinol (Oxf) 2001; 55: 391–8.

Yoshimura M, Hershman JM. Thyrotropic action of human chorionic gonadotropin. Thyroid 1995; 5: 425–34.

Zanzonico PB. Radiation dose to patients and relatives incident to ^{131}I therapy. Thyroid 1997; 7: 199–204.

11 Hypothyroidism in Pregnancy

P. Laurberg*, S. Andersen, J. Karmisholt

Department of Endocrinology and Internal Medicine, Aalborg Hospital, Aarhus University Hospital, 9000 Aalborg, Denmark

Abstract

Thyroid hormones are essential for development, and lack of thyroid hormone for more than short periods during CNS development may lead to irreversible brain damage. Moreover, abnormal levels of thyroid hormones in a pregnant woman may lead to various pregnancy complications. The most severe consequences of hypothyroidism in pregnancy are observed in states of combined maternal and foetal thyroid insufficiency as typically seen in severe iodine deficiency. Thus, large programmes have been undertaken to combat iodine deficiency. Other programmes include screening for congenital hypothyroidism to prevent brain damage caused by isolated foetal/neonatal hypothyroidism. On the other hand, no systematic programmes have been developed to prevent the damage caused by the third main type of thyroid hormone insufficiency during development: isolated maternal hypothyroidism. Detection and care depend on individual health-care providers. Evidence that untreated overt hypothyroidism in pregnancy is associated with adverse pregnancy outcome and foetal damage, and also for the beneficial effects of therapy are quite good but not sufficient for initiating universal screening in early pregnancy. Subclinical hypothyroidism is as usual more difficult, even if a number of association studies may indicate a risk of various complications. The results of intervention studies are awaited. *Current recommendations are:* active case finding in early pregnancy followed by rapid therapy of all types of thyroid insufficiency. Importantly many patients with thyroid insufficiency before pregnancy will need an adjustment of their substitution dose in early pregnancy.

11.1 Introduction

Thyroid hormones are important regulators of growth and development, and many studies have shown the deleterious effect on brain development in rats of even relatively small abnormalities in thyroid function during critical periods (Morreale de Escobar et al., 2004). Similarly, many experimental studies of the brain have illustrated how important thyroid hormones are for normal development (Bernal, 2005). Nerve cell sprouting and thereby generation of neuronal networks is nearly absent without addition of thyroid hormones to Purkinje cell cultures (Kimura-Kuroda et al., 2002) and glial cell development is also impaired (Lima et al., 2001). Part of these abnormalities may be mediated by unliganded thyroid hormone receptor type $\alpha 1$ (Wallis et al., 2008). Apart from such effects, thyroid hormone deficiency has also been shown to be important for the ability of pregnant animals to go through a normal pregnancy, and the number of surviving foetuses is lower in hypothyroid pregnant rats than in control rats (Hendrich et al., 1979).

In man, the most severe consequences of thyroid hormone deficiency on development are seen in areas of the world with severe nutritional iodine deficiency. Severe iodine deficiency leads to a lack of thyroid hormone production both in the maternal and the foetal-neonatal-infant thyroids and it is accompanied by brain damage in the child. Consequently, much effort has been devoted by national and international organisations to eradicate iodine deficiency by public health programmes (WHO, 2007).

The irreversible brain damage caused by even a few months of untreated congenital hypothyroidism is equally well accepted, and the protective effect of early diagnosis and therapy is well known from clinical practice. Accordingly, most countries have now developed public screening programmes to allow early identification and therapy of such cases.

The third area of concern, isolated maternal hypothyroidism in pregnancy, is currently not taken care of by systematic programmes in any country. There are several reasons for this. Obvious cases of cerebral damage in children caused by isolated maternal hypothyroidism in pregnancy are not a classical clinical observation in medicine (as is cretinism caused by severe iodine deficiency or by untreated congenital hypothyroidism). Another major reason is the lack of good intervention studies showing that systematic screening and therapy will benefit patients and society. Other concerns are the lack of consensus on how the common finding of small abnormalities in thyroid function should be handled, the lack of solid data on how early in pregnancy it is necessary to treat and the discussion whether a low serum free T_4 without elevated serum TSH should be treated (Pop and Vulsma, 2005; Casey et al., 2007). Moreover, the recent suggestion that all pregnant women with circulating thyroid antibodies, even those with normal thyroid function tests, might benefit from taking thyroid hormones (Negro et al., 2006) has added to the uncertainty.

As a consequence, current recommendations are to perform active case finding among pregnant women who have a higher than average risk of hypothyroidism. In a recent U.K. study this high-risk group was around 25 % of pregnant women (Vaidya et al., 2007). These women had a more than 6-fold increased risk of some degree of hypothyroidism when screened during early pregnancy. However, testing this group only would miss about one third of women with hypothyroidism. Out of the 1560 women screened, 12 patients in the low-risk group had serum TSH above 4.2 mU/L and 2 had a serum TSH > 10 mU/L. One argument for a general screening is that case-finding in high-risk patients does not work well. In a previous study Vaidya et al. (2002) reported that less than 20 % of the high-risk pregnant women in the district were screened for thyroid dysfunction, and nearly one quarter of hypothyroid women on T_4 replacement in their recent study had raised TSH at their first prenatal visit.

11.2 Current Knowledge on Maternal Hypothyroidism and Pregnancy Outcome

No prospective randomised blinded study on the effect of replacement of overt hypothyroidism has been performed in pregnant women or in other groups of patients. Therapy is based on clinical experience and it is universally accepted. The problem with this is that documentation of the exact effects of overt hypothyroidism on pregnancy outcome is far from perfect.

However, the pathophysiological evidence for an important role of maternal thyroid hormones in development is solid and many observational studies have shown an association between overt hypothyroidism in pregnancy and a number of pregnancy complications. Moreover, these complications have been observed less commonly in women who received adequate replacement to keep thyroid function normal during pregnancy.

A limitation of the retrospective and observational studies of the complications associated with maternal hypothyroidism is that it is difficult to exclude bias. The women who on retrospect turned out to have had undiagnosed hypothyroidism or thyroid insufficiency with insufficient replacement therapy during pregnancy may have represented a subgroup with a more general low compliance and with other risk factors for pregnancy complications.

A number of reviews have dealt with the association between maternal hypothyroidism and adverse pregnancy outcome (Lazarus, 2005; Anonymous, 2006; Casey and Leveno, 2006; Glinoer and Abalovich, 2007; LaFranchi et al., 2005). The types of pregnancy complications encountered in various studies are listed in Table 11.1. In a population-based study, Man et al. (1991) iden-

Table 11.1 Adverse pregnancy outcomes observed with increased frequency in some but not all studies of women with hypothyroidism in pregnancy.

No.	Adverse outcome
1	Spontaneous abortion
2	Placental abruption
3	Pregnancy induced hypertension
4	Foetal death
5	Caesarean section
6	Preterm birth
7	Perinatal mortality

tified around 3% of approximately 1400 pregnant women to be hypothyroid as judged from the diagnostic method available to them (measurement of serum butanol-extractable iodine). Much of their studies were devoted to subsequent evaluation of psychoneurological development of the progeny, but they also reported that one or another type of severe pregnancy complication was around 50% more common in the hypothyroid women.

In a clinic-based study of 16 pregnancies in 14 overtly hypothyroid women, Davis et al. (1988) reported anaemia in 31%, pre-eclampsia in 44%, placental abruption in 19% and postpartum haemorrhage in 19% of the mothers, with a 31% occurrence of low birth weight and 12% foetal death. Similarly, Leung et al. (1993) reported on a group of 23 women with overt and 45 with subclinical hypothyroidism. The dominating abnormality identified was gestational hypertension. On the other hand, Wasserstrum and Anania (1995) reported that the major complication of severe hypothyroidism in early pregnancy was foetal stress in labour leading to Caesarean section. This was independent of thyroid function in late pregnancy.

The most comprehensive population-based study of the association between hypothyroidism and pregnancy complications was performed by Casey et al (2005). They screened 17 298 women who presented for antenatal care at or before 20 weeks of pregnancy. Women who had serum TSH > 3.0 mU/L were prospectively assayed for free thyroxine. If this was below reference, women were referred to another clinic for further evaluation and therapy. A group of women identified with subclinical hypothyroidism (n = 404) (TSH > 2.74 – 5.09 mU/L depending on gestational age; 50 women had TSH > 10 mU/L) was compared with women having serum TSH within the 5 – 95 % percentiles (n = 15 689). The women with subclinical hypothyroidism had a 3-times higher risk of placental abruption (4 cases vs. 1.3 expected; RR: 3.0, CI: 1.1 – 8.2) and also a significantly higher risk of birth at or before gestational week 34 (RR: 1.8, CI 1.1 – 2.9) (but not before week 36 or week 32). There was no difference in the occurrence of maternal hypertension, in Caesarean delivery or in foetal death rate.

Allan et al. (2007) identified 209 women with serum TSH ≥ 6.0 mU/L in the 2nd trimester of pregnancy among 9403 women investigated. The women's physicians were notified when serum TSH was greater than 10 mU/L (n = 37). In the women with TSH > 6.0 mU/L the foetal death rate was significantly higher than in the remaining women (3.8% vs. 0.9%), with an 8.1% death rate in the subgroup with TSH ≥ 10 mU/L. All other complications investigated including gestational hypertension and abruptio placentae were not different between groups. Individual information on the 16 women with the highest TSH (≥ 20 mU/L) revealed that 12 of these had previously diagnosed hypothyroidism, with some suspicion of non-compliance to therapy.

Studies of women treated for hypothyroidism during pregnancy have come from several large clinical databases. Findings have been diverse: slightly higher serum TSH and fT$_4$ at newborn screening + lower birth weight and head circumference (Blazer et al., 2003), more gestational hypertension but no adverse neonatal outcomes (Wolfberg, 2005), lower birth weight and a higher frequency of Caesarean section (Idris et al., 2005), no association with pregnancy complications or perinatal outcomes, but a higher likelihood of Caesarean section (Matalon et al., 2006).

11.3   Maternal Hypothyroidism and Foetal Brain Development

A major concern is foetal brain development. Man et al. (1991) studied developmental, intellectual and motor abilities of 210 children whose mothers had normal serum butanol-extractable iodine, 15 children whose mothers had received sufficient thyroid hormone replacement for low values, and 21 children whose mothers had inadequately treated hypothyroidism. The distinction between adequate and inadequate therapy was based on the administration or not of recommended doses of thyroglobulin (Proloid) for replacement. In the adequately treated women such replacement was begun between gestational weeks 12 and 29. The mothers in the adequately and inadequately treated groups exhibited no significant difference in intelligence, years of education or chronological age. Children were investigated at eight months, four and seven years of age. Children of adequately treated mothers scored similar to controls (and siblings) although some individual abnormalities were observed. On the other hand, children of inadequately treated mothers had lower than expected developmental and intellectual scores. Apparently, at the 7 years investigation this conclusion was based on a comparison of the adequately and inadequately treated groups, and not the inadequately treated vs. the controls. Moreover, the documentation of thyroid status in the two groups of treated women is suboptimal. With these limitations, the results suggest that overt maternal hypothyroidism in the last half of pregnancy leads to impairment of foetal CNS development.

More recently and using more precise biochemical methods for evaluation of thyroid function, Haddow et al. (1999) performed a careful study of the association between elevated maternal serum TSH in the 2nd trimester of pregnancy and the neuropsychological performance of the children at age 7–9 years. Sixty-two cases were matched with 124 controls. In 15 of the 62 mothers hypothyroidism had been diagnosed before pregnancy, and 14 of these received (suboptimal) replacement therapy. The case children performed less well on all tests performed, with statistical significance between groups in two tests. Low test scores were confined to the subgroup of children whose mothers had not received any treatment for hypothyroidism during pregnancy, even if thyroid function tests were similar in treated and untreated hypothyroid mothers at the time of screening. The untreated cases scored an average of 7 IQ points lower than controls, and 19% had IQ score ≤ 85 vs. 5% among the controls.

In subsequent analyses of the data it was shown that the low IQ score in children of untreated mothers correlated significantly to maternal TSH at screening, even after adjustment for social factors (Klein et al., 2001). It was calculated that elevated maternal TSH may be associated with an IQ score > 1 SD below control in 0.09% full term live births (this was 0.01% caused by congenital hypothyroidism before screening) and that these children may constitute 0.6% among the 15% of children with IQ scores > 1 SD below the control mean.

The study suggests that untreated maternal hypothyroidism during pregnancy may dose-dependently lead to impaired intellectual development of the child. On the other hand, treated maternal hypothyroidism, even if treatment is not absolutely perfect, is not associated with such a development.

11.4 Hypothyroidism and Termination of Early Pregnancy

The focus on hypothyroidism and brain development has in some countries led to a concern about the outcome of pregnancies where pregnant women have overt hypothyroidism diagnosed in early pregnancy. Such a concern may lead some women to apt for termination of pregnancy.

For such a discussion it is important to consider that no studies have demonstrated brain damage in children if mothers were properly treated for overt hypothyroidism diagnosed in early pregnancy.

On the contrary, a joint study by Japanese and Chinese investigators (Liu et al., 1994) concluded that overt hypothyroidism diagnosed in early pregnancy (weeks 5–10) and treated with thyroxine to achieve normal TSH levels by 13–28 weeks of gestation was not associated with any measurable IQ deficit. They found normal for age IQ values in 8 children (4–10 years of age) born of mothers treated for hypothyroidism in early pregnancy. Furthermore, IQs in 7 of the children who had siblings were not different from their 9 siblings, who had not been exposed to maternal hypothyroidism.

These data are supported by a study of iodine supplementation in a severely iodine-deficient area of China (Cao et al., 1994). If mothers had received proper iodine supplements during the second half of pregnancy, this was sufficient for protection of the foetal brain.

11.5 Therapy of Hypothyroidism in Pregnancy

The thyroid hormone replacement dose necessary to keep serum TSH normal often increases during pregnancy. Alexander et al. (2004) prospectively observed women treated for hypothyroidism before and during pregnancy. To maintain preconception TSH levels, an increase in $L-T_4$ dose was necessary in 17 out of 20 pregnancies, with a medium onset of increase at 8 weeks of gestation and a mean $L-T_4$ requirement increase of 47%. A need for dose adjustment was observed already in some patients at week 5 of pregnancy, and the required increase depended on residual thyroid function.

Thus, women treated for hypothyroidism and planning pregnancy should optimally receive a dose of $L-T_4$ giving a serum TSH in the lower part of the reference range. The thyroid function should be tested already when pregnancy is diagnosed and subsequently followed regularly.

Several mechanisms probably contribute to the increase in oral $L-T_4$ requirement in early pregnancy. One factor may be the simultaneous intake of mineral supplements leading to a decrease in $L-T_4$ absorption in the gut (Chopra and Baber, 2003), but obviously more mechanisms are involved. The early increase in need of $L-T_4$ shortly after conception is probably caused by T_4 metabolism by type III deiodination in the pregnant uterus (Huang et al. 2003). In accordance with such a mechanism serum rT_3 which is a product of type III T_4 deiodination is very high in the foetal compartment from early pregnancy, and serum rT_3 is also disproportionally high compared with serum T_3 and T_4 in maternal serum in early pregnancy (Weeke et al., 1982).

Later in pregnancy, other factors such as enhanced TBG binding of T_4 and expansion of cellular pools of thyroid hormones may contribute to the higher need of $L-T_4$.

In normal pregnant women the increase in need of thyroid hormone is covered by an increase in thyroid hormone synthesis and thyroid secretion activity, which is reflected by an increase in serum thyroglobulin (Laurberg et al., 2007).

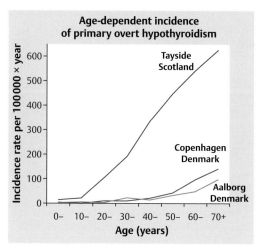

Fig. 11.**1**   Age-specific incidence rates of primary hypothyroidism in Tayside, Scotland, U.K., and in the cities of Copenhagen and Aalborg, Denmark. Overall incidence in Tayside was 3469 new cases during 1 166 216 person-years of follow-up (incidence rate 297 [95 % CI: 288 – 308] per 100 000 per year). In Denmark, the incidence rate was 27 (21 – 32) in Aalborg (96 new cases during 361 811 person-years) and 40 (32 – 48) in Copenhagen (98 new cases during 244 516 person-years). For calculation of age-specific incidence rates, all age groups in both populations were adjusted to a male/female ratio of 1/1. The graphs are based on data published by Bülow Pedersen et al. (2002) and by Flynn et al. (2004).

11.6   Conclusion

Based on experimental animal studies and the available data from studies on humans it is very likely that overt hypothyroidism with low serum fT_4 and high serum TSH in pregnancy may lead to an increase in the occurrence of pregnancy complications and to impairment of cerebral function of the child. Available evidence also indicates that if maternal overt hypothyroidism is diagnosed and treated in early pregnancy the excess risk will be eliminated. Thus, active case finding in early pregnancy is warranted. Even if the evidence is less clear, therapy is also indicated in women with serum TSH above the assay reference range but normal serum free T_4. Results of controlled intervention studies are urgently needed in order to more precisely delineate to whom and how such therapy should be given.

Even if studies of patients receiving suboptimal thyroid hormone substitution give no evidence for brain damage in the child, and results on the association between suboptimal therapy

and pregnancy outcome are not consistent, women with hypothyroidism should have a thyroid function test performed in early pregnancy and the replacement dose adjusted appropriately. Often, it is necessary to increase the replacement dose in early pregnancy to keep serum TSH within target values.

When evaluating the needs and benefits of screening for hypothyroidism in pregnancy it is pertinent to consider that the incidence of overt hypothyroidism may differ considerably between countries. In Scotland overt hypothyroidism seems to be as common in young women of reproductive age as it is in 80-year-old women in Denmark (Laurberg, 2005) (Fig. 11.**1**).

References

Alexander EK, Marqusee E, Lawrence J, Jarolim P, Fischer GA, Larsen PR. Timing and magnitude of increases in levothyroxine requirements during pregnancy in women with hypothyroidism. N Engl J Med 2004; 351: 241–9.

Allan WC, Haddow JE, Palomaki GE, Williams JR, Mitchell ML, Hermos RJ, Faix JD, Klein RZ. Maternal thyroid deficiency and pregnancy complications: implications for population screening. J Med Screen 2000; 7: 127–30.

Anonymous. Hypothyroidism in the pregnant woman. Drug Ther Bull 2006; 44: 53–6.

Bernal J. Thyroid hormones and brain development. Vitam Horm 2005; 71: 95–122.

Blazer S, Moreh-Waterman Y, Miller-Lotan R, Tamir A, Hochberg Z. Maternal hypothyroidism may affect fetal growth and neonatal thyroid function. Obstet Gynecol 2003; 102: 232–41.

Bülow Pedersen I, Knudsen N, Jørgensen T, Perrild H, Ovesen L, Laurberg P. Large differences in incidences of overt hyper- and hypothyroidism associated with a small difference in iodine intake: a prospective comparative register-based population survey. J Clin Endocrinol Metab 2002; 87: 4462–9.

Cao XY, Jiang XM, Dou ZH, Rakeman MA, Zhang ML, O'Donnell K, Ma T, Amette K, DeLong N, DeLong GR. Timing of vulnerability of the brain to iodine deficiency in endemic cretinism. N Engl J Med 1994; 331: 1739–44.

Casey BM, Dashe JS, Spong CY, McIntire DD, Leveno KJ, Cunningham GF. Perinatal significance of isolated maternal hypothyroxinemia identified in the first half of pregnancy. Obstet Gynecol 2007; 109: 1129–35.

Casey BM, Dashe JS, Wells CE, McIntire DD, Byrd W, Leveno KJ, Cunningham FG. Subclinical hypothyroidism and pregnancy outcomes. Obstet Gynecol 2005; 105: 239–45.

Casey BM, Leveno KJ. Thyroid disease in pregnancy. Obstet Gynecol 2006; 108: 1283–92.

Chopra IJ, Baber K. Treatment of primary hypothyroidism during pregnancy: is there an increase in thyroxine dose requirement in pregnancy? Metabolism 2003; 52: 122–8.

Davis LE, Leveno KJ, Cunningham FG. Hypothyroidism complicating pregnancy. Obstet Gynecol 1988; 72: 108–12.

Flynn RW, MacDonald TM, Morris AD, Jung RT, Leese GP. The thyroid epidemiology, audit, and research study: thyroid dysfunction in the general population. J Clin Endocrinol Metab 2004; 89: 3879–84.

Glinoer D, Abalovich M. Unresolved questions in managing hypothyroidism during pregnancy. BMJ 2007; 335: 300–2.

Haddow JE, Palomaki GE, Allan WC, Williams JR, Knight GJ, Gagnon J, O'Heir CE, Mitchell ML, Hermos RJ, Waisbren SE, Faix JD, Klein RZ. Maternal thyroid deficiency during pregnancy and subsequent neuropsychological development of the child. N Engl J Med 1999; 341: 549–55.

Hendrich CE, Porterfield SP, Galton VA. Pituitary-thyroid function of fetuses of hypothyroid and growth hormone treated hypothyroid rats. Horm Metab Res 1979; 11: 362–5.

Huang SA, Dorfman DM, Genest DR, Salvatore D, Larsen PR. Type 3 iodothyronine deiodinase is highly expressed in the human uteroplacental unit and in fetal epithelium. J Clin Endocrinol Metab 2003; 88: 1384–8.

Idris I, Srinivasan R, Simm A, Page RC. Maternal hypothyroidism in early and late gestation: effects on neonatal and obstetric outcome. Clin Endocrinol 2005; 63: 560–5.

Kimura-Kuroda J, Nagata I, Negishi-Kato M, Kuroda Y. Thyroid hormone-dependent development of mouse cerebellar Purkinje cells *in vitro*. Brain Res Dev Brain Res 2002; 137: 55–65.

Klein RZ, Sargent JD, Larsen PR, Waisbren SE, Haddow JE, Mitchell ML. Relation of severity of maternal hypothyroidism to cognitive development of offspring. J Med Screen 2001; 8: 18–20.

LaFranchi SH, Haddow JE, Hollowell JG. Is thyroid inadequacy during gestation a risk factor for adverse pregnancy and developmental outcomes? Thyroid 2005; 15: 60–71.

Laurberg P, Andersen S, Bjarnadóttir RI, Carlé A, Hreidarsson A, Knudsen N, Ovesen L, Pedersen I, Rasmussen L. Evaluating iodine deficiency in pregnant women and young infants – complex physiology with a risk of misinterpretation. Public Health Nutr 2007; 10: 1547–52.

Laurberg P. Global or Gaelic epidemic of hypothyroidism? Lancet 2005; 365: 738–40.

Lazarus JH. Thyroid disease in pregnancy and childhood. Minerva Endocrinol 2005; 30: 71–87.

Leung AS, Millar LK, Koonings PP, Montoro M, Mestman JH. Perinatal outcome in hypothyroid pregnancies. Obstet Gynecol 1993; 81: 349–53.

Lima FR, Gervais A, Colin C, Izembart M, Neto VM, Mallat M. Regulation of microglial development: a novel role for thyroid hormone, J Neurosci 2001; 21: 2028–38

Liu H, Momotani N, Noh JY, Ishikawa N, Takebe K, Ito K. Maternal hypothyroidism during early pregnancy and intellectual development of the progeny. Arch Intern Med 1994; 154: 785–7.

Man EB, Brown JF, Serunian SA. Maternal hypothyroxinemia: psychoneurological deficits of progeny. Ann Clin Lab Sci 1991; 21: 227–39.

Matalon S, Sheiner E, Levy A, Mazor M, Wiznitzer AJ. Relationship of treated maternal hypothyroidism and perinatal outcome. Reprod Med 2006; 51: 59–63.

Morreale de Escobar G, Obregon MJ, Escobar del Rey F. Role of thyroid hormone during early brain development. Eur J Endocrinol 2004; 151 (Suppl 3): 25–37.

Negro R, Formoso G, Mangieri T, Pezzarossa A, Dazzi D, Hassan H. Levothyroxine treatment in euthyroid pregnant women with autoimmune thyroid disease: effects on obstetrical complications. J Clin Endocrinol Metab 2006; 91: 2587–91.

Pop VJ, Vulsma T. Maternal hypothyroxinaemia during (early) gestation. Lancet 2005; 365: 1604–6.

Vaidya B, Anthony S, Bilous M, Shields B, Drury J, Hutchison S, Bilous R. Detection of thyroid dysfunction in early pregnancy: Universal screening or targeted high-risk case finding? J Clin Endocrinol Metab 2007; 92: 203–7.

Vaidya B, Bilous M, Hutchinson RS, Connolly V, Jones S, Kelly WF, Bilous RW. Screening for thyroid disease in pregnancy: an audit. Clin Med 2002; 2: 599–600.

Wallis K, Sjögren M, van Hogerlinden M, Silberberg G, Fisahn A, Nordström K, Larsson L, Westerblad H, Morreale de Escobar G, Shupliakov O, Vennström B. Locomotor deficiencies and aberrant development of subtype-specific GABAergic interneurons caused by an unliganded thyroid hormone receptor alpha1. J Neurosci 2008; 28: 1904–1915.

Wasserstrum N, Anania CA. Perinatal consequences of maternal hypothyroidism in early pregnancy and inadequate replacement. Clin Endocrinol 1995; 42: 353–8.

Weeke J, Dybkjaer L, Granlie K, Eskjaer Jensen S, Kjaerulff E, Laurberg P, Magnusson B. A longitudinal study of serum TSH, and total and free iodothyronines during normal pregnancy. Acta Endocrinol (Copenh) 1982; 101: 531–7.

WHO Secretariat, Andersson M, de Benoist B, Delange F, Zupan J. Prevention and control of iodine deficiency in pregnant and lactating women and in children less than 2-years-old: conclusions and recommendations of the Technical Consultation. Public Health Nutr 2007; 10: 1606–11.

Wolfberg AJ, Lee-Parritz A, Peller AJ, Lieberman ES. Obstetric and neonatal outcomes associated with maternal hypothyroid disease. J Matern Fetal Neonatal Med 2005; 17: 35–8.

12 Thyroid Lumps during Pregnancy – Do they Matter?

B. McIver

Mayo Clinic and Foundation, Rochester, Minnesota 55905, U.S.A.

Thyroid nodules are found frequently during pregnancy, a reflection of the fact that nodular thyroid disease (NTD) is common amongst women of child-bearing years and that pregnancy brings these women into contact with the medical profession. Thyroid gland hyperplasia, as a physiological response to the pregnancy, also may make pre-existing nodules more apparent, by increasing the prominence of the thyroid gland in the neck. Furthermore, some nodules may themselves become larger as a result of the pregnancy-associated TSH-mediated growth stimulus, which may be most prominent under conditions of iodine deficiency.

Clinically and biochemically, most pregnant women with NTD are euthyroid, reflecting the fact that solitary or multiple autonomously functioning thyroid nodules, sufficiently active to cause thyrotoxicosis, are uncommon in this age group. Nevertheless, most nodules identified during pregnancy do prove to be benign, hyperplastic nodules, sometimes arising as a response to early autoimmune thyroid disease. Indeed, the spectrum of NTD diagnosed during pregnancy is almost identical to that of nodules discovered during the non-pregnant state in women of similar age.

The principles of diagnosis and management of thyroid nodules in pregnancy should closely follow those principles already well-defined for NTD in the non-pregnant state, summarised in a variety of guidelines published in recent years by the American Thyroid Association, the American Association of Clinical Endocrinologists, and others. At a minimum, patients with a thyroid nodule should be offered assessment of thyroid functional status by measurement of serum thyrotropin (TSH) concentrations, with appropriate evaluation and management of abnormal results. Ultrasound and ultrasound-guided fine-needle aspiration biopsy (US-FNAB) should follow for euthyroid or hypothyroid patients. Isotopic scans and measurement of thyroid uptake should be avoided during pregnancy and lactation, to minimise exposure to potentially hazardous ionising radiation.

Cytologically, most nodules discovered during pregnancy are benign. Histologically, they represent colloid (adenomatous, hyperplastic) nodules, or a nodular response to autoimmune thyroid disease (nodular Hashimoto's disease). Cytological diagnosis following US-FNAB has a very high degree of accuracy, with false-negative rates well below 5%, though false-positive rates (including the category of "suspicious for follicular neoplasm") as high as 20% may be problematic.

For nodules that show cytological evidence of a benign process, further evaluation during and after pregnancy can be limited to simple clinical assessment to exclude significant, progressive growth. It is rare for such benign nodules to grow sufficiently to cause local compressive symptoms, and even less common for these patients to require surgical exploration during pregnancy. Many hyperplastic nodules stabilise, or even shrink again following pregnancy, though subsequent pregnancies may induce further nodular changes within the gland, and the incidence of NTD requiring therapy in later life is significantly higher in women presenting with a thyroid nodule during pregnancy.

For women in whom US-FNA shows evidence for malignancy, papillary thyroid carcinoma (PTC) is by far the most common histotype, followed distantly by medullary thyroid carcinoma (MTC). Cytology "suspicious for follicular neoplasm" raises concerns about follicular or Hurthle cell carcinoma (FTC or HCC), though – as in the non-pregnant state – the majority of such nodules ultimately prove to be benign adenomas or hypercellular adenomatous nodules. FTC and HCC are relatively uncommon in the age-group of this patient population, although a history of radiation exposure during childhood, or clinically suspicious features may raise higher levels of concern in specific cases.

High resolution ultrasound scanning (US) of the thyroid is entirely safe during pregnancy and can and should be used routinely to assess and to follow NTD. In addition to the assessment of the thyroid itself, the US is useful to assess regional lymph nodes, which are often involved in PTC and MTC. The presence of such regional node involvement strongly argues for a malignant diagnosis and biopsy of such abnormal nodes may provide additional diagnostic information.

Following the discovery of a thyroid malignancy during pregnancy, a careful assessment is required to determine the optimal time for surgery, in relationship to the pregnancy itself. While modern anaesthesia has made surgery feasible and relatively safe at almost any stage of pregnancy, there remains an improved margin of foetal safety by avoiding anaesthesia and surgery during the first and third trimesters. Consequently, surgery for thyroid cancer is generally undertaken either in the second trimester, or after delivery. For nodules that are "suspicious for follicular neoplasm", or PTC that is ultrasonographically localised to the thyroid gland itself, the optimal approach is likely to be one of observation by US through the pregnancy, with surgery timed shortly after delivery. For MTC, for more advanced PTC involving regional lymph nodes, or for those rare cases of thyroid carcinoma with clinical evidence suggesting locally invasive disease, second trimester surgery makes sense for those cases discovered prior to 24 weeks gestation.

For patients with a US-FNAB diagnosis "suspicious for follicular neoplasm", there can be an increase in nodule growth during pregnancy in about 20% of the cases. However, the outcome of pregnant patients diagnosed with differentiated thyroid cancer during pregnancy is identical to that of non-pregnant patients. Nevertheless, nodules that exhibit progressive growth on US during the pregnancy may be deemed worthy of earlier intervention, which can be undertaken safely during the second trimester if necessary. For nodules that do not exhibit significant growth, a delay until the postpartum period is justified, because the risk of malignancy in such nodules is very low and a delay of a few weeks before surgery has negligible impact on prognosis.

Most published series reporting outcomes in pregnant patients with PTC involve patients diagnosed during pregnancy and operated on in the postpartum phase. Although anecdotal reports sometimes suggest rapid growth of malignancy during pregnancy, larger case series suggest that outcomes in these patients are essentially identical to the excellent outcomes seen in PTC in other young patients. Certainly, close monitoring of patient diagnosed with PTC seems appropriate, with early intervention for progressive disease. Patients whose disease follows a more indolent course can safely be monitored until delivery and surgery can be scheduled electively thereafter. Fortunately, there is no need for consideration to be given to termination of pregnancy for management of thyroid carcinoma.

In contrast to PTC, there are few data available on the outcomes of patients diagnosed with MTC during pregnancy, although most practitioners recommend early surgical intervention, preferably during the second trimester. For advanced disease, or disease that shows evidence of progression on US during the pregnancy, consideration should certainly be given to immediate intervention, irrespective of the stage of pregnancy.

The availability of US and US-FNAB have revolutionised our approach to the diagnosis and management of NTD during pregnancy, permitting both accurate diagnosis and careful follow-up. Most cases of NTD can be safely followed through the pregnancy and treated definitively in the postpartum phase. Those few cases that exhibit more aggressive histology, show evidence of advanced disease, or demonstrate rapid growth can safely be managed during the pregnancy. As a consequence, with very few exceptions, the outcomes for women diagnosed with NTD during pregnancy are excellent.

References

Choe W. McDougall IR. Thyroid cancer in pregnant women: diagnostic and therapeutic management. Thyroid 1994; 4: 433 – 5.

Morris PC. Thyroid cancer complicating pregnancy. Obstetr Gynecol Clin N Am 1998; 25: 401 – 5.

Session IV

After Delivery – Mother and Child

Chairperson: F. Péter (Budapest)

13 Postpartum Thyroid Disease

J. H. Lazarus

Centre for Endocrine and Diabetes Sciences, Cardiff University, University Hospital of Wales, Heath Park, Cardiff CF14 4XN, U. K.

Abstract

Thyroid dysfunction occurs commonly postpartum due to the changing immune status from Th2 to Th1. Up to 40% of new onset Graves' hyperthyroidism has been reported to present in the postpartum period. Postpartum thyroiditis (PPT) occurs in 5–9% of women and is almost always associated with positive TPO antibodies as detected at 14 weeks gestation, found in 10% of pregnant women. Fifty percent of these women present with postpartum thyroid dysfunction (PPTD) characterised by hyper-/hypo-/hyper-hypothyroidism and 20–30% of these develop permanent hypothyroidism. Apart from positive TPO antibodies other risk factors include type 1 diabetes mellitus, family history of thyroid or other autoimmunity and goitre. While there is agreement on the fact that there is an immune aetiology of PPT the exact mechanisms are not clear. There is some HLA haplotype restriction. In addition, there is a role for complement activation as well as alterations in the cellular lymphocyte population. The phenomenon of fetal microchimerism has been suggested to play a part but this is not completely confirmed. Treatment of PPT is by levothyroxine for the hypothyroidism. Selenium administration to anti-TPOAb positive women in gestation has been reported to reduce the incidence of PPT, hypothyroidism and TPO antibody positivity postpartum but this intriguing study requires confirmation. Currently, the best predictor of PPT is the presence of TPO antibodies observed in early gestation. With improvements in assay methodology for TPO antibodies together with a reduction in cost of the assay, routine screening for TPO antibodies in early pregnancy should be considered.

13.1 Introduction

In addition to changes in circulating thyroid hormone concentrations observed during gestation (Glinoer, 1997), pronounced alterations in the immune system are evident (Weetman, 1999). The cellular changes consist of a change from a Th1 state to a predominance of cytokines such as IL-4 consistent with a Th2 status (Wegmann et al., 1993). On the humoral side the titre of antithyroid peroxidase antibodies (anti-TPOAb), found in 10% of pregnant women at 14–16 weeks gestation, decreases markedly during the 2nd and 3rd trimesters. At birth the Th2 status abruptly reverts back to the non-pregnant Th1 position and this is accompanied by a dramatic rebound in the titre of anti-TPOAb which reaches a maximum between 3 and 6 months postpartum ('immune rebound phenomenon'). If thyrotropin receptor stimulating antibodies (TSHRAb) are present in early pregnancy they behave in a similar manner through gestation and the postpartum period. These immunological changes at delivery and postpartum (Davies, 1999) set the scene for the

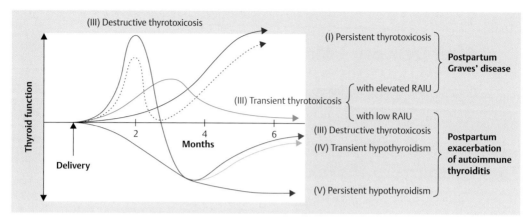

Fig. 13.**1**   Thyroid dysfunction occurring after pregnancy [from Amino et al. (2002)].

development of postpartum thyroid disease. Various types of clinical thyroid dysfunction may arise following delivery (Fig. 13.**1**). The changes in postpartum thyroid dysfunction may be transient or permanent and may be due to destructive or stimulating disease.

13.2   Graves' Disease

Several groups have reported that the incidence of Graves' hyperthyroidism is particularly high following delivery due to the immunological switch referred to above (Jansson et al., 1987; Glinoer, 2005). Up to 40% of Graves' hyperthyroidism in Japanese women of childbearing age were recorded during the postpartum period (Tada et al., 1994). However, the incidence of postpartum Graves' hyperthyroidism is not always as high as this in other countries and a recent Italian study (Chiovato et al., 2008) did not support a role for the postpartum period as a major risk factor for the first occurrence of Graves' disease. The reasons may be related to methods of ascertainment or to variable environmental factors such as ambient iodine concentration.

13.3   Postpartum Thyroiditis

In 1948 H.E.W. Roberton, a general practitioner in New Zealand, described the occurrence of lassitude and other symptoms of hypothyroidism relating to the postpartum period (Robertson, 1948). These complaints were treated successfully with thyroid extract. The syndrome remained generally

unrecognised until the 1970s when reports from Japan (Amino et al., 1976) and Canada (Ginsberg and Walfish. 1977) rediscovered the existence of postpartum thyroiditis (PPT) and recognised the immune nature of the condition (for reviews, see Muller et al., 2001; Lazarus et al., 2002; Stagnaro-Green, 2004; Lazarus and Premawardhana, 2008). Postpartum thyroiditis is essentially sporadic thyroiditis in the postpartum period. The term postpartum thyroiditis relates to destructive thyroiditis occurring during the first twelve months postpartum and not to Graves' disease although the two conditions may be seen concurrently.

13.3.1   Incidence and Risk Factors

Due to wide variations in the number of women studied, the frequency of thyroid assessment postpartum, diagnostic criteria employed and differences in hormone assay methodology a variable incidence (from 3–17%) has been reported worldwide (Table 13.1). The data in this table are also approximate as the calculations have been performed on different proportions of the base population. However, there is a general concensus that the disease occurs in 5–9% of unselected postpartum women and the clinical characteristics of PPT are similar in different areas with different prevalences, e.g., Brazil (Barca et al., 2000), Turkey (Bagis et al., 2001) and Greece (Kita et al., 2002). Risk factors for the development of PPT are outlined in Table 13.**2**. Women with type 1 diabetes have a three-fold incidence of PPT compared to non-diabetics (Gerstein, 1993). PPT is also more likely to occur in a woman who has had a previous episode (Lazarus et al., 1997).

Table 13.**1** Worldwide epidemiology of postpartum thyroiditis [see Lazarus and Premawardhana (2008) for references. Adapted with permission].

Country	Year	Base population	% PPT	First author (year)
Japan	1982	507	5.5	Amino (1982)
Sweden	1984	644	6.5	Jansson (1984)
U.S.A.	1986	216	1.9	Freeman (1986)
Denmark	1987	694	3.9	Lervang (1987)
U.S.A.	1987	238	6.7	Nikolai (1987)
U.S.A.	1988	1034	3.3	Hayslip (1988)
U.S.A.	1988	261	21.1	Vargas(1988)
U.K.	1988	901	16.7	Fung (1988)
Thailand	1990	812	1.1	Rajatanavin (1990)
Denmark	1990	1163	3.3	Rasmussen (1990)
Italy	1991	372	8.7	Roti (1991)
Canada	1992	1376	5.9	Walfish (1992)
U.S.A.	1992	552	8.8	Stagnaro-Green(1992)
U.K.	1992	1248	5.0	Harris (1992)
Netherlands	1993	382	7.2	Pop (1993)
Netherlands	1998	448	5.2	Kuijpens (1998)
Australia	1999	1816	10.3	Kent (1999)
Spain	2000	757	7.5	Lucas (2000)
Brazil	2000	830	14.6	Barca (2000)
Japan	2000	4072	6.5	Sakaihara (2000)
Iran	2001	1040	11.4	Shahbazian (2001)
Turkey	2001	876	5.5	Bagis (2001)
Czech Republic	2002	650	2.8	Hauerova (2002)
India	2002	120	7	Zargar (2002)
Greece	2002	1594	2.4	Kita (2002)
China	2003	119	5.6–23.1	Li (2003)

Table 13.**2** Risk factors for postpartum thyroiditis.

No.	Risk factor
1	Previous episode of PPTD
2	History of AITD (e.g., Hashimoto)
3	Diabetes mellitus type I
4	Recurrent miscarriages
5	Goitre
6	Family history of AITD

13.3.2 Clinical Features

PPT with thyroid dysfunction (i.e., postpartum thyroid dysfunction – PPTD) is characterised by an episode of transient hyperthyroidism followed by transient hypothyroidism. The former presents at about 14 weeks postpartum followed by transient hypothyroidism at a median of 19 weeks. Very occasionally the hypothyroid state is seen before the hyperthyroidism. The thyroid dysfunction that occurs in up to 50% of TPO antibody positive women ascertained around 14 weeks gestation comprises 19% with hyperthyroidism alone, 49% hypothyroidism alone and the remaining 32% hyper- followed by hypothyroidism (i.e., biphasic). Not all women manifest both thyroid states and the hyperthyroid episode may escape detection as it may be of short duration. PPTD is almost always associated with the presence of antithyroid antibodies, usually anti-TPO antibodies which rise in titre after 6 weeks postpartum. In fact the titre of TPO antibodies at 14 weeks gestation correlates with an increasing risk of the development of PPTD. The anti-Tg antibody occurs in about 15% and is the sole antibody in less than 5%. However, postpartum thyroid dysfunction has been described in small numbers of women who have not been shown to have circulating thyroid antibodies (Kuipens et al., 1998). Although the clinical manifestations of the hyperthyroid state are not usually severe, lack of energy and irritability are particularly prominent even in thyroid antibody positive women who do not develop thyroid dysfunction. In contrast, the symptomatology of the hypothyroid phase may be profound. Many classic hypothyroid symptoms occur before the onset of thyroid hormone reduction and persist even when recovery is seen in hormone levels (Lazarus et al., 1996). Postpartum thyroiditis can also occur in women receiving T_4 therapy before pregnancy (Caixas et al., 1999) and after miscarriage (Marqusee et al., 1997). Quantitative evaluation of postpartum depression by the author's group has shown an increase of mild to moderate symptomatology in thyroid antibody positive women even when they remain euthyroid during the postpartum period and this may present as early as 6 weeks postpartum (Harris et al., 1992). However, the association of postpartum depression and postpartum thyroiditis has not been confirmed by others (Kent et al., 1999) perhaps due to differences in population sampling.

Thyrotoxicosis in the postpartum period may be due to a recurrence or the development of new Graves' disease or to the hyperthyroid phase of postpartum thyroiditis. Symptoms of hyperthyroidism are much more evident in Graves' disease.

As postpartum hyperthyroidism is a destructive process radioiodine uptake will be very low at early and late times after isotope administration. TSH receptor antibodies are not seen unless there is coexisting Graves' disease. Hyperthyroidism due to postpartum thyroiditis is diagnosed by a suppressed TSH together with an elevated FT_4 or FT_3, or elevated FT_3 and FT_4, with either set of criteria occurring on more that one occasion. If possible a normal range of thyroid hormone concentrations should be derived in the postpartum period as they fall into a narrower range than the general population. Antibodies to thyroxine and T_3 may cause confusion in diagnosis but they are infrequent. Hypothyroidism in the postpartum period occurs at a median of 19 weeks but has been observed as late as 36 to 40 weeks after birth. The symptoms are often dramatic and may develop before the decrease in thyroid function is noted. The most frequent symptoms have been found to be lack of energy, aches and pains, poor memory, dry skin and cold intolerance.

Hypothyroidism may be defined as either TSH > 3.6 mU/L together with FT4 < 8 pmol/l or FT3 < 4.2 pmol/L or TSH greater than 10 mU/L on one or more occasion. The use of thyroid ultrasonography has demonstrated diffuse or multifocal echogenicity reflecting the abnormal thyroid morphology and consistent with the known lymphocytic infiltration of the thyroid (Adams et al., 1992). The destructive nature of the thyroiditis is also shown by the increase in urinary iodine excretion in the hyperthyroid as well as the hypothyroid phase of the illness (Othman et al., 1992). In addition there is evidence that an early rise in serum thyroglobulin (a further indicator of thyroid destruction) may help in the identification of those women at risk of PPT (Parkes et al., 1994) although it is also elevated in Graves' disease. Interestingly, neither IL-6 (Ahmad et al., 1998) nor high sensitivity C-reactive protein (Pearce et al., 2003) are helpful in the diagnosis of the condition.

13.3.3   Aetiology of Postpartum Thyroiditis

There have been many immunogenetic studies of the HLA haplotype restriction in PPT (Lazarus and Premawardhana, 2008). A higher incidence of HLA-A26, -BW46 and -BW67 with significantly lower frequencies of HLA-BW62 and -CW7 in women with postpartum hypothyroidism was noted (Tachi et al., 1988; Kologlu et al., 1990) as well as an increased incidence of HLA-A1 and -B8 (Kologlu et al., 1990). Increased frequencies of HLA-DR3, DR4 and DR5 have been reported in patients with PPT (Lazarus and Premawardhana, 2008). This variation may reflect ethnic differences as well as variations in sample number and methodology. Interestingly a negative association between PPT and DR2 together with the increased frequency of DR3 was observed. The frequency of HLA-DQ7 is also raised in PPT probably due to the increase in DR5 since both DR11 and DR12 are in linkage disequilibrium with DQ7.

Some studies suggest that the incidence of PPT may be related to iodine deficiency (Li et al., 2003) and subsequent iodine supplementation (Shahbazian et al., 2001). Iodide administration can aggravate the disease (Kämpe et al., 1990) but most studies show no effect of iodine intake or administration on the incidence (Othman et al., 1992; Reinhardt et al., 1998; Zargar et al., 2002; Triggiani et al., 2004). A randomised placebo-controlled double blind trial in Denmark (Nøhr et al., 2000) confirmed that iodine supplementation in gestation does not change the incidence in a moderate iodine-deficient population.The overall conclusion is that while some data suggest moderate alterations in incidence related to iodine status, the majority of studies do not show any effect of administered iodine or ambient iodine concentration. This is important in underpinning the strategy of iodine supplementation in pregnancy to benefit the foetus.

From the immunological point of view there is abundant immunogenetic evidence as well as data from humoral and cellular studies that postpartum thyroiditis is an immunologically related disease (Muller et al., 2001). Biopsy of the thyroid in this syndrome shows lymphocytic infiltration similar to that seen in Hashimoto's thyroiditis (Mizukami et al., 1993). Amino et al. (1976) first documented the association of postpartum thyroiditis with high titres of antithyroid antibodies and the dramatic rise of antimicrosomal antibody titre after delivery was confirmed in a large series (Fung et al., 1988). There is also a rise in postpartum thyroglobulin antibody titre in women who have been found to be TgAb positive in early pregnancy. TgAb is less prevalent than TPOAb in PPT, being present in only around 15% of the cases; however, it has been noted to be the only antibody present in 2% of the patients. Furthermore, gestation and the postpartum period are characterised by fluctuations in the immune response and the postpartum increase appears to be a reflection of a general enhancement of immunoglobulin synthesis. This pattern of transient antibody increase in microsomal antibody levels was observed also for serum total IgG and IgG subclass levels but not other immunoglobulins (Lazarus and Premawardhana, 2008). Although the antibody response is dramatic its precise role in the immunopathogenesis of the condition remains to be determined. Probably, the antibody titre is merely a marker of disease and the immunological damage is mediated by lymphocyte and complement-associated mechanisms.

Complement has been shown to be involved in the pathogenesis of autoimmune thyroid disease by the demonstration of terminal complement complexes (TCC) around thyroid follicles in such patients (Weetman et al., 1989). However, despite the presence of circulating bioactive TPOAbs, the extent of complement activation is inadequate to cause detectable increases in peripheral blood TCC, suggesting that the complement system is not the only factor in the pathogenesis of PPT (Okosleme et al., 2002). Nevertheless, there is activation of the complement system by thyroid directed autoantibodies (Parkes et al., 1994), and complement activation is related to the extent of the thyroiditis (Pakes et al., 1996) and correlates with the severity of the thyroid dysfunction (Parkes et al., 1995).

During pregnancy maternal immune reactions are regulated to prevent rejection of the foetal allograft such that the cytokine profile is a T helper 2 (Th2) pattern which switches back to the Th1 state postpartum (Wegmann et al., 1993; Davies, 1999).

Early postpartum (within three months) changes in T cell subsets have been described similar to those seen in Hashimoto's disease (Muller et al., 2001). The peripheral T lymphocyte subset ratio CD4/CD8 is higher in TPO antibody positive women who developed postpartum thyroid dysfunction compared to similar antibody positive women who did not (Stagnaro-Green et al., 1992). Peripheral circulating lymphocyte populations during and after pregnancy show generalised activation of immune activity at 36 weeks gestation in TPO antibody positive women who develop postpartum thyroid dysfunction, compared to those who do not; furthermore the former group had lower plasma cortisol concentrations pre-delivery (Kokandi et al., 2003). Thus there may be less immunological suppression at 36 weeks in TPOAb-positive women destined to develop PPTD possibly due to lower levels of cortisol at this time. The immunological determinants of PPTD may in part occur antenatally although the mechanism(s) for this is (are) still unclear. Another mechanism for postpartum immune stimulation may be that of foetal microchimerism (defined as the presence of foetal cells in maternal tissues during and after pregnancy) as a potential immunomodulatory factor in the development of postpartum thyroiditis (Badenhoop, 2004). It is suggested that the loss of placental immune suppression postpartum may allow activation of intrathyroidal foetal immune cells. Subsequent immune stimulation would initiate or exacerbate autoimmune thyroid disease including postpartum thyroiditis.

13.4 Management of PPT

13.4.1 Prevention

The evidence that cigarette smoking is a contributory factor in the development of PPT is mixed. Early studies (Fung et al., 1988) did not find an association but a large Swedish epidemiological study concluded that smoking may increase the risk of thyroiditis occurring in the postpartum period (Galanti et al., 2007). These data require confirmation from other studies but it is clearly beneficial for women to stop smoking during pregnancy and the prevention of PPT in a susceptible person is another reason to do so. Further prevention may be possible by the administration of selenium during gestation. In a prospective randomised placebo-controlled study Negro et al. (2007) showed that the incidence of both PPT and permanent hypothyroidism were significantly lower in a group of TPOAb-positive women receiving selenomethionine during pregnancy than control TPOAb-positive women (Fig. 13.2). Interestingly, the titre of TPO antibodies was also reduced in line with known effects of selenium (Gärtner et al., 2002).

13.4.2 Treatment

The hyperthyroid phase is relatively asymptomatic and usually requires no specific therapy. If symptoms of tachycardia and palpitations are troublesome or if other symptoms of hyperthyroidism such as sweating or anxiety are present then beta-adrenoreceptor blocking agents may be used. Propanolol is the drug of choice but if nightmares develop a more cardioselective β-blocker may be used. If this class of drug is contraindicated verapamil may be effective for cardiac symptoms. Antithyroid drugs are not indicated as the condition is a destructive thyroiditis. In contrast, patients may experience persistent and troublesome symptoms related to the hypothyroid period and treatment with levothyroxine should be given starting with 0.1 mg per day and increasing as necessary. At this stage it will not be clear whether the patient has developed transient or permanent hypothyroidism. In this instance levothyroxine should be given for one year and

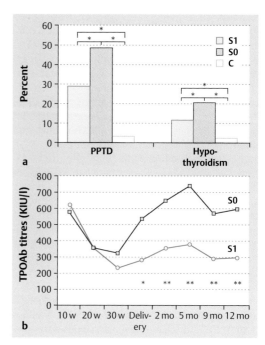

Fig. 13.2 Effect of selenium or placebo administration to TPOAb-positive women in pregnancy on the incidence of **a** PPT and **b** positive thyroid antibodies (from Negro et al., 2007).

the patient then reviewed to determine the thyroxine requirement by stopping therapy for 4–6 weeks prior to a thyroid function test. Patients who have been known to have transient thyroid dysfunction postpartum should be checked at least annually as 50% of them will develop hypothyroidism after 7 years. This is in contrast to TPOAb-positive women who have not experienced any thyroid dysfunction postpartum whose rate of hypothyroidism at 7 years follow-up is only 5% (Premawardhana et al., 2000). Clearly these patients require less intensive surveillance. While the hyperthyroidism of PPT always persistence of hypothyroidism occurs in 20–30% of cases (Lazarus and Premawardhana, 2008). Recurrence of transient PPT has been observed in up to 70% in subsequent pregnancies.

13.5 Conclusion

Postpartum thyroid disease, namely Graves' hyperthyroidism and the various clinical presentations of postpartum thyroiditis are common clinical events in the postpartum period. Postpartum thyroiditis represents a unique experiment of nature where the development of an autoimmune syndrome may be observed during a relatively short time period. Moreover, in many cases the immune perturbations resolve and the patient remains euthyroid. While there have been advances in our understanding of the humoral and cellular immune changes during and after pregnancy, the complete immunopathological picture is not yet available. We need to know more about the immunogenetics as well as appreciating the effects of pregnancy hormones on the immune response during gestation. The phenomenon of microchimerism has been mentioned but more understanding of this process in regard to PPT is required. These studies may be difficult in patients and normal pregnant women because of ethical considerations but the opportunity should be taken to perform further studies on appropriate animal models.

In view of the high incidence of clinical postpartum thyroiditis together with the accompanying medical and psychiatric symptomatology, it would seem logical that an appropriate screening programme should exist. The presence of thyroid antibodies in early pregnancy at least alerts the clinician to the possibility of the condition even if their presence is only a 50% predictor of thyroid dysfunction at best. Further clinical features are required to improve the predictive power of TPO-antibodies in this setting. For example, the measurement of serum thyroglobulin and biological active TPO-antibody may improve the prediction of thyroid dysfunction, perhaps to 75–80%.

References

Adams H, Jones MC, Othman S et al. The sonographic appearances in postpartum thyroiditis. Clin Radiol 1992; 45: 311–8.

Ahmad L, Parkes A, Lazarus JH et al. Interleukin-6 levels are not increased in women with postpartum thyroid dysfunction. Thyroid 1998; 8: 371–5.

Amino N, Miyai KJ, Onishi T et al. Transient hypothyroidism after delivery in autoimmune thyroiditis. J Clin Endocinol Metab 1976; 42: 296–301.

Amino N, Tada H, Hadaka Y. Thyroid disease after pregnancy: postpartum thyroiditis. In: Oxford Textbook of Endocrinology and Diabetes. Wass JAH and Shalet SM, eds. Oxford: Oxford University Press, 2002: 527–32.

Badenhoop K. Intrathyroidal michrochimerism in Graves' disease or Hashimoto's thyroiditis: regulation of tolerance or alloimmunity by fetal-maternal immune interactions? Eur J Endocrinol 2004; 150: 421–3.

Bagis T, Gokeel A, Saygili ES. Autoimmune thyroid disease in pregnancy and the postpartum period: relationship to spontaneous abortion. Thyroid 2001; 11: 1049–53.

Barca MF, Knobel M, Romimori E, Cardia MS, Medeiros-Neto G. Prevalence and characteristis of postpartum thyroid dysfunction in Sao Paulo, Brazil. Clin Endocrinol (Oxf) 2000; 53: 21–31.

Caixas A, Albareda M, Garcia-Patterson A et al. Postpartum thyroiditis in women with hypothyroidism antedating pregnancy. J Clin Endoc Metab 1999; 84: 4000–5.

Chiovato L, Rotondi M, Pirali B et al. The postpartum period and the onset of Graves', disease: an overestimated risk factor Eur J Endoc 2008; in press.

Davies TF. The thyroid immunology of the postpartum period. Thyroid 1999; 9: 675–84.

Fung HY, Kologlu M, Collinson K et al Postpartum thyroid dysfunction in Mid Glamorgan. Br Med J 1988; 296: 241–4.

Galanti HR,Cnattingius S,Granath F et al. Smoking and environmental iodine as risk factors for thyroiditis among parous women. Eur J Epidemiol 2007; 22: 467–72.

Gärtner R, Gasnier BC, Dietrich JW, Krebs B, Angstwurm MW. Selenium supplementation in patients with autoimmune thyroiditis decreases thyroid peroxidase antibodies concentrations. J Clin Endocr Metab. 2002; 87: 1687–91.

Gerstein HC. Incidence of postpartum thyroid dysfunction in patients with type 1 diabetes mellitus. Ann Intern Med 1993; 118: 419–23.

Ginsberg J, Walfish PG. Postpartum transient thyrotoxicosis with painless thyroiditis. Lancet 1977; 1: 1125–8.

Glinoer D. Thyroid disease during pregnancy. In: Werner and Ingbar's The Thyroid, 9th ed., Braverman LE, Utiger RD, eds. Philadelphia: Lippincott Williams and Wilkins 2005: 1086–108.

Glinoer D. The regulation of thyroid function in pregnancy: pathways of endocrine adaptation from physiology to pathology. Endocr Rev 1997; 18: 404–33.

Harris B, Othman S, Davies J et al. Association between postpartum thyroid dysfunction and thyroid antibodies and depression. Br Med J 1992; 305: 152–6.

Jansson R, Dahlberg PA, Winsa B et al. The postpartum period constitutes an important risk for the development of clinical Graves' disease in young women. Acta Endocrinologica 1987; 116: 321–5.

Kämpe O, Jansson R, Karlsson FA. Effects of L-thyroxine and iodide on the development of autoimmune postpartum thyroiditis. J Clin Endoc Metab 1990; 70: 1014–8.

Kent GN, Stuckey BG, Allen JR et al. Postpartum thyroid dysfunction: clinical assessment and relationship to psychiatric affective morbidity. Clin Endocrinol (Oxf) 1999; 51: 429–38.

Kita M, Goulis DG, Avramides A. Post-partum thyroiditis in a Mediterranean population: a prospective study of a large cohort of thyroid antibody positive women at the time of delivery. J Endocrinol Invest 2002; 25: 513–9.

Kokandi AA, Parkes AB, Premawardhana LDKE et al. Association of postpartum thyroid dysfunction with antepartum hormonal and immunological changes. J Clin Endocr Metab 2003; 88; 1126–32.

Kologlu M, Fung H, Darke C et al. Postpartum thyroid dysfunction and HLA status. Eur J Clin Invest 1990; 20: 56–60.

Kuijpens JL, De Hann-Meulman M, Vader HL, Pop VJ, Wiersinga WM, Drexhage HA. Cell-mediated immunity and postpartum thyroid dysfunction: a possibility for the prediction of disease? J Clin Endoc Metab1998; 83: 1959–66.

Lazarus JH, Ammari F, Oretti R, Parkes AB, Richards CJ, Harris B. Clinical aspects of recurrent postpartum thyroiditis. Br J Gen Pract 1997; 47: 305–8.

Lazarus JH, Hall R, Othman S et al. The clinical spectrum of postpartum thyroid disease. Quart J Med 1996; 89: 429–35.

Lazarus JH, Premawardhana LDKE, Parkes AB. Postpartum thyroiditis. Autoimmunity 2002; 35: 169–73.

Lazarus JH, Premawardhana LDKE. Postpartum Thyroiditis. In: Contemporary Endocrinology: Autoimmune Diseases in Endocrinology. AP Weetman (ed), Humana Press Inc. New Jersey, USA, 2008: 177–92.

Li D, Li CY, Teng WP. Prevalence of postpartum thyroiditis in three different iodine intake areas. Zhonghua Fu Chan Ke Za Zhi 2003; 38: 216–8.

Marqusee E, Hill JA, Mandel SJ. Thyroiditis after pregnancy loss. J Clin Endoc Metab 1997; 82: 2455–7.

Mizukami Y, Michigishi T, Nonomura A et al Postpartum thyroiditis – a clinical, histological and immunologic study of 15 cases. Am J Clin Pathol 1993; 100: 200–5.

Muller AF, Drexhage HA, Berghout A. Postpartum thyroiditis and autoimmune thyroiditis in women of childbearing age: recent insights and consequences for antenatal and postnatal care. Endocr Rev 2001; 22: 605–30.

Negro R, Greco G, Mangieri T et al. The influence of selenium supplementation on postpartum thyroid status in pregnant women with thyroid peroxidase antibodies. J Clin Endocr Metab 2007; 92: 1263–8.

Nøhr SB, Jørgensen A, Pedersen KM, Laurberg P. Postpartum thyroid dysfunction in pregnant thyroid peroxidase antibody-positive women living in an area with mild to moderate iodine deficiency: is iodine supplementation safe? J Clin Endocr Metab. 2000; 85: 3191–8.

Okosieme OE, Parkes AB, McCullough B et al. Complement activation in postpartum thyroiditis. Quart J Med 2002; 95: 173–9.

Othman S, Phillips DIW, Lazarus JH et al. Iodine metabolism in postpartum thyroiditis. Thyroid 1992; 2: 107–11.

Parkes AB, Adams H, Othman S. The role of complement in the pathogenesis of postpartum thyroiditis. Ultrasound echogenicity and the degree of complement induced thyroid damage. Thyroid 1996; 6: 177–82.

Parkes AB, Black EG, Adams H et al. Serum thyroglobulin – an early indicator of autoimmune postpartum thyroiditis. Clin Endocrinol 1994; 41: 9–14

Parkes AB, Othman S, Hall R. The role of complement in the pathogenesis of postpartum thyroiditis: relationship between complement activation and disease presentation and progression. Eur J Endocrinol 1995; 133: 210–5.

Parkes AB, Othman S, Hall R et al. The role of complement in the pathogenesis of postpartum thyroiditis. J Clin Endocr Metab 1994; 79: 53–6

Pearce EN, Bogazzi F, Martino E et al. The prevalence of elevated serum C-reactive protein levels in inflammatory and noninflammatory thyroid disease. Thyroid 2003; 13: 643–8.

Premawardhana LDKE, Parkes AB, Ammari F et al. Postpartum thyroiditis and long-term thyroid status: prognostic influence of thyroid peroxidase antibodies and ultrasound echogenicity. J Clin Endocr Metab 2000; 85: 71–5.

Reinhardt W, Kohl S, Hollmann D et al. Efficacy and safety of iodine in the postpartum period in an area of mild iodine deficiency. Eur J Med Res 1998; 83: 203–10.

Roberton HEW. Lassitude, coldness, and hair changes following pregnancy, and their response to treatment with thyroid extract. Br Med J 1948; 2: 93–4.

Shahbazian HB, Sarvghadi F, Azizi F. Prevalence and characteristics of postpartum thyroid dysfunction in Tehran. Eur J Endocrinol 2001; 145: 397–401.

Stagnaro-Green A. Postpartum thyroiditis. Best Pract Res Clin Endocrinol Metab 2004; 18: 303–16.

Stagnaro-Green A, Roman SH, Cobin RH et al. A Prospective study of lymphocyte-initiated immunosuppression in normal pregnancy: Evidence of a T-cell etiology for postpartum thyroid dysfunction. J Clin Endocr Metab 1992; 74: 645–53

Tachi J, Amino N, Tamaki H et al. Long term follow-up and HLA association in patients with postpartum hypothyroidism. J Clin Endoc Metab 1988; 66: 480–4.

Tada H, Hidaka Y, Tsuruta E et al. Prevalence of post-partum onset of disease within patients with Graves' disease of child-bearing age. Endocr J 1994; 41: 325 – 7

Triggiani V, Ciampolillo A, Guastamacchia E, Licchelli B. Prospective study of post-partum thyroid immune dysfunctions in type 1 diabetic women and in a healthy control group living in a mild iodine deficient area. Immunopharmacol Immunotoxicol 2004; 26: 215 – 24.

Weetman AP. The immunology of pregnancy. Thyroid 1999; 9: 643 – 6.

Weetman AP, Cohen SB, Oleesky DA, Morgan BP. Terminal complement complexes and C1/C1 inhibitor complexes in autoimmune thyroid disease Clin Exp Immunol 1989; 77: 25 – 30.

Wegmann TG, Lin H, Guilbert L, Mosmann TR. Bidirectional cytokine interactions in the maternal-fetal relationship: Is successful pregnancy a Th2 phenomenon? Immunology Today 1993; 14: 353 – 6.

Zargar AH, Shah IH, Masoodi SR, Laway BA et al. Postpartum thyroiditis in India: prevalence of postpartum thyroiditis in Kashmir Valley of Indian subcontinent. Exp Clin Endocrinol Diabetes 2002; 110: 171 – 5.

14 Genetics of Congenital Hypothyroidism

A. M. Macchia, P. E. Ferrara

Dipartimento di Endocrinologia ed Oncologia Molecolare e Clinica,
Università degli Studi di Napoli Federico II, Via S. Pansini, 5 80131 Napoli Italy

Abstract

Primary congenital hypothyroidism (CH) is the most frequent endocrine metabolic disease in infancy, with an incidence of about 1/3000 live births. With the exception of the rare cases of central hypothyroidism, CH is characterised by the presence of elevated TSH levels in response to reduced thyroid hormone production. In 15% of cases, the disease is caused by inborn errors in the mechanisms required for thyroid hormone synthesis and are indicated with the term of dyshormonogenesis. In the remaining 85%, CH is due to alterations occurring during the gland organogenesis, which result in a thyroid gland that is absent (thyroid agenesis or athyreosis), severely reduced in size (thyroid hypoplasia) or located in an unusual position (thyroid ectopy). All these entities are grouped under the term "thyroid dysgenesis" (TD). Thyroid dyshormonogenesis shows the classical Mendelian recessive inheritance and very frequently leads to enlargement of the gland (goitre), presumably as a consequence of the elevated TSH levels. Among the genes causing dyshormonogenesis, initially the role of the thyroid peroxidase and thyroglobulin genes were described. More recently, also other genes have been demonstrated to be involved, including pendrin (*PDS*, in Pendred syndrome), the sodium iodide symporter (*NIS*), and *THOX2* (thyroid oxidase 2) gene. TD occurs mostly as a sporadic disease. However a genetic cause of the disease has been demonstrated in about 5% of the studied cases. Genes associated with TD include several thyroid transcription factors expressed in the early phases of thyroid organogenesis (*NKX2.1/TITF1, FOXE1/TITF2, PAX8, NKX2.5*) as well as genes, like the thyrotropin receptor gene (*TSHR*) expressed in the late phases of the gland morphogenesis. The more recent aspects of the genetics of congenital hypothyroidism will be reviewed, providing inputs for the discussion.

14.1 Introduction

Congenital hypothyroidism (CH) is the most frequent endocrine-metabolic disease in infancy, with an incidence of about 1/3–4000 newborns (Toublanc, 1992; Klett, 1997). With the exception of rare cases due to hypothalamic or pituitary defects, CH is characterised by elevated TSH in response to reduced thyroid hormone levels.

In the majority of the cases (80–85%), primary permanent CH is due to alterations occurring during the gland's organogenesis, which result in a thyroid that is absent (thyroid agenesis or athyreosis), hypoplastic (thyroid hypoplasia) or located in an unusual position (thyroid ectopy). All these entities are grouped under the term "thyroid dysgenesis" (TD) (Fisher and Klein, 1981). In about 15% of the cases the disease is caused by inborn errors in the molecular steps required for the biosynthesis of thyroid hormones, and often it is associated with an enlargement of the gland (goitre), presumably as a consequence of the elevated TSH levels (Madeiros-Neto and Starbury, 1994). Finally, congenital hypothyroidism of central origin is rare; it is caused by hypothalamic or pituitary diseases, with a reduced efficiency of thyrotropin-releasing hormone (TRH) or of thyrotropin (TSH) (Grüters et al., 2004).

CH is essentially a sporadic disease, however, dyshormonogenetic defects are often inherited as a recessive character, while TD shows a familial occurrence in a small but significant proportion of cases (Castanet et al., 2001). TD presents a clear female prevalence (Castanet et al., 2001; Lorey and Cunningham, 1992) and epidemiological studies demonstrated a different incidence of the disease in different ethnic groups (Lorey and Cunningham, 1992; Knobel and Medieros-Neto, 2003) suggesting that the genetic background plays a role in this affection. Also in favour of genetic factors involved in the pathogenesis of TD is the finding that, among the first degree relatives

Table 14.**1** Developmental steps of thyroid morphogenesis.

Embryonic day		Stage of morphogenesis	Morphology	Differentiation markers			Controller genes
Mouse	Human			Tg, TPO, Tshr	NIS	Throid hormones	Titf1/Nkx2-1, Foxe1, Pax8, Hhex
			Undifferentiated endoderm	–	–	–	–
E8–8,5	E20–22	Thyroid anlage appears	Thyroid anlage	–	–	–	+
E9.5	E24	Thyroid bud migration begins	Thyroid bud	–	–	–	+
E11.5–13.5	E30–40	Thyroglossal duct disappears		–	–	–	+
E13.5	E45–50	Thyroid migration is complete	Expansion of thyroid primordium	–	–	–	+
E14.5–15	E60	Fusion with ultimobranchial bodies	Definitive bilobated shape	+	–	–	+
E16	E70	Onset of folliculogenesis	Folliculogenesis	+	+	–	+
E16.5	E75	Beginning of hormone synthesis	Completion of organogenesis	+	+	+	+
			Undifferentiated endoderm	–	–	–	–

of patients with sporadic CH with TD, there is a significantly higher rate of asymptomatic thyroid developmental anomalies compared to the normal populations (Leger et al., 2002). Against the notion of heritable TD is the finding that, in 12 of 13 monozygotic twin pairs, there is discordance for TD (Perry et al., 2002), suggesting that post-zygotic events must be evoked in the pathogenesis of many cases of TD.

14.2 Thyroid Dysgenesis

In about 85% of the cases, permanent congenital hypothyroidism is caused by an alteration in the morphogenesis of the thyroid (Fisher and Klein, 1981).

Most of the critical events in thyroid organogenesis take place in the first 60 days of gestation in man or the first 15 days in mice (Table 14.1). For this reason, most thyroid developmental abnormalities result from morphogenetic errors during this period. Mutations in the genes involved in thyroid development give rise to animal models with thyroid dysgenesis (De Felice and Di Lauro, 2007), and mutations in the same genes have been identified also in a small number of patients with congenital hypothyroidism associated with TD (Table 14.**2**).

Table 14.**2** Pathogenesis of thyroid dysgenesis as consequence of mutations in the genes described in the text.

Stage of thyroid organogenesis	Expected phenotype	Genetic lesions in human diseases	Genetic lesions in mouse models
Specification of thyroid anlage	Agenesis	Unknown	Unknown
Survival of precursor cells	Athyreosis	FOXE1 mutations, NKX2-5 mutations	Foxe1 knock-out, Titf1/Nkx2-1 knock-out, Pax8 knock-out, Hhex knock-out
Migration	Ectopic thyroid	NKX2-5 mutations	Foxe1 knock-out
Expansion of cell population	Hypoplasia	PAX8 mutations, TITF1/NKX2-1 mutations, TSHRr mutations, TSH induced genes	Tshr knock-out, Tshr$^{hyt/hyt}$ mouse, Tshr$^{dw/dw}$ mouse
Specification of thyroid anlage	Agenesis	Unknown	Unknown

14.3 Athyreosis

The absence of thyroid follicular cells in orthotopic or ectopic location is called athyreosis or agenesis of the gland. More precisely, the term agenesis should be used to define the absence of the gland due to a defective initiation of thyroid morphogenesis, while athyreosis indicates a dysgenesis characterised by the disappearance of the thyroid due to alterations in any step following the specification of the thyroid anlage. So far, the absence of thyroid was reported in patients with CH associated with FOXE1 defects (Clifton-Bligh et al., 1998; Castanet et al., 2002), in one subject carrying a mutation in PAX8 (Macchia et al., 1998) and in one patient with NKX2–5 mutation (Dentice et al., 2006).

14.3.1 FOXE1 and Its Mutations

Foxe1 (formerly called TTF-2 for thyroid transcription factor-2) is a transcription factor containing a forkhead domain. The gene encoding for this transcription factor is named Foxe1 in mice and FOXE1 in humans, and the human gene maps to chromosome 9q22 (Macchia et al., 1999), and encodes for a 42 kDa protein that is phosphorylated and contains an alanine stretch of variable length (Macchia et al., 1999; Hishinuma et al., 2001; Carre et al., 2007; Santarpia et al., 2007).

Foxe1$^{-/-}$ mice are born at the expected Mendelian ratio but die within 48 hours after birth. These mice display a severe cleft palate (probably responsible for the perinatal death), absence or ectopy of the thyroid, and hypothyroidism (De Felice et al., 1998). At E8.5, the mice show normal budding of the thyroid anlage, but at E9.5 the thyroid precursor cells are unable to migrate downward, suggesting that – during embryonic life – Foxe1 has a specific role in controlling the migration of thyroid follicular cell precursors.

Bamforth-Lazarus syndrome (Bamforth et al., 1989) is a clinical entity characterised by cleft palate, bilateral choanal atresia, spiky hair and athyreosis. Two homozygous mutations in FOXE1 gene have been described in two pairs of siblings affected by this syndrome (Clifton-Bligh et al., 1998; Castanet et al., 2002) and in one patient with syndromic congenital hypothyroidism but not athyreosis (Baris et al., 2006). All the affected members carry homozygous missense mutations in conserved amino acids within the Foxe1 forkhead domain. The mutant proteins were tested *in vitro* and have shown a reduction in both DNA binding and transcriptional activity.

By contrast to what is observed in mice, ectopic thyroid associated with FOXE1 mutations has not yet been described in humans.

14.4 Ectopic Thyroid

During embryonic life, the developing thyroid migrates, leaving behind the foramen caecum. The ectopic thyroid is the consequence of a failure in the descent of the developing thyroid from the thyroid anlage region to its definitive location in front of the trachea, and an ectopic thyroid can be found in any location along the path of migration from the foramen caecum to the mediastinum.

Gene targeting experiments have demonstrated that Foxe1 is required for thyroid migration and that mice homozygous for *Foxe1* mutations show a sublingual thyroid.

In humans more than 50% of TD cases are associated with an ectopic thyroid; however, up to now, only three heterozygous mutations in the *NKX2–5* gene have been associated to the human ectopic thyroid (Dentice et al., 2006).

14.4.1 NKX2–5 and Its Mutations

Nkx2–5 is another member of the *Nkx2* family, present in the thyroid anlage at early developmental stages. The thyroid bud appears smaller in *Nkx2-5$^{-/-}$* embryos when compared to the WT, suggesting that *Nkx2–5* is required during thyroid development (Dentice et al., 2006).

NKX2–5 is essential for normal heart morphogenesis, myogenesis, and function (Tanaka et al., 2001), and several loss of function mutations in *NKX2–5* have been described in patients with congenital heart diseases (Schott et al., 1998; Hirayama-Yamada et al., 2005). Recently we have identified three mutations in four subjects with TD (three patients with thyroid ectopy and one with athyreosis) (Dentice et al., 2006). Functional studies have demonstrated that these mutants exhibited a significant functional impairment, with reduction of transactivation properties and dominant negative effect. The patients were all heterozygous and the mutations were inherited from one of the parents. These data suggested that *NKX2–5* is a novel gene involved in the pathogenesis of congenital hypothyroidism with ectopy or athyreosis of the thyroid gland, and *NKX2–5* mutations have a variable penetrance and clinical significance.

14.5 Hypoplasia

The presence of hypoplastic thyroid has been reported in about 5% of cases of TD. This can be the consequence of a defect in any of the genes involved in both the early (*TITF1, FOXE1, PAX8*) as well as the late steps of development (*TSHR*). Thyroid hypoplasia is probably a genetically heterogeneous dysgenesis; indeed, mutations in *TITF1,*

PAX8 or *TSHR* gene have been reported in patients with thyroid hypoplasia.

14.5.1 NKX2–1/TITF1 and Its Mutations

NKX2–1/TITF1 (TTF-1 for thyroid transcription factor-1, or T/EBP) is a homeodomain transcription factor. The human gene, named *TITF1*, maps to chromosome 14q13 and is formed by 3 exons.

Knock-out *Titf1* homozygous mice die at birth and are characterised by impaired lung morphogenesis, lack of thyroid and pituitary and severe alterations in the ventral region of the forebrain (Kimura et al., 1996). Analyses during development demonstrate that the thyroid anlage forms in its correct position but at an early stage the morphogenesis of the gland is impaired, suggesting that *Titf1* is required for the survival and subsequent differentiation of the follicular cells. Detailed functional studies revealed a decreased coordination and mild hyperthyrotropinemia in *Titf1/Nkx2-1$^{+/-}$* mice (Pohlenz et al., 2002; Moeller et al., 2003).

Patients with *NKX2–1/TITF1* loss-of-function mutations are affected by choreoathetosis, hypothyroidism, and pulmonary alterations with incomplete penetrance and the variability of the phenotype (De Felice and Di Lauro, 2004). So far, twenty mutations in the *NKX2–1* gene have been identified in patients with this clinical picture (reviewed in Provenzano et al., 2008). When tested *in vitro*, all the mutated forms of *Titf1/Nkx2–1* show neither functional activity nor a dominant negative effect on the wild-type form, suggesting that the haploinsufficiency is responsible for the pathological phenotype.

14.5.2 PAX8 and its Mutations

Pax8 (paired box gene 8) is a member of a family of transcription factors characterised by the presence of the paired domain (Prd). The gene encoding Pax8 (called *Pax8* in mice and *PAX8* in humans) is located on chromosome 2 in both humans and mice (Plachov et al., 1990; Stapleton et al., 1993).

Pax8 null mice are born at expected frequencies but show growth retardation, and die within 2–3 weeks unless treated with thyroid hormone (Mansouri et al., 1998). In Pax8 null embryos the thyroid anlage forms, evaginates from the endoderm and migrates into the mesenchyme. However, by E11 the thyroid bud is smaller compared to wild type, and at E12.5 thyroid follicular cell are not detectable (Mansouri et al., 1998). Thus, during morphogenesis Pax8 is required for the survival of the thyroid precursor cells and to maintain the tissue-specific gene expression program.

The involvement of *PAX8* has been described in sporadic and familial cases of CH with TD (Macchia et al., 1998; Vilain et al., 2001; Congdon et al., 2001; Komatsu et al., 2001; de Sanctis et al., 2004; Al Taji et al., 2007). An *in vitro* transfection assay demonstrated that the mutated proteins are unable to bind DNA and drive transcription of the *TPO* promoter. All affected individuals are heterozygous for the mutations and in the familial cases transmission is autosomal dominant with a variable penetrance and expressivity. In humans, both *PAX8* alleles are necessary for correct thyroid morphogenesis and a reduced dosage of the gene product (haploinsufficiency) causes dysgenesis; in contrast, the *Pax8+/−* mice display a normal phenotype (Mansouri et al., 1998).

Of note, in mice the combination of partial deficiencies in the *Titf1* and *Pax8* genes results in a small thyroid gland, elevated TSH, reduced thyroglobulin biosynthesis, and high occurrence of hemiagenesis (Amendola et al., 2005). The observed phenotype is strain specific, and the pattern of transmission indicates that at least two other genes, in addition to *Titf1* and *Pax8*, are necessary to generate the condition. These results show that TD can be of multigenic origin in mice and strongly suggest that a similar pathogenic mechanism may also be observed in humans.

14.5.3   TSH Receptor (*TSHR*) and Its Mutations

In late stages of thyroid organogenesis, the binding of TSH to its receptor (TSHR) triggers a signalling pathway that regulates many functions of the adult thyroid but also during thyroid organogenesis.

The TSHR is a member of the family of G protein-coupled receptors and is expressed in thyroid follicular cells and in few other tissues. Expression of TSHR is detected in the developing thyroid after the final migration of the precursor cells, when final functional differentiation of the gland starts (Lazzaro et al., 1991).

The role of *TSHR* gene in TSH unresponsiveness associated with CH and no goitre was hypothesised almost forty years ago, but only the identification of *Tshr^{hyt/hyt}* mice, affected by a primary hypothyroidism with elevated TSH and hypoplastic thyroid, as consequence of a loss-of-function mutation in the *Tshr* gene (Beamer et al., 1981; Stuart et al., 1994) and the production of *Tshr−/−* mice (Marians et al., 2002) offered a useful model for this autosomal recessive form of CH.

In patients the first mutations were identified in three siblings (Sunthornthepvarakui et al., 1995) characterised by high TSH and normal thyroid hormone levels in the serum. The siblings were compound heterozygous, carrying a different mutation in each of the two alleles. After this report other mutations in the *TSHR* gene have been identified in several patients with thyroid hypoplasia and increased TSH secretion. Among the molecular defects causing TD, mutations in the *TSHR* gene represent the most frequent finding. Athyreosis or ectopic thyroid has never been found in patients carrying TSHR mutations, confirming that the TSHR-induced pathway is not involved in the early stages of thyroid development. All the affected individuals are homozygous or compound heterozygous for loss-of-function mutations, and consistently, in the familial forms, the disease is inherited as an autosomal recessive trait.

14.6   Hemiagenesis

Thyroid hemiagenesis is a dysgenesis in which one thyroid lobe fails to develop. The prevalence of this morphological abnormality ranges from 0.05% to 0.2% in healthy children, with the absence of the left lobe in almost all the cases (Maiorana et al., 2003). Thyroid function tests are within the normal range in subjects with thyroid hemiagenesis (Maiorana et al., 2003).

The molecular mechanisms leading to the formation of the two thyroid symmetrical lobes are still unclear. Indeed, *Shh−/−* mice embryos can display either a non-lobulated gland (Alt et al., 2006) or hemiagenesis of the thyroid (Fagman et al., 2004). Hemiagenesis of the thyroid is also a frequent observation in mice double heterozygous for *Titf1+/−*, *Pax8+/−* (Amendola et al., 2005). However, in humans, candidate genes responsible for the hemiagenesis of the thyroid have not yet been described.

Table 14.**3**   Genes known to be responsible for dyshormonogenetic congenital hypothyroidism.

Gene	Chromosomal localisation	No. of exons	Protein function	Inheritance	Human phenotype
Sodium iodide symporter (*NIS*)	19p13 – p12	15	Transports iodide across the membrane of the follicular thyroid cell	AR	From moderate to severe CH; sometimes euthyroid goitre
Thyroperoxidase (*TPO*)	2p25	16	Catalyses the oxidation, organification, and coupling reactions	AR	Goitre and CH due to a total iodide organification defect
Dual oxidases (*DUOX1* and *DUOX2*)	15q15.3	34/34	H_2O_2 generation in the follicle	AD and AR	Permanent hypothyroidism (from mild to severe); transient and moderate hypothyroidism
Pendrin (*PDS*)	7q31	21	Transport of iodide across apical membrane into the follicular lumen	AR	"*Pendred syndrome*": goitre, moderate hypothyroidism and deafness
Thyroglobulin (*TG*)	8q24	42	Support for thyroid hormone synthesis	AD and AR	Goiter and CH (from moderate to severe)
Iodotyrosine deiodinase (*DEHAL1*)	6q25.1	6	Nitroreductase-related enzyme capable of deiodinating iodotyrosines	AR	Hypothyroidism with variable age of diagnosis

14.7   Dyshormonogenesis

In about 15% of cases, CH is due to hormonogenesis defects caused by mutations in thyroid hormone synthesis, secretion or recycling. These cases are clinically characterised by the presence of goitre, and the molecular mechanisms in most of these forms have been characterised (Madeiros-Neto and Stanbury, 1994).

In the follicular thyroid cells, iodide is actively transported and concentrated by the sodium iodide symporter present in the baso-lateral membrane. Subsequently it is oxidised by the hydrogen peroxide generation system (thyroperoxidase, pendrin) and bound to tyrosine residues in thyroglobulin to form iodothyrosine (iodide organification). Some of these iodotyrosine residues (monoiodotyrosine and diiodotyrosine) are coupled to form the hormonally active iodothyronines, T_4 and T_3, and, when needed, thyroglobulin

is hydrolysed and hormones are released in the blood. There is also a small part of the iodotyronines that is hydrolysed, and the iodine is recovered by the action of specific enzymes, the intrathyroidal dehalogenases.

Defects in any of these steps lead to dyshormonogenesis, which manifests as congenital hypothyroidism and goitre. Except in rare cases, all mutations in these genes appear to be inherited in an autosomal recessive fashion (Table 14.**3**).

14.7.1   Sodium Iodide Symporter

The sodium iodide symporter (NIS) is a member of the sodium/solute symporter family that actively transports iodide across the membrane of the thyroid follicular cells. The human gene (*SLC5A5*) maps to chromosome 19p13.2-p12. It has 15 exons and encodes a 643-amino acid protein expressed primarily in the thyroid, but also in the breast, colon, and ovary. The inability of the thyroid gland to accumulate iodine was one of the early known causes of CH and, before the cloning of NIS, a clinical diagnosis of hereditary iodide transport defect had been made for several decades on the basis of goitrous hypothyroidism and absent thyroidal radioiodine uptake. To date, several mutations inherited in an autosomal recessive manner have been described, with a clinical picture characterised by hypothyroidism of variable severity (from severe to fully compensated) and goitre not always present (Dohan et al., 2003; Park and Chatterjee, 2005).

14.7.2   Thyroperoxidase

The most frequent cause of dyshormonogenesis is thyroperoxidase (TPO) deficiency. TPO is the enzyme that catalyses the oxidation, organification, and coupling reactions. The human TPO gene is located on chromosome 2p25 and spans approximately 150 kb and encodes for a 933-amino acid, membrane-bound, glycated, haem-containing protein, located on the apical membranes of the thyroid follicular cell. Defects in the TPO gene have been reported to cause congenital hypothyroidism by a total iodide organification defect, and mutations have been identified in the all exons of the TPO gene (Madeiros-Neto and Stanbury, 1994; Park and Chatterjee, 2005; LaFrancji, 1999).

If untreated, patients with organification defects presented variable degrees of mental retardation, very large goitre and hypothyroidism. In some cases hypothyroidism was compensated, mostly in patients with partial defects.

14.7.3   DUOX1 and DUOX2

Recently two new proteins involved in the H_2O_2 generation of the apical membrane of the follicular thyroid cell have been identified (De Deken et al., 2000). These proteins, initially named THOX1 and THOX2 (for thyroid oxidase), map on chromosome 15q15.3, only 16 kb apart from each other and in opposite transcriptional orientations. In 2001, since these proteins contain two distinct functional domains, it has been suggested that their names be changed into DUOX (dual oxidase).

DUOX1 and DUOX2 are glycoproteins with seven putative transmembrane domains. Their function remained unclear until Grasberger and Refetoff identified a factor, named DUOXA2 (Gorbman, 1986), which allows the transition of

DUOX2 from the endoplasmic reticulum to the Golgi. The coexpression of this factor with DUOX2 in HeLa cells is able to reconstitute the H_2O_2 production *in vitro*. A similar protein (DUOXA1) is necessary for the complete maturation of the DUOX1, and, of note, both DUOXA genes map in the 16 kb that separates the *DUOX1* and *DUOX2* genes on chromosome 15.

Several mutations have been reported in patients with congenital hypothyroidism with a very variable phenotype (Moreno and Visser, 2007; Ohye et al., 2008). In fact, it seems that, in order to produce congenital permanent hypothyroidism, a severe alteration of both alleles of *DUOX2* gene is required. The presence of some residual activity in one of the alleles may produce a less severe phenotype, whereas monoallelic severe inactivation of the *DUOX2* gene is associated with transient congenital hypothyroidism. In addition, the phenotype of monoallelic inactivation seems to be modulated by other factors, including environmental conditions (such as iodine insufficiency) or lifetime events (pregnancy, immediate postnatal life).

So far, no mutation in the *DUOX1* gene has been identified in patients with CH, suggesting that a putative DUOX1 phenotype may rather be related to a defect in defense against infections.

In contrast, very recently a biallelic inactivation in the dual oxidase maturation factor 2 (*DUOXA2*) gene was identified in a patient with congenital hypothyroidism, indicating also this gene as a potential candidate for CH (Zamproni et al., 2008).

14.7.4   Pendrin

In 1896, Vaughan Pendred described a syndrome characterised by congenital neurosensorial deafness and goitre due to a mild organification defect. The disease is transmitted as an autosomal recessive disorder. Patients have a moderately enlarged thyroid gland, are usually euthyroid and show only a partial discharge of iodide after the administration of thiocyanate or perchlorate. The impaired hearing is not constant, and is due to a cochlear defect that corresponds to the Mondini's type of developmental abnormality of the cochlea.

In 1997, the *PDS* gene was cloned and the predicted protein of 780 amino acids (86 kDa) was called pendrin. The *PDS* gene maps to human chromosome 7 q, contains 21 exons, and it is expressed in the cochlea and in the thyroid. Pendrin has been localised to the apical membrane of thyroid follicular cells, but its function is still not clear. It has been hypothesised that pendrin transports iodide across the apical membrane of the thyrocyte into the colloid space.

A number of mutations in the *PDS* gene have been described in patients with Pendred syndrome. Despite the goitre, individuals are likely to be euthyroid and only rarely present congenital hypothyroidism. However, TSH levels are often in the upper limit of the normal range, and hypothyroidism of variable severity may eventually develop (Glaser, 2003).

14.7.5 Thyroglobulin

Thyroglobulin is a homodimer protein synthesised exclusively in the thyroid. The human gene is located on chromosome 8q24 and the coding sequence is divided into 42 exons. Thyroglobulin defects are associated with congenital hypothyroidism from moderate to severe degrees, and usually serum thyroglobulin concentrations are low. Several mutations in the thyroglobulin gene were reported in patients with CH and also in animals including Afrikander cattle (p. R697X), Dutch goats (p. Y296X), cog/cog mouse (p. L2263P) and rdw rats (p. G2300R) (Rivolta and Targovnik, 2006).

14.7.6 DEHAL1

Iodine in the follicular thyroid cells, in addition to the active transport from the blood due to the NIS activity, derives also from the deiodination of monoiodotyrosine and diiodotyrosine (Roche et al., 1952). The gene encoding this enzymatic activity was recently identified (Moreno et al., 2001) and named DEHAL1. The human gene maps to chromosome 6q25.1 and it consists in six exons encoding a protein of 293 amino acids with a nitroreductase-related enzyme capable of deiodinating iodotyrosines.

In the past it was suggested that DEHAL1 mutations could be responsible for congenital hypothyroidism, but only very recently four patients with three mutations in the *DEHAL1* gene have been reported (Moreno et al., 2008). The disease was transmitted as an autosomal recessive character, and the patients presented hypothyroidism with a high phenotypic variability with regard to the time of expression of the disease. Goitre and hypothyroidism were present in all patients with different ages of onset. The two patients born af-

ter the introduction of the screening programme for congenital hypothyroidism were not identified by the screening. There is also a variable severity of the clinical picture, and this can derive from the molecular effects of the mutation (complete absence or partial activity of the protein), but also from environmental factors, such as iodine.

The prevalence of iodotyrosine deiodinase defects among persons with hereditary hypothyroidism is currently unknown, and it is possible to speculate that borderline expression during the neonatal period and a possible masking of this defect as a non-autoimmune goitre might lead to underdiagnosis of the *DEHAL1* defect (61).

Also the DEHAL1 mutations should be considered as a possible cause for congenital hypothyroidism and goitre, and, of note, they may be unidentified by the screening programme, producing severe consequences in these patients.

14.8 Central Hypothyroidism

Central hypothyroidism is the less frequent form of CH. It has been estimated to occur with an incidence of 1 in 50 000 newborn, and it is generally associated to an alteration in the hypothalamus or pituitary development. Several defects of the hypothalamic-pituitary axis can be responsible for central hypothyroidism.

14.8.1 TRH and TRH Receptors

In mice, homozygous deletion of the TRH produced a phenotype characterised by hypothyroidism and hyperglycaemia (Yamada et al., 1997). Only few cases of patients with reduced TRH have been described in the literature (Niimi et al., 1982; Katakami et al., 1984).

Similarly, mice lacking the TRH receptor appear almost normal, with some growth retardation, and a considerable decrease in serum T_3, T_4, and prolactin (PRL) levels but not in serum TSH (Rabeler et al., 2004). So far only one family with a compound heterozygous loss of function mutation of TRH receptor has been described (Collu et al., 1997).

14.8.2 TSH

Mutations in the TSH beta gene are a rare cause of congenital hypothyroidism, and in all the reported cases, the mutations were homozygous or compound heterozygous. Available data have been recently reviewed by Miyai. The phenotype is very variable and it may range from a very mild hypothyroidism to severe forms associated to mental retardation in cases of delayed treatment. Patients with a mutation in the TSH-beta are characterised by the presence of low levels of circulating TSH that will not be stimulated by TSH. In addition, also cases of an immunologically reactive but biologically inactive TSH have been reported (Miyai, 2007).

14.8.3   Developmental Defects of the Pituitary

Congenital hypothyroidism can also be the consequence of combined defects in the development of the pituitary gland.

These rare forms are characterised by multiple hormone deficiencies, however, the clinical manifestations can be variable in terms of hormonal involvements, severity and time course of manifestations. Potentially, these forms can be caused by genetic alterations in several genes, including *PIT1, PROP1, HESX1, LHX3, LHX4* and *SOX3* (Grüters et al., 2004; Miyai, 2007).

14.9   Conclusions

Starting from 1974, a screening programme for CH was initiated in almost every country in the Western world permitting the identification and early treatment of the majority of cases of CH. This allowed the possible transmission of the disease, because of the reduced likelihood of the untreated CH patients to have progeny. Despite an early treatment, to date CH still seems a sporadic disease, and familial occurrence is rare. A clear Mendelian recessive inheritance is present in the majority of forms of dyshormonogenesis, although several lines of evidence indicate that TD can also be a genetic and inheritable condition, mutations in genes important in the morphogenesis of the thyroid have been reported only in few patients. Such a low frequency of mutations in TD can be an underestimate because the molecular analyses to search for mutations in the studied genes have been limited to the coding region of these genes. Therefore, alterations in regulatory non-coding regions may also lead to a disease phenotype. In addition, it should be considered that TTIF1, FOXE1, PAX8 and NKX2-5 are transcription factors able to modulate target downstream genes that ultimately activate the organogenesis of the thyroid. Some cases of TD could be due to mutations in the as yet unidentified gene targets for these transcription factors. Similarly, genes upstream of these transcription factors and genes important in the initial specification of thyroid bud have not been identified, and alterations in these genes can potentially be involved in the pathogenesis of TD. In addition, as suggested from the discordance for TD in monozygotic twins, it is possible that epigenetic mechanisms might be involved at early stages of morphogenesis, causing somatic mutations in every gene mentioned above and being responsible for TD. Finally, as suggested from a recent report (Amendola et al., 2005), at least in some cases, TD could be a multigenic condition. The phenotypic variability observed in patients affected by heterozygous mutations in either *PAX8, TITF1* or *NKX2-5* genes strongly suggests that other unidentified modifier genes are involved in the diseases.

Despite such difficulties, we believe that TD can be considered a genetic disease, and the mutational screening is now starting to be applied to large population of patients with CH. The first results of mutational screening on blood spots recently appeared in the literature (Camilot et al., 2007) with the identification of three heterozygous mutations in the TSHR gene and an unknown heterozygous substitution in PAX8 which could interfere with the start of transcription.

References

Al Taji E, Biebermann H, Limanova Z, Hnikova O, Zikmund J, Dame C et al. Screening for mutations in transcription factors in a Czech cohort of 170 patients with congenital and early-onset hypothyroidism: identification of a novel PAX8 mutation in dominantly inherited early-onset non-autoimmune hypothyroidism. Eur J Endocrinol 2007; 156: 521–9.

Alt B, Elsalini OA, Schrumpf P, Haufs N, Lawson ND, Schwabe GC et al. Arteries define the position of the thyroid gland during its developmental relocalisation. Development 2006; 133: 3797–804.

Amendola E, De Luca P, Macchia PE, Terracciano D, Rosica A, Chiappetta G et al. A mouse model demonstrates a multigenic origin of congenital hypothyroidism. Endocrinology 2005; 146: 5038–47.

Bamforth JS, Hughes IA, Lazarus JH, Weaver CM, Harper P. Congenital hypothyroidism, spiky hair, and cleft palate. J Med Genet 1989; 26: 49–60.

Baris I, Arisoy AE, Smith A, Agostini M, Mitchell CS, Park SM et al. A novel missense mutation in human TTF-2 (FKHL15) gene associated with congenital hypothyroidism but not athyreosis. J Clin Endocrinol Metab 2006; 91: 4183 – 7.

Beamer WJ, Eicher EM, Maltais LJ, Southard JL. Inherited primary hypothyroidism in mice. Science 1981; 212: 61 – 3.

Camilot M, Teofoli F, Vincenzi M, Federici F, Perlini S, Tato L. Implementation of a congenital hypothyroidism newborn screening procedure with mutation detection on genomic DNA extracted from blood spots: the experience of the Italian northeastern reference center. Genet Test 2007; 11: 387 – 90.

Carre A, Castanet M, Sura-Trueba S, Szinnai G, Van Vliet G, Trochet D et al. Polymorphic length of FOXE1 alanine stretch: evidence for genetic susceptibility to thyroid dysgenesis. Hum Genet 2007; 122: 467 – 76.

Castanet M, Park SM, Smith A, Bost M, Leger J, Lyonnet S et al. A novel loss-of-function mutation in TTF-2 is associated with congenital hypothyroidism, thyroid agenesis and cleft palate. Hum Mol Genet 2002; 11: 2051 – 9.

Castanet M, Polak M, Bonaiti-Pellie C, Lyonnet S, Czernichow P, Leger J. Nineteen years of national screening for congenital hypothyroidism: familial cases with thyroid dysgenesis suggest the involvement of genetic factors. J Clin Endocrinol Metab 2001; 86: 2009 – 14.

Clifton-Bligh RJ, Wentworth JM, Heinz P, Crisp MS, John R LJ, Ludgate M et al. Mutation of the gene encoding human TTF-2 associated with thyroid agenesis, cleft palate and choanal atresia. Nat Genet 1998; 19: 399 – 401.

Collu R, Tang J, Castagne J, Lagace G, Masson N, Huot C et al. A novel mechanism for isolated central hypothyroidism: inactivating mutations in the thyrotropin-releasing hormone receptor gene. J Clin Endocrinol Metab 1997; 82: 1561 – 5.

Congdon T, Nguyen LQ, Nogueira CR, Habiby RL, Medeiros-Neto G, Kopp P. A novel mutation (Q40P) in PAX8 associated with congenital hypothyroidism and thyroid hypoplasia: evidence for phenotypic variability in mother and child. J Clin Endocrinol Metab 2001; 86: 3962 – 7.

De Deken X, Wang D, Many M, Costagliola S, Libert F, Vassart G et al. Cloning of two human thyroid cDNAs encoding new members of the NADPH oxidase family. J Biol Chem 2000; 275: 23227 – 33.

De Felice M, Di Lauro R. Murine models for the study of thyroid gland development. Endocr Dev 2007; 10: 1 – 14.

De Felice M, Di Lauro R. Thyroid development and its disorders: genetics and molecular mechanisms. Endocr Rev 2004; 25: 722 – 46.

De Felice M, Ovitt C, Biffali E, Rodriguez-Mallon A, Arra C, Anastassiadis K et al. A mouse model for hereditary thyroid dysgenesis and cleft palate. Nat Genet 1998; 19: 395 – 8.

de Sanctis L, Corrias A, Romagnolo D, DI Palma T, Biava A, Borgarello G et al. Familial PAX8 small deletion (c.989_992delACCC) associated with extreme phenotype variability. Clin Endocrinol Metab 2004; 89: 5669 – 74.

Dentice M, Cordeddu V, Rosica A, Ferrara AM, Santarpia L, Salvatore D et al. Missense mutation in the transcription factor NKX2 – 5: a novel molecular event in the pathogenesis of thyroid dysgenesis. J Clin Endocrinol Metab 2006; 91: 1428 – 33.

Dohan O, De la Vieja A, Paroder V, Riedel C, Artani M, Reed M et al. The sodium/iodide symporter (NIS): characterization, regulation, and medical significance. Endocr Rev 2003; 24: 48 – 77.

Esperante SA, Rivolta CM, Miravalle L, Herzovich V, Iorcansky S, Baralle M et al. Identification and characterization of four PAX8 rare sequence variants (p. T225 M, p. L233 L, p. G336S and p. A439A) in patients with congenital hypothyroidism and dysgenetic thyroid glands. Clin Endocrinol (Oxf) 2008; 68: 828 – 35.

Fagman H, Grande M, Gritli-Linde A, Nilsson M. Genetic deletion of sonic hedgehog causes hemiagenesis and ectopic development of the thyroid in mouse. Am J Pathol 2004; 164: 1865 – 72.

Fisher DA, Klein A. Thyroid development and disorders of thyroid function in the newborn. New Engl J Med 1981; 304: 702 – 12.

Glaser B. Pendred syndrome. Pediatr Endocrinol Rev 2003; 1 (Suppl 2): 199 – 204.

Gorbman A. Comparative anatomy and physiology. In: Ingbar SI, Braverman LE, eds. The Thyroid. Philadelphia; 1986: 43 – 52.

Grüters A, Krude H, Biebermann H. Molecular genetic defects in congenital hypothyroidism. Eur J Endocrinol 2004; 151 (Suppl 3): 39 – 44.

Hirayama-Yamada K, Kamisago M, Akimoto K, Aotsuka H, Nakamura Y, Tomita H et al. Phenotypes with GATA4 or NKX2.5 mutations in familial atrial septal defect. Am J Med Genet A 2005; 135: 47 – 52.

Hishinuma A, Ohyama Y, Kuribayashi T, Nagakubo N, Namatame T, Shibayama K et al. Polymorphism of the polyalanine tract of thyroid transcription factor-2 gene in patients with thyroid dysgenesis. Eur J Endocrinol 2001; 145: 385 – 9.

Katakami H, Kato Y, Inada M, Imura H. Hypothalamic hypothyroidism due to isolated thyrotropin-releasing hormone (TRH) deficiency. J Endocrinol Invest 1984; 7: 231 – 3.

Kimura S, Hara Y, Pineau T, Fernandez-Salguero P, Fox C, Ward J et al. The T/ebp null mouse: thyroid-specific enhancer-binding protein is essential for the organogenesis of the thyroid, lung, ventral forebrain, and pituitary. Genes Dev 1996; 10: 60 – 9.

Klett M. Epidemiology of congenital hypothyroidism. Exp Clin Endocrinol Diabetes 1997; 105: 19–23.

Knobel M, Medeiros-Neto G. An outline of inherited disorders of the thyroid hormone generating system. Thyroid 2003; 13: 771–801.

Komatsu M, Takahashi T, Takahashi I, Nakamura M, Takahashi I, Takada G. Thyroid dysgenesis caused by PAX8 mutation: the hypermutability with CpG dinucleotides at codon 31. J Pediatr 2001; 139: 597–9.

LaFranchi S. Congenital hypothyroidism: etiologies, diagnosis, and management. Thyroid 1999; 9: 735–40.

Lazzaro D, Price M, De Felice M, Di Lauro R. The transcription factor TTF-1 is expressed at the onset of thyroid and lung morphogenesis and in restricted regions of the foetal brain. Development 1991; 113: 1093–104.

Leger J, Marinovic D, Garel C, Bonaiti-Pellie C, Polak M, Czernichow P. Thyroid developmental anomalies in first degree relatives of children with congenital hypothyroidism. J Clin Endocrinol Metab 2002; 87: 575–80.

Lorey FW, Cunningham GC. Birth prevalence of primary congenital hypothyroidism by sex and ethnicity. Hum Biol 1992; 64: 531–8.

Macchia PE, Mattei M, Lapi P, Fenzi G, Di Lauro R. Cloning, chromosomal localization and identification of polymorphisms in the human thyroid transcription factor 2 gene (TITF2). Biochimie 1999; 81: 433–40.

Macchia PE, Lapi P, Krude H, Pirro MT, Missero C, Chiovato L et al. PAX8 mutations associated with congenital hypothyroidism caused by thyroid dysgenesis. Nat Genet 1998; 19: 83–6.

Madeiros-Neto G, Stanbury JB. Inherited disorders of the thyroid system. Boca Raton, CRC Press; 1994.

Maiorana R, Carta A, Floriddia G, Leonardi D, Buscema M, Sava L et al. Thyroid hemiagenesis: prevalence in normal children and effect on thyroid function. J Clin Endocrinol Metab 2003; 88: 1534–6.

Mansouri A, Chowdhury K, Gruss P. Follicular cells of the thyroid gland require *Pax8* gene function. Nat Genet 1998; 19: 87–90.

Marians RC, Ng L, Blair HC, Unger P, Graves PN, Davies TF. Defining thyrotropin-dependent and -independent steps of thyroid hormone synthesis by using thyrotropin receptor-null mice. Proc Natl Acad Sci USA 2002; 99: 15776–81.

Miyai K. Congenital thyrotropin deficiency – from discovery to molecular biology, postgenome and preventive medicine. Endocr J 2007; 54: 191–203.

Moeller LC, Kimura S, Kusakabe T, Liao XH, Van Sande J, Refetoff S. Hypothyroidism in thyroid transcription factor 1 haploinsufficiency is caused by reduced expression of the thyroid stimulating hormone receptor. Mol Endocrinol 2003; 17: 2295–302.

Moreno JC, Klootwijk W, van Toor H, Pinto G, D'Alessandro M, Leger A et al. Mutations in the iodotyrosine deiodinase gene and hypothyroidism. N Engl J Med 2008; 358: 1811–8.

Moreno JC, Pauws E, van Kampen AH, Jedlickova M, de Vijlder JJ, Ris-Stalpers C. Cloning of tissue-specific genes using serial analysis of gene expression and a novel computational substraction approach. Genomics 2001; 75: 70–6.

Moreno JC, Visser TJ. New phenotypes in thyroid dyshormonogenesis: hypothyroidism due to DUOX2 mutations. Endocr Dev 2007; 10: 99–117.

Niimi H, Inomata H, Sasaki N, Nakajima H. Congenital isolated thyrotropin releasing hormone deficiency. Arch Dis Child 1982; 57: 877–8.

Ohye H, Fukata S, Hishinuma A, Kudo T, Nishihara E, Ito M et al. A novel homozygous missense mutation of the dual oxidase 2 (DUOX2) gene in an adult patient with large goiter. Thyroid 2008; 18: 561–6.

Park SM, Chatterjee VK. Genetics of congenital hypothyroidism. J Med Genet 2005; 42: 379–89.

Perry R, Heinrichs C, Bourdoux P, Khoury K, Szots F, Dussault JH et al. Discordance of monozygotic twins for thyroid dysgenesis: implications for screening and for molecular pathophysiology. J Clin Endocrinol Metab 2002; 87: 4072–7.

Plachov D, Chowdhury K, Walther C, Simon D, Guenet JL, Gruss P. Pax8, a murine paired box gene expressed in the developing excretory system and thyroid gland. Development 1990; 110: 643–51.

Pohlenz J, Dumitrescu A, Zundel D, Martine U, Schonberger W, Koo E et al. Partial deficiency of thyroid transcription factor 1 produces predominantly neurological defects in humans and mice. J Clin Invest 2002; 109: 469–73.

Provenzano C, Veneziano L, Appleton R, Frontali M, Civitareale D. Functional characterization of a novel mutation in TITF-1 in a patient with benign hereditary chorea. J Neurol Sci 2008; 264: 56–62.

Rabeler R, Mittag J, Geffers L, Ruther U, Leitges M, Parlow AF et al. Generation of thyrotropin-releasing hormone receptor 1-deficient mice as an animal model of central hypothyroidism. Mol Endocrinol 2004; 18: 1450–60.

Rivolta CM, Targovnik HM. Molecular advances in thyroglobulin disorders. Clin Chim Acta 2006; 374: 8–24.

Roche J, Michel R, Michel O, Lissitzky S. Enzymatic dehalogenation of iodotyrosine by thyroid tissue; on its physiological role. Biochim Biophys Acta 1952; 9: 161–9.

Santarpia L, Valenzise M, Di Pasquale G, Arrigo T, San Martino G, Ciccio MP et al. TTF-2/FOXE1 gene polymorphisms in Sicilian patients with permanent primary congenital hypothyroidism. J Endocrinol Invest 2007; 30: 13 – 9.

Schott JJ, Benson DW, Basson CT, Pease W, Silberbach GM, Moak JP et al. Congenital heart disease caused by mutations in the transcription factor NKX2–5. Science 1998; 281 (5373): 108 – 11.

Stapleton P, Weith A, Urbanek P, Kozmik Z, Busslinger M. Chromosomal localization of 7 Pax genes and cloning of a novel family member, Pax-9. Nature Genet 1993; 3: 292 – 8.

Stuart A, Oates F, Hall C, Grumbles R, Fernandez L, Taylor N et al. Identification of a point mutation in the thyrotropin receptor of the hyt/hyt hypothyroid mouse. Mol Endocrinol 1994; 8: 129 – 38.

Sunthornthepvarakui T, Gottschalk ME, Hayashi Y, Refetoff S. Brief report: resistance to thyrotropin caused by mutations in the thyrotropin-receptor gene. N Engl J Med 1995; 332: 155 – 60.

Tanaka M, Schinke M, Liao HS, Yamasaki N, Izumo S. Nkx2.5 and Nkx2.6, homologs of *Drosophila tinman*, are required for development of the pharynx. Mol Cell Biol 2001; 21: 4391 – 8.

Toublanc JE. Comparison of epidemiological data on congenital hypothyroidism in Europe with those of other parts in the world. Horm Res 1992; 38: 230 – 5.

Vilain C, Rydlewski C, Duprez L, Heinrichs C, Abramowicz M, Malvaux P et al. Autosomal dominant transmission of congenital thyroid hypoplasia due to loss-of-function mutation of PAX8. J Clin Endocrinol Metab 2001; 86: 234 – 8.

Yamada M, Saga Y, Shibusawa N, Hirato J, Murakami M, Iwasaki T et al. Tertiary hypothyroidism and hyperglycemia in mice with targeted disruption of the thyrotropin-releasing hormone gene. Proc Natl Acad Sci USA 1997; 94: 10862 – 7.

Zamproni I, Grasberger H, Cortinovis F, Vigone MC, Chiumello G, Mora S et al. Biallelic inactivation of the dual oxidase maturation factor 2 (DUOXA2) gene as a novel cause of congenital hypothyroidism. J Clin Endocrinol Metab 2008; 93: 605 – 10.

15 Genetic Polymorphism in Autoimmune Thyroid Disease

M. Marga[1,3]*, P. Tretjakovs[1,2]

[1] Institute of Experimental and Clinical Medicine, University of Latvia, 4 Ojara Vaciesa str., Riga, LV-1004, Latvia
[2] Faculty of Medicine, University of Latvia, 1 Sarlotes str., Riga, LV-1001, Latvia
[3] Endocrinology & Diabetes, Medicine Division, Bedford Hospital NHS Trust, Kempston Road, Bedford, MK42 9SJ, U.K.

Abstract

Autoimmune thyroid diseases (AITD) are common autoimmune disorders affecting up to 2–4% of women and 1% of men in the general population. The current model of pathogenesis presents AITD as a result of the impact of hormonal and environmental factors (cigarette smoking, adverse psychosocial events, intercurrent infections and dietary iodine intake) on the background of genetic susceptibility. The phenotype of AITD comprises a wide range of interrelated conditions such as hyperthyroid Graves' disease (GD), Hashimoto's thyroiditis, atrophic autoimmune hypothyroidism, postpartum thyroiditis (PPT) and thyroid-asociated orbitopathy (TAO). Moreover, the cluster of different AITD phenotypes within an individual indicates a common pathophysiological basis. There are also numerous factors such as amelioration of GD during pregnancy, occurrence of PPT, and proven impact of gonadal steroids on the modulation of experimental AITD in animals contributing to the female predominance of the development of the disease. There have been various epidemiological family and twin studies, confirming a genetic influence on the development of AITD. The various techniques used in the last two decades have contributed to the identification of several genetic regions linked to AITD. The putative AITD susceptibility genes include both immune-modifying genes and thyroid-specific genes. The interaction of AITD predispositional loci and their impact on the diverse phenotype and course of the disease remains to be proven by further studies.

16　Iodine Status and TSH in Neonatal Thyroid Screening

P. P. A. Smyth[1]*, R. Burns[1], P. D. Mayne[2], D. F. Smith[1], M. Higgins[3], A. Staines[3], C. O'Herlihy[3]

[1] UCD Conway Institute of Biomolecular and Biomedical Research, School of Medicine and Medical Science, University College Dublin, Dublin, Ireland
[2] Children's University Hospital, Dublin, Ireland
[3] National Maternity Hospital, Holles Street, Dublin, Ireland

Abstract

The most commonly employed method of assessing population iodine status is the measurement of urinary iodine excretion (UI). However, some reports have made use of the results of neonatal blood-spot TSH screening programmes with an increased proportion (> 3%) of blood TSH values > 5.0 mU/L being indicative of iodine deficiency. A decline in median UI excretion in a young Irish female population, both pregnant and non-pregnant, prompted a study examining blood TSH from infants from The National Neonatal Screening Programme (n = 73 019) during seven separate years between 1995 and 2006. After 1995–1996 the proportion of individual blood TSH values > 5.0 mIU/L did not exceed 3% and a significant declining trend in the proportion of blood TSH > 5.0 mIU/L was observed in subsequent years (p < 0.01). While excluding severe iodine deficiency, these analyses failed to detect the slight but highly significant (p < 0.001) trend towards increasing blood TSH values in the study population between 1999 and 2006 which was greater in summer than in winter months (p < 0.001). UI excretion in Ireland over the period 1988–2006 supported the seasonal variation in TSH and confirmed a borderline iodine-deficient population with relatively stable UI (summer median ranging from 70–83 µg/L; winter 82–137 µg/L over the period 1988–2003). Since then a worrying decline in UI, most marked in the summer months, was observed with a median UI of 61–83 µg/L between 1988 and 1999; falling to 45.0 µg/L in 2004 and to 42.5 µg/L in 2005 with UI values < 50 µg/L (64.5% and 73.9%, respectively in summer; winter equivalent: 21.4–23.8%). These findings suggest that evaluation of neonatal blood TSH trends may reflect alterations in maternal iodine nutrition, particularly in areas where UI is not routinely measured. Early detection of such trends gives the possibility of identifying the problem before it can lead to potential long-term foetal consequences. The findings assume greater importance in the light of the declining UI reported from many developed countries previously considered iodine replete.

16.1　Introduction

Measurement of urinary iodine excretion (UI), with subsequent derivation of the median value and distribution of individual values and various concentration intervals is the most commonly used index for the assessment of a population's iodine status (WHO, 1994; WHO Secretariat, 2007). Other traditional measures employed include determination of goitre prevalence or thyroid volume by palpation or ultrasound. Other less commonly employed indices are the study of the results of blood spot TSH or Tg values obtained in screening programmes for neonatal hypothyroidism (Zimmermann et al., 2006)]. These approaches, in common with measurement of UI, are not suitable for use as an individual test to diagnose iodine deficiency but can yield an indication of overall population iodine status. Although the primary purpose of neonatal blood-spot TSH screening is the detection of congenital hypothyroidism, the finding of an increased proportion (> 3%) of blood TSH values > 5.0 mIU/L has been used as an index of iodine deficiency (WHO, 1994). While this threshold was derived from subjects residing in an iodine-sufficient area and its validity restated in a comprehensive literature review by Delange (1999), the numerical value of 3% > 5.0 mIU/L is not absolute. A recently observed decline in UI in both pregnant women and young female controls in Ireland has prompted a study of neonatal blood TSH to determine what effect this decline might have on neonatal thyroid function. The observed decline in UI mirrored that recently reported from the U.S.A., Australia and New Zealand (Hollowell et al., 1998; Dunn, 1998; Caldwell et al., 2005; Thomson et al., 2001; Gunton et al., 1999). The reason for such a decline is unclear but may reflect changes in food preferences, agricultural practices or the use of food iodine supplementation (Leung et al., 2007). The objective of this study was to examine blood TSH from infants from a national cohort born to mothers during seven separate years between 1995 and 2007 to determine if any alteration was observed in the percentage of values > 5.0 mIU/L and whether any trend in neonatal blood TSH was apparent (Sullivan et al., 1997; Copeland et al., 2002).

16.2   Subjects

16.2.1   Urinary Iodine Excretion (UI)

Results of UI on various groups of Irish females (n = 53 – 1063) selected for specific studies over the years 1988 – 2007 were used to indicate changes in dietary iodine intake. These subjects were selected opportunistically and can only serve as an indication of broad population trends rather than providing an accurate index of contemporary dietary iodine intake. Unlike the blood TSH values detailed below, urine samples designated as being collected in winter or summer were not all sampled in the specific months of January and August but over the specified season.

16.2.2   Neonatal Blood TSH

As part of the National Neonatal Screening Programme, a heel-prick blood sample was taken from all infants born in Ireland between 72 and 120 hours post-partum and all samples were sent for analysis to the National Newborn Screening Laboratory at the Children's University Hospital, Temple Street, Dublin. The records reviewed were held on paper and values had to be manually transcribed from daily TSH assay work-sheets with distributions recorded in histograms created in Microsoft Excel. For this reason it was necessary to be selective in terms of years chosen for study. This selection was therefore made on the basis of individual years in which data on UI excretion in pregnant Irish women were available

commencing in 1995 and continuing to 2006 (Nawoor et al., 2006; Symth et al., 1997). Blood TSH data for these and intervening years were selected on the basis of available TSH assay sheets. In view of the known seasonal variation in urinary iodine excretion in Ireland (Hetherton and Smyth, 1993), individual months in winter (January, n = 35079) and in summer (August, N = 37940) were selected to represent the individual years in each of seven years between 1995 – 2006 in which some UI data were available. The two months were combined (n = 73019) to provide the annualised figures in this report.

16.3   Methods

16.3.1   Urinary Iodine (UI) Estimation

Urinary iodine (UI) was measured using the ammonium persulphate digestion microplate method as described by Ohashi et al. (2000). Results were expressed as μgI/L urine (μg/L). Quality control was assessed under the Centre for Disease Control (CDC, Atlanta, Georgia, USA) EQUIP programme. Study group values were expressed as medians and % of individual values indicative of iodine deficiency (< 50 μg/L) as recommended by the WHO (1994).

16.3.2   Neonatal TSH

Blood TSH was measured by dissociation enhanced fluoroimmunoassay (DELFIA) on an Auto DELFIA analyser. The analytical methods used did not change over the period of study. While this assay is designed to detect the gross increases in blood TSH experienced by infants with congenital hypothyroidism and is less accurate at detecting changes closer to the lowest standard employed, the large number of specimens analysed in this study permitted the examination of possible trends in blood TSH at lower values including those at the limits of assay sensitivity.

16.3.3   Statistical Methods

Statistical analysis was carried out using the chi-squared (χ^2) tests and a robust regression procedure based on an original method described by Huber (1981) and implemented by Venables and Ripley (2002) in the 'MASS' package of the R programming language (R-Development-Core-Team, 2007). This is a variant of linear regression, fitted

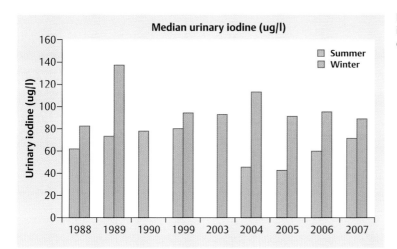

Fig. 16.**1** Median urinary iodine excretion by season over the years 1988–2007.

by the method or iterative re-weighted least squares, which is very resistant to outliers in the data. Trend analysis was carried out using the chi-squared test for trend in proportions.

16.4 Results

16.4.1 Urinary Iodine Excretion (UI)

The results of median UI (µg/L) measured in the various groups of female subjects in summer and winter months are shown in Fig. 16.**1**. The overall borderline iodine status of the study groups is demonstrated by the finding that on only two occasions (winter 1989 and winter 2004) did the median UI value exceed 100 µg/L. This finding confirms earlier reports of seasonal variation in UI in that winter values were consistently higher than their summer equivalents. While there was no sequential change in winter UI over the study period, the summer median showed a modest trend towards higher values between 1988 and

1990 (61.5–80.0 µg/L) but declined dramatically in 2004 and 2005 (45–42.5 µg/L) and showed a modest recovery (59.5–71.0 µg/L) in 2006–2007. These changes were mirrored by findings for the % of values < 50 µg/L which reached highs of 64.5% and 73.3% in 2004 and 2005 before reaching the still unacceptably high values of 44.4% and 34.0% in 2006 and 2007.

16.4.2 Neonatal TSH

The number of subjects investigated during the months of January and August combined together with the % of blood TSH values > 5.0 mIU/L are shown in Table 16.**1**. In total 73 019 values were assessed. Comparing differences in the proportion of neonatal blood TSH values > 5.0 mIU/L demonstrated a significant difference only between the sequential years 1995 and 1996 (p = 0.02). However, analysing the data showed a highly significant downward trend (p < 0.01) in the proportion of values > 5.0 mIU/L. As trends in the distribution of lower levels of blood TSH were

Table 16.**1** Percentage of individual neonatal blood TSH values > 5 mIU/L from 1995–2006. Significance refers to the difference between an individual year and its preceding year. n. s. = not significant.

Year	1995	1996	1999	2003	2004	2005	2006
% > 5 mIU/L	3.64	2.99	2.62	2.53	2.64	2.42	2.35
N	9466	9286	9703	10074	11226	11437	11827
Statistical significance		p = 0.02	n. s.	n. s.	n. s.	n. s.	n. s.

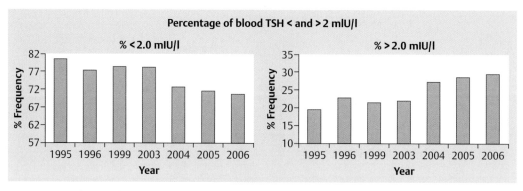

Fig. 16.**2** Distribution of neonatal TSH > 2.0 mIU/L sampled over the years 1995 to 2006.

Table 16.**2** Mean and median neonatal blood TSH by month and year.

Month	TSH mIU/L	1995	1996	1999	2003	2004	2005	2006
Aug	N	4822	4555	5081	4842	5944	6290	6406
	Median	0.83	1.23	1.30	1.11	1.38	1.36	1.45
	Mean ± SD	1.37 ± 2.20	1.84 ± 11.04	1.84 ± 5.29	1.60 ± 3.60	1.89 ± 6.41	1.76 ± 4.22	1.80 ± 2.61
Jan	N	4644	4731	4622	5232	5282	5147	5421
	Median	0.97	1.13	1.12	1.12	1.27	1.38	1.31
	Mean ± SD	1.49 ± 1.72	1.74 ± 7.66	1.74 ± 8.29	1.66 ± 6.59	1.64 ± 2.14	1.97 ± 9.77	1.61 ± 1.93

being sought, the distribution over the study years of values < and > 2.0 mIU/L was examined. As shown in Fig. 16.2 a highly significant (p < 0.001) increase in the proportion of blood TSH values > 2.0 mIU/L was observed rising from 19.5 % in 1995 to 29.3 % in 2006. The corresponding downward trend in the % of values < 2.0 mIU/L was also highly significant as early as 1996 (rising from 19.5 % to 22.5 %) and was maintained up to 2006 (29.3 %) (p < 0.001 compared to 1995 in all cases). The increases between 2004 and 2006 (27.1 %; 28.36 %; 29.3 %) were not significantly different. Table 16.2 shows the mean and median values for blood TSH by month and year. It should be noted that there is quite a variation between mean and median reflecting the very high values obtaining in congenital hypothyroidism.

Fig. 16.3 shows a histogram of the annual % frequency distribution of neonatal blood TSH values over the seven years studied between 1995 and 2006 (January and August values combined) which demonstrates that paradoxically the proportion of values from 0 – 1.0 mIU/L was greatest between 1995 and 1996 despite the presence of

a relatively large number of values > 5.0 mIU/L (3.64 % in 1995) and apart from 2003 showed a decline thereafter. From 1.0 – 2.0 mIU/L the trend was upwards and continued in the cohort of values from 2.0 – 4.0 mIU/L. From 2003 the distribution began to shift to the right with a median blood TSH of 1.11 mIU/L moving to 1.33 mIU/L in 2004 and to 1.37 and 1.38 mIU/L in 2005 and 2006, respectively. This trend to the right was not reflected by an increase in the proportion of blood TSH values > 5.0 mIU/L with such elevated values in 2004 – 2006 being 2.64 %, 2.42 % and 2.35 %, respectively.

This increase in mean blood TSH concentration over time and the variation in blood TSH levels by month was examined further using regression analysis. To ensure that this analysis is not unduly affected by the few large values observed in each month, a robust regression method was used. The regression of the effect of month alone confirms a significant difference (p < 0.001) between blood TSH levels in January and August, specifically mean blood TSH levels are slightly lower (by an average of 0.0559 mIU/L) in January than in Au-

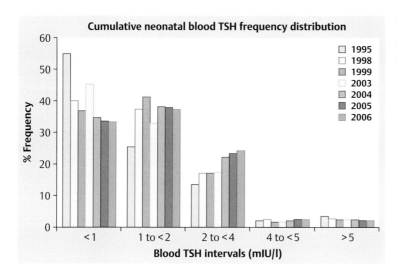

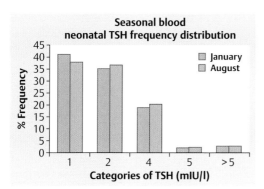

Fig. 16.**4**   Seasonal % frequency distribution of neonatal blood TSH values 1995–2006.

gust. The frequency distribution of TSH levels between January and August is shown in Fig. 16.**4**.

The change in the distribution of blood TSH values was not accompanied by any significant trend in the incidence of congenital hypothyroidism in the Irish population which, as shown in Fig. 16.**5**, varied from 57.7/100 000 (1 : 1735) subjects tested in 1995 to a minimum of 32.5/100 000 (1 : 3075) in 2003 (p = 0.06). The overall incidence for the 7 years was 44.2/100 000 (1 : 2619) subjects. The variation from year to year in incidence rates results from the small absolute number of CHT cases detected.

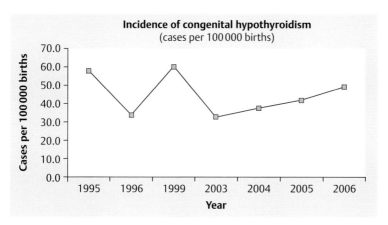

Fig. 16.**5**   Incidence of confirmed congenital hypothyroidism (CHT) in the individual years of the study period.

16.5   Discussion

The dietary iodine status of a population is best and most readily established by sampling UI concentration in a sufficiently large cohort (WHO-Secretariat, 2007). However the effects of any deficit in iodine intake on individual thyroid function and general health are more difficult to quantify. It is well established that the foetus and neonate are at greatest risk from the ill effects of iodine deficiency (Glinoer and Delange, 2000). Although maternal UI values < 50 µg/L are generally accepted as being indicative of iodine deficiency, this state cannot be readily established on the basis of a single UI measurement, whether with a casual specimen or even a 24-h collection (Als et al., 2000; Knudsen et al., 2000). Differences in daily dietary intake can result in considerable swings in UI excretion. In the case of pregnant mothers, continuation of iodine supply to the foetus/neonate is dependent not only on dietary intake but also on placental transport and possibly storage. In addition, the adequacy of preconception iodine stores may determine the ability of the mother in achieving the dual role of maintaining both her own and her offspring's thyroid function. The present study demonstrates that although UI seemed to vary between the study years, the median values were consistently lower than those recommended by the WHO with the % of individual values < 50 µg/L putting a significant number of women and their babies at potential risk of iodine deficiency. There was no evident explanation for these relatively low values which had declined from a median first trimester pregnancy UI of 135 µg/L (20% < 50 µg/l) reported by our group in 1997 (Smyth et al., 1997). Thyroid function tests were not performed on these subjects but it was possible to seek an impact of apparently declining antenatal dietary iodine intake (Nawoor et al., 2006) on neonatal thyroid function by examining the records of neonatal blood TSH measured over the period 1995–2006 as part of the Irish National Neonatal Screening Programme. Neonatal blood TSH values have been used as an index of iodine deficiency by examining the number of individuals having blood TSH > 5.0 mIU/L; the threshold for iodine deficiency being > 3% (WHO; 1994). If our findings are classified according to this definition (WHO, 1994), then the female reproductive Irish population was iodine-deficient in 1995 (3.64% > 5 mIU/L) and borderline deficient in 1996 (2.99% > 5 mIU/L) but thereafter remained relatively iodine-sufficient (the propor-

tion of blood TSH > 5.0 mIU/L being relatively constant, 2.35–2.62%), although there was a significant trend towards a lower proportion of values > 5 mIU/L over the entire period.

Despite the observed decline in blood TSH > 5.0 mIU/L there is strong evidence for a steady tendency towards higher, but not significantly elevated, blood TSH values in the study population underlying the weakness inherent in using % of TSH values > 5 mIU/L as an index of iodine deficiency. This shift toward values at the higher end of the normal range was quite consistent in the years studied from 1996 to 2006 with the exception of 2003 and was highly significant. Interestingly the greatest increase in the proportion of blood TSH values > 2.0 mIU/L occurred after 2003 and coincided with the report of a steep decline in maternal UI (Nawoor et al., 2006) and supports a link between falling maternal iodine intake and foetal thyroid function.

The present study shows that on a population basis there is a relationship between falling maternal urinary iodine values and higher neonatal blood TSH results. Although the findings demonstrate that readily available neonatal blood-spot TSH data can be utilised to detect the effects of altered trends in maternal iodine nutrition, even in areas considered iodine replete, they do not support the conventional wisdom on the use of blood TSH as an index of iodine deficiency solely on the exclusive basis of the proportion of values > 5.0 mIU/L. While this cut-off point was derived from subjects residing in an iodine-sufficient area (WHO, 2001) and its validity restated in reviews by Sullivan et al. (1997) and Delange (1999), the figure of 3% > 5.0 mIU/L is not absolute and may be affected by factors such as the use of iodine-containing antiseptics (Copeland et al., 2002; McElduff et al., 2005).

No ready explanation is available for the shift to the right in blood TSH distribution in the absence of an increase in blood TSH values > 5.0 mIU/L. This trend may reflect the fact that iodine intake is sufficient to maintain thyroid hormones at a suboptimal level with very modest increases in TSH. Whether such a suboptimal thyroid status is sufficient to maintain normal brain development is unclear. As indicated in this study, the shift to the right in blood TSH distribution may provide an early indication of thyroid hormone insufficiency resulting from diminished iodine intake. These data also provide initial evidence of a seasonal variation in neonatal TSH, with the babies born in summer months, during which dietary iodine intake in Ireland is low (Hetherton and Smyth, 1993), having significantly higher values than those born in winter. With the exception of severe iodine deficiency or excess, there is seldom a significant correlation between individual UI and serum TSH in adults (Thomson et al., 2001; Teng et al., 2006). The possible pitfalls of over interpreting the fall in TSH have been outlined by Laurberg et al. (2007). These findings illustrate the complexity of the relationship between dietary iodine intake and thyroid function with lower iodine paradoxically being associated with hyperthyroidism and higher values with hypothyroidism. However, in the present study there is strong evidence, based on the large number of samples assayed, for a tendency towards higher but not significantly elevated blood TSH coinciding with a decline in UI. Sustained low iodine is of course associated with decreased thyroid hormone levels with potentially serious consequences in the foetus or neonate (Glinoer and Delange, 2000).

In the case of neonatal blood TSH we are suggesting the use of trends in addition to, rather than instead of, numerical values. Of course, measurement of UI continues to provide the best index for the study of iodine deficiency (WHO, 1994). However, in view of the importance of thyroid hormones for the developing brain and the possible consequences of even a minor degree of hypothyroxinaemia for neuropsychological development and subsequent intellectual capacity, it would seem desirable to evaluate neonatal blood TSH data, when available, to reflect altered trends in maternal iodine nutrition, particularly in areas where UI is not routinely measured. Early detection of such trends gives the possibility of identifying the problem before it can lead to potential long-term foetal consequences. The findings assume greater importance in light of the declining UI reported from many developed countries previously considered to be iodine replete.

Acknowledgements

The authors gratefully acknowledge the helpful advice in preparing this manuscript of Professor Glen F. Maberly of the Department of International Health, Rollins School of Public Health, Emory University, Atlanta GA, USA and the late Professor Francois Delange, Universite Libre de Bruxelles, Belgium.

References

Als C, Helbling A, Peter K, Haldimann M, Zimmerli B, Gerber H. Urinary iodine concentration follows a circadian rhythm: a study with 3023 spot urine samples in adults and children. J Clin Endocrinol Metab 2000; 85: 1367–9.

Caldwell KL, Jones R, Hollowell JG. Urinary iodine concentration: United States National Health And Nutrition Examination Survey 2001–2002. Thyroid 2005; 15: 692–9.

Copeland DL, Sullivan KM, Houston R, May W, Mendoza I, Salamatullah Q et al. Comparison of neonatal thyroid-stimulating hormone levels and indicators of iodine deficiency in school children. Public Health Nutrition 2002; 5: 81–7.

Delange F. Neonatal thyroid screening as a monitoring tool for the control of iodine deficiency. Acta Paediatr Suppl. 1999; 88: 21–4.

Dunn JT. What's happening to our iodine? J Clin Endocrinol Metab 1998; 83: 3398–400.

Glinoer D, Delange F. The potential repercussions of maternal, fetal, and neonatal hypothyroxinemia on the progeny. Thyroid 2000; 10: 871–87.

Gunton JE, Hams G, Fiegert M, McElduff A. Iodine deficiency in ambulatory participants at a Sydney teaching hospital: is Australia truly iodine replete? Med J Aust.1999; 171: 467–70.

Hetherton A, Smyth P. Status of iodine deficiency in Ireland. In: Delange F, Dunn J, Glinoer D, eds.: Iodine Deficiency in Europe – A Continuing Concern. New York: Plenum Press, 1993: 317–22.

Hollowell JG, Staehling NW, Hannon WH, Flanders DW, Gunter EW, Maberly GF, et al. Iodine nutrition in the United States. Trends and public health implications: iodine excretion data from National Health and Nutrition Examination Surveys I and III (1971–1974 and 1988–1994). J Clin Endocrinol Metab 1998; 83: 3401–8.

Huber P. Robust Statistics. New York: Wiley, 1981.

Knudsen N, Christiansen E, Brandt-Christensen M, Nygaard B, Perrild H. Age- and sex-adjusted iodine/creatinine ratio. A new standard in epidemiological surveys? Evaluation of three different estimates of iodine excretion based on casual urine samples and comparison to 24 h values. Eur J Clin Nutrition 2000; 54: 361–3.

Laurberg P, Andersen S, Bjarnadottir RI, Carle A, Hreidarsson A, Knudsen N et al. Evaluating iodine deficiency in pregnant women and young infants – complex physiology with a risk of misinterpretation. Public Health Nutrition 2007; 10 (12A): 1547–52; discussion 53.

Leung AM, Braverman LE, Pearce EN. A dietary iodine questionnaire: correlation with urinary iodine and food diaries. Thyroid 2007; 17: 755–62.

McElduff A, McElduff P, Wiley V, Wilcken B. Neonatal thyrotropin as measured in a congenital hypothyroidism screening program: influence of the mode of delivery. J Clin Endocrinol Metab 2005; 90: 6361 – 3.

Nawoor Z, Burns R, Smith DF, Sheehan S, O'Herlihy C, Smyth PP. Iodine intake in pregnancy in Ireland – a cause for concern? Ir J Med Sci 2006; 175: 21 – 4.

Ohashi T, Yamaki M, Pandav CS, Karmarkar MG, Irie M. Simple microplate method for determination of urinary iodine. Clin Chem 2000; 46: 529 – 36.

R-Developement-Core-Team. R: A language and environment for statistical computing. R Foundation for statistical computing, Vienna, Austria, 2007.

Smyth PP, Hetherton AM, Smith DF, Radcliff M, O'Herlihy C. Maternal iodine status and thyroid volume during pregnancy: correlation with neonatal iodine intake. J Clin Endocrinol Metab 1997; 82: 2840 – 3.

Sullivan KM, May W, Nordenberg D, Houston R, Maberly GF. Use of thyroid stimulating hormone testing in newborns to identify iodine deficiency. J Nutr 1997; 127: 55 – 8.

Teng W, Shan Z, Teng X, Guan H, Li Y, Teng D et al. Effect of iodine intake on thyroid diseases in China. N Engl J Med 2006; 354: 2783 – 93.

Thomson CD, Woodruffe S, Colls AJ, Joseph J, Doyle TC. Urinary iodine and thyroid status of New Zealand residents. Eur J Clin Nutrition 2001; 55: 387 – 92.

Venables W, Ripley B. Modern Applied Statistics with S. 4th ed., Berlin, Heidelberg: Springer, 2002.

WHO U, ICCIDD. Assessment of iodine deficiency disorders and monitoring their elimination: a guide for programme managers. 2nd ed., Geneva: World Health Organisation/NHD/011. 2001.

WHO U, ICCIDD. Indicators for assessing iodine deficiency disorders and their control through salt iodization. Geneva: World Health Organisation/NUT/946. 1994.

WHO-Secretariat, Andersson M, de Benoist B, Delange F, Zupan J. Prevention and control of iodine deficiency in pregnant and lactating women and in children less than 2-years-old: conclusions and recommendations of the Technical Consultation. Public Health Nutrition 2007; 10: 1606 – 11.

Zimmermann MB, de Benoist B, Corigliano S, Jooste PL, Molinari L, Moosa K et al. Assessment of iodine status using dried blood spot thyroglobulin: development of reference material and establishment of an international reference range in iodine-sufficient children. J Clin Endocrinol Metab 2006; 91: 4881 – 7.

17 Neonatal Thyroid Screening and Child Development

F. Azizi*, A. Amouzegar

Endocrine Research Center, Research Institute for Endocrine Sciences, Shahid Beheshti University of Medical Sciences, P. O. Box: 19395–4763, Tehran, I. R. Iran

Abstract

Thyroid hormone is essential for normal brain development. Neonates born with congenital hypothyroidism are at risk of brain damage and mental retardation, which can be prevented by timely diagnosis and treatment; the disorder results from an abnormality in thyroid gland development or in thyroid hormonogenesis. Transient hypothyroidism and central or secondary/tertiary hypothyroidism are other forms of neonatal hypothyroidism. Since the advent of newborn screening programmes in 1974, in many countries the diagnosis of congenital hypothyroidism is now provided in the first 2 weeks of life. The aim of therapy is to ensure normal growth and development by maintaining the serum FT_4 level in the upper half of and the serum TSH level within the reference ranges. Growth rate, adult height and sexual development are normal in affected children for whom levothyroxine therapy is consistently maintained. However, minor differences in intelligence, school achievement and neuropsychological tests may occur in treated congenital hypothyroid patients as compared to control groups of classmates and siblings. Residual defects include impaired visuospatial processing and selective sensorimotor or memory defects. Factors associated with outcome of management, such as aetiology of hypothyroidism, severity of the disease at the time of diagnosis, age at the onset of therapy, starting dose levels of levothyroxine, treatment adequacy and compliance, and moderating variables such as gender, genetic, social and environmental influences have been studied and have shed more light on the proper management of congenital hypothyroidism, so that today newborns with congenital hypothyroidism may have a better intellectual and neurological prognosis. Further research is needed to determine the optimal starting doses for the different aetiologies and subsequent long-term management, in particular during adulthood and during pregnancy in women with congenital hypothyroidism.

17.1 Introduction

Thyroid hormones are responsible for normal growth and development during pre- and postnatal life. Congenital hypothyroidism (CH) is the most common cause of neonatal thyroid disorder that is caused by a defect in thyroid structure or hormonogenesis. It affects about one newborn infant in 3500. However, higher incidences have been reported from some countries.

CH causes life-long cognitive and motor and somatic deficits. CH-screening programmes now allow for early identification and treatment. As a result, affected children now show normal or near normal physical, neurological and psychological development. Nevertheless, because affected children still undergo a brief but circumscribed period of thyroid hormone insufficiency, they are at risk for subtle selective impairments (Rovet, 2002; Bernal et al., 2003; Raiti and Newns, 1971; Klein et al., 1972; Tillotson et al., 1994; Derksen-Lubsen and Berkerk, 1996; Bernal and Nunez, 1995).

Neonatal screening programmes for congenital hypothyroidism (CH) were initiated in the 1970s to ensure early treatment in order to prevent mental retardation. With screening, the developmental prognosis is considerably improved, but follow-up studies still report developmental delay compared to controls (Heyerdahl and Oerbeck, 2003; Dalivia et al., 2000). There are limited data available to show the long-term social, emotional and behavioural consequences of early treated CH.

Table 17.**1** The classification and prevalence of congenital hypothyroidism.

Classification	Prevalence
Thyroid dysgenesis; Agenesis; Hypogenesis; Ectopia	1 : 1000 – 1 : 4000
Thyroid dyshormonogenesis; Thyroid-stimulating hormone unresponsiveness; Iodide trapping defect; Organification defect; Defect in thyroglobulin; Iodotryrosine deiodinase deficiency	1 : 40 000
Transient hypothyroidism; Drug induced hypothyroidism; Maternal antibody induced hypothyroidism; Idiopathic hypothyroidism	1 : 40 000
Hypothalamic-pituitary hypothyroidism; Hypothalamic-pituitary anomaly; Panhypopituitarism; Isolated thyroid-stimulating hormone deficiency; Thyroid hormone resistance	1 : 100 000

17.2 Methods

MEDLINE and EMBASE were searched using the terms "neonatal screening", "hypothyroidism", "child development". All English articles were reviewed from 1972 until May, 2008.

17.3 Results and Discussion

17.3.1 Embryogenesis of Thyroid Gland

Congenital hypothyroidism is due to thyroid agenesis, hypoplasia and ectopic thyroid. These defects occur on about the 16th and 17th day of the embryonic period. Primordium of the thyroid gland begins as a thickening of epithelium in the pharyngeal floor, and descends down the neck along the thyroglossal duct. It reaches the lower section of the neck by the 7th week of gestation. Its upper segment undergoes involution, while the lower segment gives rise to the thyroid gland. The thyroid presents with iodine by the 8th week of intrauterine life and, in the 10th week the potential for iodothyronine production develops. A defect in each of these processes or formation of extrathyroid aberrations of thyroid tissue provides the possibility for developmental anomalies of the thyroid gland, which lead to deficient hormonal function (Pniewska-Siark et al., 2006) (Table 17.**1**).

17.3.2 Neurological Development

Many factors may influence neuropsychological outcome in congenital hypothyroidism (Table 17.**2**).

Table 17.**2** Factors that may affect the neuropsychological development in patients with congenital hypothyroidism.

No.	Disease-Related Variables
1	Aetiology of hypothyroidism
2	Skeletal maturity
3	Thyroid hormone levels at diagnosis
4	Age at onset of therapy
5	Starting dose of levothyroxine
6	Time to achieve normalisation
7	Subsequent treatment and outcome
8	Compliance and treatment adequacy
9	Gender, social, genetic and environmental factors

17.3.3 Motor Activities

Screening programmes for congenital hypothyroidism (CH) have dramatically improved the neuropsychological prognosis in affected children. Children with severe neonatal hypothyroidism (serum thyroxine level less than 2 µg/dL) have significantly lower neurological scores compared to CH affected children with less severe disease and normal controls; for the latter group, the most affected functions are imbalance, extremity coordination, fine motor activity, quality of movements, associated movements, and head movements; these children hence have underdeveloped neuromotor skills (Bargagna et al., 2000).

Screening programs have eliminated mental retardation. However, children with congenital hypothyroidism, even treated early in life, may still have subtle specific deficits in cognitive performances, visuospatial abilities, defective language abilities, learning disabilities, selective attention and memory problems. As all these disorders are potentially disabling conditions, this makes neuropsychological follow-up mandatory; selected tests of motor proficiency are indicated at 3 and 5 years of age to detect those defects in motor skills that appear to more specifically affected children (Rovet and Daneman, 2003; Connelly et al., 2001; Kempers et al., 2007)

17.3.4 IQ Defects

Although the global IQ of congenitally hypothyroid children may not differ from those of their siblings or those of control children, some studies report mild decreases in global IQ level in these children in comparison to controls. The New England Congenital Hypothyroidism Collaboration detected normal school performance in all aspects among children affected by congenital hypothyroidism. However, others have reported subtle difficulties in school performance (Rovet and Ehrlich, 2000; New England Congenital Hypothyroidism Collaborative, 1990).

17.3.5 Language Disorders

Language disorders were observed in half of CH children between 3 and 5 years of age, those however with severe neonatal hypothyroidism have moderately severe defects (Gottschalk et al., 1994). A problem-oriented, simplified neuropsychological follow-up of early-treated children with CH should not systematically include the frequent repetition of time-consuming and expensive psychometric tests because individual IQ scores are in the normal range in almost all CH children and can be differentiated from those of normal controls only on a population-statistic basis. Language performances may be affected in CH children, and should be always checked at 3 and 5 years of age. Children with even mild language disorders or delayed language achievements are candidates for regular reevaluation every 6 months and, if no spontaneous improvement is observed, they should receive specific rehabilitation treatment. No further evaluation is warranted in CH children with normal tests at age 5 years (Bargagna et al., 2000).

17.3.6 Learning Disabilities

Early treated CH is associated with mild delays in several fundamental achievement skills.

Learning disorders in many items such as writing, reading, listening, reasoning and mathematics are also problematic. Besides these, they may have selective learning disorders such as dysgraphia, dyscalculia and dyslexia. The poorest academic performance and behaviour problems have been detected in children with severe hypothyroidism or when long intervals are needed to achieve euthyroidism. Educational achievement in early-treated CH children is usually reported to be quite favourable; however arithmetic and reading comprehension may be weaker than normal; while some studies had shown that they achieved similar school performances in early adolescence compared to that of subjects in the national population (Rovet and Ehrlich, 2000: Légert et al., 2001), others had indicated school-related learning problems and underachievement (Rovet, 1999; Connelly et al., 2001; Kooistra et al., 1994; Fuggle et al., 1991; Gottschalk et al., 1994; Rovert et al., 1992; Kooistra et al., 1996; Rovet and Alvarez, 1996; Rover and Ehrlich, 2000; Bargagna et al., 1999; Glorieux et al., 1992; Rochiccioli et al., 1992).

Careful monitoring of the adequacy of treatment is thus required throughout childhood to reduce the risk of low school performance, and that is especially true in children subjected to poor social conditions (Rovet and Ehrlich, 2000; Légert et al., 2001).

17.3.7 Longitudinal Growth and Final Height and Sexual Maturation

Linear growth and final height are normal in children with congenital hypothyroidism treated from the first weeks of life (Buchwer et al., 1985; Moschini et al., 1986; Moreno et al., 1989). Severe hypothyroidism at diagnosis causes a significant delay of increase in length during the first year of life (Siragusa et al., 1996), but these children reach a normal final height if they are treated within the first month of life (Aronson et al., 1990). However, treatment delay in patients diagnosed before the introduction of systematic neonatal screening gave rise to short stature and adult height that was shorter than observed following the introduction of screening (Salerno et al., 2001). Patients with CH have a normal sexual maturation when treated appropriately. Puberty begins within a normal age and progresses normally in both sexes (Dickerman and De Vries, 1997).

17.3.8   Time of Screening and Treatment

Serum free T_4 and TSH levels are used as biochemical markers for neonatal screening for congenital hypothyroidism. The screening test involves the detection of raised levels of thyroid-stimulating hormone (TSH) and/or low levels of thyroxine (T_4) in filter paper blood samples collected shortly after birth. Children are screened for TSH on days 3–5: if TSH levels are > 40 mU/L, they are recalled for repeat TSH and free T_4 levels by postnatal days 7–10. Treatment begins immediately in those whose repeat TSH shows levels above 40 mU/L. When TSH is below 20 mU/L, they are followed only; children with values above 20 mU/L are scanned and, if the scan suggests a thyroid abnormality, they receive treatment (Rovet and Daneman, 2003). Although hypothyroidism should be treated as soon as possible after birth, in some studies with controversial results, this treatment contributes minimally to outcomes (New England Congenital Hypothyroidism Collaborative, 1994; Tilotson et al., 1994).

17.3.9   Treatment dose

Today the daily oral dose of levothyroxine is all that is needed for treatment of congenital hypothyroidism. The American Academy of Pediatrics (AAP) promotes 10–15 µg/kg/day in order to normalise thyroid hormone levels as soon as possible (American Academy of Pediatrics, 1993). There is no clear evidence that the starting dose of levothyroxine has any positive effect on cognition or development, growth and behaviour; however, there is weak evidence for increased behavioural problems in children given a high starting of levothyroxine (Hrytsiuk et al., 2002; Oerbeck et al., 2005).

17.4   Conclusions

Since the advent of newborn screening programmes in 1974, in many countries the diagnosis of congenital hypothyroidism is now provided in the first 2 weeks after birth. Minor differences in school achievement and neuropsychological tests may occur in treated congenital hypothyroid patients as compared to controls. Many factors are associated with the outcome of management

Table 17.**3**   Unsettled questions related to congenital hypothyroidism.

No.	Question
1	What constitutes optimal treatment?
2	Could children with severe hypothyroidism develop normally with optimal treatment?
3	Could prenatal hypothyroidism per se affect later developmental outcome?
4	Which specific neuropsychological and neurological functions are affected by thyroid dysfunction at different ages, prenatal and postnatal?
5	What is the optimal management during adulthood, in particular during pregnancy?

of CH, which should be sought during various phases of management of such patients (Table 17.**3**). Further research is needed for treatment of CH with different aetiologies and their long-term management, in particular, during adulthood.

References

American Academy of Pediatrics, Section on Endocrinology and Committee on Genetics, and American Thyroid Association Committee on Public Health. Newborn screening for congenital hypothyroidism: recommended guidelines. Pediatrics 1993; 91: 1203–92.

Aronson R, Ehrlich RM, Bailey JD, Rovet JF. Growth in children with congenital hypothyroidism detected by neonatal screening. J Pediatr 1990; 116: 33–7.

Bargagna S, Canepa G, Costagli C, Dinetti D, Marcheschi M, Millepiedi S, Montanelli L, Pinchera A, Chiovato L. Neuropsychological follow-up in early-treated congenital hypothyroidism: a problem-oriented approach. Thyroid 2000; 10: 243–9.

Bargagna S, Dinetti D, Pinchera A, et al. School attainments in children with congenital hypothyroidism detected neonatal screening and treated early in life. Eur J Endocrinol 1999; 140: 407–13

Bernal J, Guadano-Ferraz A, Morte B. Perspectives in the study of thyroid hormone action on brain development and function. Thyroid 2003 13: 1005–12

Bernal J, Nunez J. Thyroid hormones and brain development. Eur J Endocr 1995; 133: 390–8

Bucher H, Prader A, Illig R. Head circumference, height, bone age and weight in 103 children with congenital hypothyroidism before and during thyroid hormone replacement. Helv Paediatrica Acta 1985; 40: 305–16.

Connelly JF, Rickards AL, Coakley JC et al. Newborn screening for congenital hypothyroidism, Victoria, Australia, 1977–1997 (part II): treatment, progress, and outcome. J Pediatr Endocrinol Metab 2001; 14: 1611–34

Daliva AL, Linder B, DiMartino-Nardi J, Saenger P. Three-year follow-up of borderline congenital hypothyroidism. J Pediatr 2000; 136: 53–6.

Derksen-Lubsen G, Verkerk PH. Neuropsychologic development in early treated congenital hypothyroidism: analysis of literature data. Pediatr Res 1996; 39: 561–6.

Dickerman Z, De Vries L. Prepubertal and pubertal growth, timing and duration of puberty and attained adult height in patients with congenital hypothyroidism (CH) detected by the neonatal screening program for CH – a longitudinal study. Clinic Endocrinol 1997; 47: 649–54.

Fuggle PW, Grant DB, Smith I et al. Intelligence motor skills and behaviour at 5 years in early-treated congenital hypothyroidism. Eur J Pediatr 1991; 150: 570–4

Glorieux J, Dussault J, Van Vliet F. Intellectual development at age 12 years in children with congenital hypothyroidism diagnosed by neonatal screening. J Pediatr 1992; 121: 581–4

Gottschalk B, Richman R, Lewandowski L. Subtle speech and motor deficits of children with congenital hypothyroidism treated early. Dev Med Child Neurol 1994; 36: 216–20

Heyerdahl S, Oerbeck B. Congenital hypothyroidism: developmental outcome in relation to levothyroxine treatment variables. Thyroid 2003; 13: 1029–38.

Hrytsiuk I, Gilbert R, Logan S, Pindoria S, Brook CG. Starting dose of levothyroxine for the treatment of congenital hypothyroidism. Arch Pediatr Adolesc Med 2002; 156: 485–91.

Kempers MJ, van der Sluijs Veer L, Nijhuis-van der Sanden RW, Lanting CI, Kooistra L, Wiedijk BM, Last BF, de Vijlder JJ, Grootenhuis MA, Vulsma T. Neonatal screening for congenital hypothyroidism in the Netherlands: cognitive and motor outcome at 10 years of age. J Clin Endocrinol Metab 2007; 92: 919–24.

Klein AH, Meltzer S, Kenny FM · Improved prognosis in congenital hypothyroidism treated before age three months. J Pediatr 1972; 81: 912–5.

Kooistra L, Laane C, Vulsma T et al. Motor and cognitive development in children with congenital hypothyroidism: a long-term evaluation of the effects of neonatal treatment. J Pediatr 1994; 124: 903–9

Kooistra L, van der Meere JJ, Vulsma T et al. Sustained attention problems in children with early treated congenital hypothyroidism. Acta Paediatr 1996; 85: 425–9

Léger J, Larroque B, Norton J, on behalf of AFDPHE. Influence of severity of congenital hypothyroidism and adequacy of treatment on school achievement in young adolescents: a population-based cohort study. Acta Paediatr 2001; 90: 1249–56.

Moreno L, Ythier H, Loeuille GA, Lebeq MF, Dhondt JL & Farriaux JP. Etude de la croissance et de la maturation osseuse au cours de l'hypotyroïdie congenitale depistée en période néonatale. A propos de 82 observations. Archives Françaises de Pediatrie 1989; 46: 723–8.

Moschini P, Costa P, Marinelli E, Maggioni G, Sorcini Carta M, Fazzini C et al. Longitudinal assessment of children with congenital hypothyroidism detected by neonatal screening. Helv Paediatrica Acta 1986; 41: 415–24.

New England Congenital Hypothyroidism Collaborative. Elementary school performance of children with congenital hypothyroidism. J Pediatr 1990; 116: 27–32.

New England Congenital Hypothyroidism Collaborative. Correlation of cognitive test scores and adequacy of treatment in adolescents with congenital hypothyroidism. J Pediatr 1994; 124: 383–7.

Oerbeck B, Sundet K, Kase BF, Heyerdahl S. Congenital hypothyroidism: no adverse effects of high dose thyroxine treatment on adult memory, attention, and behaviour. Arch Dis Child 2005; 90: 132–7.

Pniewska-Siark B, Jeziorowska A, Bobeff I, Lewiński A. Analysis of physical and mental development of children with aplasia, hypoplasia and ectopy of the thyroid gland. Endocr Regul 2006; 40: 7–14.

Raiti S, Newns GH. Cretinism: early diagnosis and its relation to mental prognosis. Arch Dis Child 1971; 46: 692–4.

Rochiccioli P, Roge B, Dechaux E et al. School achievement in children with hypothyroidism detected at birth and search for predictive factors. Horm Res 1992; 38: 236–40.

Rovet JF. Congenital hypothyroidism: an analysis of persisting deficits and associated factors. Child Neuropsychol 2002; 8: 150–62.

Rovet JF. Long-term neuropsychological sequelae of early-treated congenital hypothyroidism: effects in adolescence. Acta Paediatr Suppl 1999; 88 (432): 88–95.

Rovet J, Alvarez M. Thyroid hormone and attention in children with congenital hypothyroidism. J Pediatr Endocrinol Metab 1996; 9: 63–6.

Rovet J, Daneman D. Congenital hypothyroidism. A review of current diagnostic and treatment practices in relation to neuropsychologic outcome. Pediatr Drugs 2003; 5: 141–9.

Rovet JF, Ehrlich R. Psychoeducational outcome in children with early-treated congenital hypothyroidism. Pediatrics 2000; 105 515–22

Rovet J, Ehrlich R, Sorbara D. Neurodevelopment in infants and preschool children with congenital hypothyroidism: etiological and treatment factors affecting outcome. J Pediatr Psychol 1992; 17: 187–213.

Salerno M, Micillo M, Di Maio S, Capalbo D, Ferri P, Lettiero T, Tenore A. Longitudinal growth, sexual maturation and final height in patients with congenital hypothyroidism detected by neonatal screening. Eur J Endocrinol 2001; 145: 377–83.

Siragusa V, Terenghi A, Rondanini GF, Vigone MC, Galli L, Weber G et al. Congenital hypothyroidism: auxological retrospective study during the first six years of age. J Endocrinol Invest 1996; 19: 224–9.

Tillotson SL, Fuggle PW, Smith I, Ades A, Grant D. Relation between biochemical severity and intelligence in early-treated congenital hypothyroidism. A threshold effect. Br Med J 1994; 309: 440–5.

Session V

Clinical Cases and Guidelines

Chairpersons: V. Pirags (Riga), J. Lazarus (Cardiff)

18 Guidelines on Thyroid Disease in Pregnancy

M. Abalovich

Sarmiento 2012, 2 A (CP 1044), Buenos Aires, Argentina

Abstract

From the early stages of pregnancy, the maternal thyroid must increase its hormone production, thus allowing not only to keep the maternal euthyroidism but also to secure the necessary hormone levels for proper foetal development. However, this balance might become lost, if there is an insufficient iodine contribution or if different pathologies affecting the gland prevent the achievement of such a balance. Therefore, it is of particular interest to elaborate recommendations permitting an adequate management of the thyroid alterations during pregnancy and postpartum, tending to achieve an adequate maternal and foetal/neonatal health. For this purpose, and commissioned by the Endocrine Society (USA), guidelines were recently elaborated and the recommendations were published. Some of the conclusions stemming from these recommendations are as follows. 1) Foetal and maternal hypothyroidism (overt and subclinical) should be diagnosed and adequately treated, because of the complications that it may cause on mother and foetus. 2) Overt hyperthyroidism (mainly caused by Graves' disease) may provoke alterations for the mother and the offspring; treatment with antithyroid drugs effects their prevention, although it may also cause unwanted side-effects on the foetus. 3) The hyperemesis gravidarum may be associated to hyperthyroidism but, unlike what has been mentioned in item 2), this is temporary and treatment with antithyroid drugs is seldom required. 4) Although a positive association exists between the presence of thyroid antibodies and pregnancy loss, universal screening for thyroid antibodies and possible treatment with levothyroxine (only one adequate trial has demonstrated the benefit of the intervention) cannot be recommended. 5) Fine-needle aspiration cytology should be performed for dominant thyroid nodules. If there is a differentiated thyroid carcinoma diagnosis, surgery should be offered during pregnancy but, if the decision is to postpone surgery till after delivery, this does not usually worsen the prognosis. [131]Iodine administration must be avoided during pregnancy and lactation. 6) Women should increase their iodine intake during pregnancy and breast-feeding. 7) Since there is not sufficient information so as to recommend universal screening for thyroid dysfunction in women during pregnancy and postpartum, case finding targeted to specific groups of patients who are at increased risk is recommended.

18.1 Introduction

To cover the physiological necessities during pregnancy, the maternal thyroid must increase its hormone production by approximately 50% with regards to the one observed prior to conception. It is necessary for the gland to adapt itself to a new balance, balance which is often achieved without difficulty in iodine-sufficient areas; however, this does not happen when the hormone production is limited, as can be observed in moderately or severely iodine-insufficient areas.

Iodine deficiency (ID), known to affect over 1.2 billion individuals, can provoke not only maternal hypothyroidism or hypothyroxinaemia but also affect the offspring, causing a deficit in their thyroid function and/or alterations in their mental development. Thus, it is essential to establish patterns to achieve an adequate iodine nutrition status during pregnancy and its adequate supervision.

In iodine-sufficient areas, the main cause of maternal hypothyroidism is the autoimmune (Hashimoto's) thyroiditis; there is some controversy about subclinical hypothyroidism (SCH) deserving a consideration different from that for overt hypothyroidism (OH). Likewise, the impact that thyroid autoimmunity in euthyroid women may have on pregnancy generates uncertainty. A higher risk of miscarriages and prematurity in this condition has been described, and the benefits of levothyroxine treatment are a subject of debate.

The finding of inhibited TSH during pregnancy forces the diagnosis of hyperthyroidism, mainly provoked by Graves' disease. It is important not to mistake it for gestational thyrotoxicosis with hyperemesis gravidarum or inhibited levels that a certain number of normal pregnant women might present, because hyperthyroidism due to Graves' disease, untreated or inadequately treated, may cause complications to mother and foetus. The thyroid dysfunction may not be the only problem affecting the pregnant woman. Thyroid nodules, already known or previously ignored, can be diagnosed and, in this sense, the discussion on the management of thyroid cancer during pregnancy acquires special interest.

After delivery, the woman may present with alterations of her thyroid function (postpartum thyroiditis), especially those with positive antithyroid antibodies. The dysfunction is typically transient but it is also linked with permanent hypothyroidism. Finally, considering the complications that an unknown thyroid dysfunction may cause during pregnancy and postpartum, the discussion remains open on whether thyroid function screening should be universally done on all pregnant women or only on those groups at high risk.

Hence, it is absolutely essential to establish guidelines for the management of thyroid pathology during pregnancy and postpartum, that are useful for endocrinologists, obstetricians, specialists in reproduction, internists, etc., taking into consideration that interdisciplinary team work is of fundamental relevance for this kind of patients.

18.2   Methods

In 2005, an international task force was created under the Endocrine Society auspices, and with Dr. L. de Groot as the chairman, to elaborate an evidence-based guideline for the management of thyroid pathology during pregnancy and postpartum. Representatives from the main thyroid societies in the world, from the Association of American Clinical Endocrinologists and the Endocrine Society itself were summoned. After two-years' work, the guidelines have been published (Abalovich et al., 2007a) and reprinted (Abalovich et al., 2007b).

The first step was to work out clinically relevant questions on the following issues:
1. hypothyroidism and pregnancy: maternal and foetal aspects,
2. hyperthyroidism and pregnancy: maternal and foetal aspects,
3. gestational hyperemesis and hyperthyroidism,
4. autoimmune thyroid disease and miscarriage,
5. thyroid nodules and cancer,
6. iodine nutrition during pregnancy,
7. postpartum thyroiditis,
8. screening for thyroid dysfunction during pregnancy.

Once the questions were posed, the evidence, which would allow elaborating the recommendations, was searched for. Hereby, mainly original works published in English in the last twenty years were reviewed. The recommendations were classified according to the grades of the U.S. Preventive Services Task Force (USPSTF), taking into account the strength of evidence and magnitude of net benefit, as follows:
A) strongly recommends,
B) recommends,
C) no recommendation for or against,
D) recommends against,
I) evidence is insufficient to recommend for or against.

Likewise, the USPSTF grades of quality of the evidence were considered as follows:
– Good: evidence included consistent results from well-designed, well-conducted studies.

– Fair: evidence is sufficient but limited by the number or the consistency of the studies.
– Poor: evidence is insufficient.

In addition to the USPSTF grading, the appropriate level of the recommendation was indicated by the GRADE system: 0–1–2 (strong, moderate, low).

The recommendations stated in this chapter correspond to the literature (Abalovich, 2007a).

18.3 Questions – Evidence – Recommendations

18.3.1 Hypothyroidism and Pregnancy: Maternal and Foetal Aspects

18.3.1.1 What Risks does Hypothyroidism Imply for Mother and Foetus?

Untreated or inadequately treated hypothyroidism during pregnancy may lead to obstetric maternal complications, such as incremented miscarriage prevalence, anaemia, gestational hypertension, premature rupture of membranes, placental abruption and postpartum haemorrhages. The adequate treatment with thyroxine prevents the risk of these complications (Montoro et al., 1981; Davis et al., 1988; Leung et al., 1993; Abalovich et al., 2002). Additionally, untreated maternal hypothyroidism may cause complications for the foetus and the newborn such as: prematurity, low birth weight, neonatal respiratory distress and foetal and perinatal death (Montoro et al.,1981; Davis et al., 1988; Leung et al., 1993; Allan et al., 2000; Abalovich et al., 2002; Casey et al., 2005; Stagnaro-Green et al., 2005). The above-mentioned complications, both maternal and foetal, more often appear in pregnant women with OH than with SCH. Besides, there is strong evidence that the maternal thyroid hormone is an important factor contributing to the development of the foetal brain. This acquires special relevance during the first trimester of pregnancy, when the foetal thyroid does not yet produce thyroid hormone and the contribution to the foetus depends solely on the maternal transfer through the placenta (Morreale de Escobar et al., 2004). Different studies have demonstrated there is a significant risk of alterations in the neuropsychological development, IQ scores and school learning abilities in the offspring of women who suffered hypothyroidism or hypothyroxinaemia, at least during the first trimester of pregnancy. (Haddow et al., 1999; Pop et al., 1999; Rovet, 2004).

Recommendation 1.1: Both maternal and foetal hypothyroidism are known to have serious adverse effects on the foetus. Therefore, maternal hypothyroidism should be avoided. USPSTF recommendation level A, evidence fair, grade 1.

18.3.1.2 What Happens when Hypothyroidism is Diagnosed before Pregnancy?

There is a known association between OH and SCH and decreased fertility, although hypothyroidism does not preclude the possibility to conceive (Abalovich et al., 2002). Thus, it is very important to establish an adequate treatment or adjust the thyroxine dose before pregnancy to reach TSH levels that will secure the euthyroidism of female patients in childbearing age. In this sense, TSH levels not higher than 2.5 mIU/L seem adequate, although some authors consider that they should not be higher than 0.7 mIU/L especially in thyroidectomised patients (Rotondi et al, 2004).

Recommendation 1.2: If hypothyroidism has been diagnosed before pregnancy, we recommended adjustment of the preconception T_4 dose to reach a TSH level not higher than 2.5 mIU/L before pregnancy. USPSTF recommendation level I, evidence poor.

18.3.1.3 What Happens with the Levothyroxine Doses when the Hypothyroidism is Treated before Pregnancy?

Most women receiving levothyroxine prior to pregnancy (up to an 80%) have to increase the dose during pregnancy (Mandel et al.,1990; Kaplan, 1992; Alexander et al., 2004). Different reasons can explain the requirement increase: the precocious increase in thyroxine-binding globulin (TBG), the larger distribution volume of thyroid hormones, the increased placental transport and metabolism of maternal T_4. In addition to this, the stimulus that the chorionic gonadotrophic hormone (hCG) exerts on the maternal thyroid should be added. The need to adjust the dosage can manifest early during pregnancy (4–6 weeks), though a smaller percentage of women can manifest at later stages (Mandel, 2004). The magnitude of the increment (30–50%) depends on the hypothyroidism aetiology: women without residual functional thyroid tissue (radioiodine ablation, total thyroidectomy, congenital agenesis) require a greater increment in thyroxine dosage than women with Hashimoto's thyroiditis, who usually have some residual thyroid tissue. (Kaplan, 1992). Some authors have observed that the offspring of women with suboptimally treated hypothyroidism may be at risk for selective cognitive deficits (Rovet, 2004). That is why some thyrodologists propose incrementing the LT_4 dose by approximately 30% as soon as pregnancy becomes known (Alexander et al., 2004).

Recommendation 1.3: The thyroxine dose often needs to be incremented by 4–6 weeks gestation and may require a 30–50% increment in dosage. USPSTF recommendation level A, evidence good, grade 1.

18.3.1.4 How is Hypothyroidism Diagnosed, Treated and Monitored during Pregnancy?

In order to diagnose primary hypothyroidism during pregnancy, it is necessary to determine when TSH is considered high. It is not useful to take the values above for the method top limit (4 mIU/L) for 28% of SCH patients would not be diagnosed (Dashe et al., 2005). On the other hand, it seems more useful to establish "trimester-specific" normal values. Serum TSH levels above 2.5 mIU/L (first trimester) and 3.1–3.5 (second and third trimester) may already be indicative of hypothyroidism (Panesar et al., 2001). In order to differentiate OH from SCH and diagnose hypothyroxinaemia, it is imperative to have reliable T_4 values during pregnancy. The free T_4 determination should be interpreted carefully because the values vary during gestation and the different assays may be influenced due to changes in the transport proteins. It has been proposed to set "laboratory-specific" and "trimester-specific" ranges. Considering the existing difficulties with free T_4, some authors have proposed the measurement of total T_4 in pregnancy, multiplying the non-pregnant range by 1.5-fold (Mandel et al., 2005). Treatment with levothyroxine must be initiated (approximately 2.0–2.4 µg/kg/day) as soon as OH is diagnosed during pregnancy. Serum TSH and free T_4 (or total T_4) should be measured approximately 1 month after the initiation of treatment. Once the tests of thyroid function have

been normalised by treatment they should be monitored every 6–8 weeks.

Recommendation 1.4: If OH is diagnosed during pregnancy, thyroid function tests should be normalised as rapidly as possible. Thyroxine dosage should be titrated to rapidly reach and thereafter maintain serum TSH concentrations of less than 2.5 mIU/L in the first trimester (or 3 mIU/L in the second and third trimesters) or to trimester-specific normal ranges. Thyroid function tests should be re-measured within 30–40 days. USPSTF recommendation level A, evidence good, grade 1.

18.3.1.5 What Happens when a Woman has Thyroid Autoimmunity during Pregnancy?

It has been proved that women with thyroid autoimmunity (TAI) who are euthyroid in early pregnancy have a significant risk of developing hypothyroidism during gestation. Of the 87 euthyroid TPOAb-positive women studied by Glinoer et al. (1994), 40% had a serum TSH ≥ 3 mIU/L (almost half of them exceeding 4 mIU/L) at parturition. Recently, in a prospective work, Negro et al. (2006) observed that the percentages of miscarriages and premature deliveries were higher in euthyroid TPO Ab-positive pregnant women than in TPO Ab-negative ones.

Recommendation 1.5: Women with TAI who are euthyroid in the early stages of pregnancy are at risk of developing hypothyroidism and should be monitored for elevation of TSH above the normal range. USPSTF recommendation level A, evidence good, grade 1.

18.3.1.6 Does Subclinical Hypothyroidism Deserve a Different Consideration from Overt Hypothyroidism?

Though less frequently than OH, SCH may give rise to complications in the mother, the foetus and the neonate: miscarriage, prematurity, gestational hypertension, placental abruption and neonatal respiratory distress syndrome (Leung et al., 1993; Abalovich et al., 2002; Casey et al., 2005; Stagnaro Green et al., 2005). Besides, 47 out of the 62 hypothyroidal women described having children with IQ deficits, and suffered from SCH

(Haddow et al, 1999). The levothyroxine treatment has been able to diminish the frequency of abortions and prematurity in SCH pregnant women and in euthyroid pregnant patients with TPOAb-positive and TSH levels higher (although within the normal range) than those with TPOAb-negative (Abalovich et al., 2002; Negro et al., 2006).

Recommendation 1.6: SCH has been shown to be associated with an adverse outcome for both the mother and offspring. Thyroxine treatment has been shown to improve obstetric outcome, but has not been proved to modify long-term neurological development in the offspring. However, given that the potential benefits outweigh the potential risks, thyroxine replacement in women with SCH is recommended. For obstetric outcome, USPSTF recommendation level B, evidence fair, grade 1. For neurological outcome, USPSTF recommendation level I, evidence poor.

18.3.1.7 What Happens with Levothyroxine after Delivery?

After parturition, most patients need to decrease the levothyroxine dosage received during pregnancy. It must be taken into account that patients with evidence of thyroid autoimmunity are at risk of developing postpartum thyroiditis, and this could justify the differences in the pre- and post-pregnancy thyroxine requirements (Caixas et al., 1999).

Recommendation 1.7: After delivery, most hypothyroid women need to decrease the thyroxine dosage received during pregnancy. USPSTF recommendation level A, evidence good, grade 1.

18.3.2 Hyperthyroidism and Pregnancy: Maternal and Foetal Aspects

18.3.2.1 What Happens if a Subnormal Serum TSH Concentration is Detected during Gestation?

The simple finding of subnormal serum TSH levels during the first trimester of pregnancy should not be interpreted as a diagnosis of hyperthyroidism. The median serum TSH level in said span has been estimated at 0.8 mIU/L with a lower limit of 0.03 mIU/L (2.5th percentile) (Panesar et al., 2001) and it is considered that 18% of normal pregnant women may present TSH inhibited levels. This matches the peaks in the hCG level and the consequent increase of free T_4 although within the normal range. Besides, over 60% of patients with hyperemesis gravidarum may present subnormal TSH even with high free T_4 (gestational thyrotoxicosis). It is important to differentiate this from hyperthyroidism provoked by Graves' disease due to the complications that untreated or inadequately treated overt hyperthyroidism may cause on mother and foetus: gestational hypertension, heart failure, thyroid storm, placental abruption, miscarriage, prematurity, foetal and perinatal death, low birth weight, congenital malformations and neonatal hyperthyroidism (Chan and Mandel, 2007).

Recommendation 2.1: If a subnormal serum TSH concentration is detected during gestation, hyperthyroidism must be differentiated from both normal physiology of pregnancy and hyperemesis gravidarum because of the adverse effects of overt hyperthyroidism on the mother and foetus. Differentiation of Graves' disease from gestational thyrotoxicosis is supported by the presence of clinical evidence of autoimmunity, a typical goitre and the presence of TRAb. USPSTF recommendation level A, evidence good, grade 1.

18.3.2.2 What about the Treatment for Hyperthyroidism during Gestation?

The treatment of choice for overt hyperthyroidism during pregnancy is antithyroid drugs (ATD). Propyltiouracil (PTU) and methimazole (MMI) are the substances commonly used. Both go through the placenta alike (Mortimer et al., 1997) and exert similar effects on the maternal and foetal function. The doses should be appropriate for the maternal hyperthyroidism control but not excessive for the foetus; this is generally achieved by keeping the maternal free T_4 levels in the non-pregnant normal upper limit.

ATD have been involved in generating congenital malformations, more frequently MMI has been more linked to the production of aplasia cutis, choanal and oesophageal atresia, hypothelia and athelia, hypospadia, etc., than PTU (aorta atresia, choanal atresia) (Cheron et al., 1981; Di

Gianantonio et al., 2001). Nevertheless some authors argue whether it is the ATD or the untreated hyperthyroidism during the first trimester that causes the teratogenicity (Momotani et al.,1984).

When, for different reasons, ATD cannot be used or fail in their therapeutic function or severe hyperthyroidism should persist, subtotal thyroidectomy may be indicated, preferably during the second trimester so as to reduce risks and a few days pre-treatment with β-blocker and potassium iodide. Therapy with ^{131}I must not be given during pregnancy. However, accidental administration may occur. If this happens after the first trimester, the foetus is at high risk of presenting hypothyroidism requiring intrauterine thyroid hormone replacement and treatment throughout his life (Stoffer and Hamburger, 1976).

Recommendation 2.2.1: For overt hyperthyroidism due to Graves' disease or hyperfunctioning thyroid nodules, ATD therapy should be either initiated (for those with new diagnoses) or adjusted (for those with a prior history) to maintain the maternal thyroid hormone for free T_4 in the upper non-pregnant reference range. USPSTF recommendation level A, evidence good, grade 1.

Recommendation 2.2.2: Because available evidence suggests that MMI may be associated with congenital malformations, PTU should be used as a first-line drug, if available, especially during the first-trimester organogenesis. MMI may be prescribed if PTU is not available, or if a patient cannot tolerate or has an adverse response to PTU. USPSTF recommendation level B, evidence fair, grade 1.

Recommendation 2.2.3: Subtotal thyroidectomy may be indicated during pregnancy as a therapy for maternal Graves' disease if 1) a patient has a severe adverse reaction to ATD therapy, 2) persistently high doses of ATD are required, or 3) a patient is non-adherent to ATD therapy and has uncontrolled hyperthyroidism. The optimal timing for surgery is in the second trimester. USPSTF recommendation level I, evidence poor.

Recommendation 2.2.4: ^{131}I should not be given to a woman who is or may be pregnant. If inadvertently treated, the patient should be promptly informed of the radiation danger to the foetus, including thyroid destruction if treated after the 12th week of gestation. USPSTF recommendation level A, evidence good, grade 1. There are not data for or against recommending termination of pregnancy after ^{131}I exposure. USPSTF recommendation level I, evidence poor.

18.3.2.3 Should Subclinical Hyperthyroidism be Treated during Pregnancy?

It has been recently published that pregnancy complications and perinatal morbidity or mortality were not increased in women with subclinical hyperthyroidism (Casey, 2006).

Recommendation 2.3: There is no evidence that treatment of subclinical hyperthyroidism improves pregnancy outcome and treatment could potentially affect foetal outcome. USPSTF recommendation level I, evidence poor.

18.3.2.4 Should Thyroid Receptor Antibodies (TRAb) be Measured during Pregnancy in a Woman with Graves' Disease? What about the Newborns?

Between 1% and 5% of mothers with Graves' disease may present neonatal hyperthyroidism, though larger percentages have been described (Peleg et al., 2002). The neonatal disease is due to the transplacental crossing of high titres of stimulating TRAb, independently from the maternal thyroid functional state. Thus, the detection of high TRAb levels in the second half of the pregnancy constitutes an important predicting factor of foetal hyperthyroidism, added to the detection of tachycardia and foetal goitre, intrauterine growth retardation, etc. Determining a cut-off in the TRAb measurement for the prognosis is not easy for it depends on the assay used and if the TRAb binding is measured or, specifically, the stimulating fraction.

Recommendation 2.4.1: Because thyroid receptor antibodies freely cross the placenta and can stimulate the foetal thyroid, these antibodies should be measured by the end of the second trimester in mothers with current Graves' disease or with a history of Graves' disease and treatment with ^{131}I or thyroidectomy before pregnancy or with a previous neonate with hyperthyroidism. Women who have a negative TRAb and do not require ATD, have a very low risk of foetal or neonatal thyroid dysfunction. USPSTF recommendation level B, evidence fair, grade 1.

Recommendation 2.4.2: All newborns of mothers with Graves' disease should be evaluated by a medical care provider for thyroid dysfunction and treated if necessary. USPSTF recommendation level B, evidence fair, grade 1.

18.3.2.5 Should Foetal Ultrasound be Performed in Women with Graves' Disease?

Luton et al. (2005) performed ultrasound evaluations of foetal thyroid and bone age on 71 pregnant patients with Graves' disease. The presence of foetal goitre, accelerated bone aging and high maternal TRAb titres corresponded to the foetal hyperthyroidism diagnosis. On the other hand, the presence of foetal goitre in mothers receiving ATD led to the diagnosis of foetal hypothyroidism due to transplacental ATD crossing.

Recommendation 2.5: In women with elevated TRAb or in women treated with ATD, foetal ultrasound should be performed to look for evidence of foetal thyroid dysfunction, which could include growth restriction, hydrops, presence of goitre, advanced bone age or cardiac failure. USPSTF recommendation level B, evidence fair, grade 1.

18.3.2.6 Umbilical Blood Sampling in Women with Thyroid Disease in Pregnancy: Is it Necessary?

Umbilical cord blood sampling carries a risk of foetal loss of 1 – 2 % (Van Kamp et al., 2005).

Recommendation 2.6: Umbilical blood sampling should be considered only if the diagnosis of foetal thyroid disease is not reasonably certain from the clinical data and the information gained would change the treatment. USPTF recommendation level B, evidence fair, grade 2.

18.3.3 Gestational Hyperemesis and Hyperthyroidism

It is estimated that between 30 % and 65 % of women with hyperemesis gravidarum may present hyperthyroidism. It corresponds to clinical and/or biochemical thyrotoxicosis in the first trimester of gestation with posterior spontaneous remission, associated with hyperemesis, dehydration, 5 % weight loss and ketonuria. Thyrotoxicosis appears during gestations, with no symptoms between these. There is usually no goitre or this is very small. There is no evidence of clinical or biochemical autoimmunity. Few are the cases where hyperthyroidism requires a specific treatment (Goodwin et al., 1992).

Recommendation 3.1: Thyroid function tests should be measured in all patients with hyperemesis gravidarum. USPTF recommendation level B, evidence poor, grade 2.

Recommendation 3.2: Few women with hyperemesis gravidarum will require ATD treatment. USPSTF recommendation level A, evidence good, grade 1. Overt hyperthyroidism believed to be due to coincident Graves' disease should be treated with ATD. USPSTF recommendation level B, evidence fair, grade 1. Gestational hyperthyroidism with clearly elevated thyroid hormone levels (free T_4 above the reference range or total $T_4 > 150$ % of the top normal pregnancy value and TSH < 0.1 mIU/L) and evidence of hyperthyroidism may require treatment as long as clinically necessary. USPSTF recommendation level I, evidence poor.

18.3.4 Autoimmune Thyroid Disease and Miscarriage

18.3.4.1 Is Levothyroxine Treatment Useful for Thyroid Antibody-Positive Euthyroid Women?

It has been demonstrated that the miscarriage risk is higher in TPOAb-positive euthyroid pregnant women and in non-pregnant TPOAb-positive ones with recurrent abortion (Prummel and Wiersinga, 2004). But even though TSH levels and free T_4 are within normal ranges, it has been observed that TSH levels are statistically higher and free T_4 levels are lower in women with positive thyroid antibodies (Bagis et al., 2001). Recently a prospective and randomised trial has been published showing a decrease in miscarriage and preterm delivery rates in TPOAb-positive euthyroid pregnant women treated with levothyroxine (Negro et al, 2006).

Recommendation 4: Although a positive association exists between the presence of thyroid antibodies and pregnancy loss, universal screening for thyroid antibodies and possible treatment cannot be recommended at this time. As of this date, only one adequately designed intervention trial has demonstrated a decrease in the miscarriage rate in thyroid antibody-positive euthyroid women. USPSTF recommendation level C, evidence fair, grade 2.

18.3.5 Thyroid Nodules and Cancer

18.3.5.1 What is the Management of Thyroid Nodules and Cancer during Pregnancy?

The number and the volume of the preexisting nodules may increase during pregnancy (Kung et al., 2002.).

As in non-pregnant women, fine needle aspiration (FNA) biopsy guided by ultrasound constitutes the main diagnostic procedure to be used in nodules larger than 1 cm. It is not simple to determine the prevalence of thyroid cancer in pregnancy considering the low number of data and the limitations of the studies. Homogeneous groups of pregnant and non-pregnant women with differentiated thyroid cancer have been studied. Pregnancy did not produce an increment in local recurrence, metastases or death by cancer

(Moosa and Mazzaferri, 1997). Thyroidectomised women during pregnancy (ideally during the 2nd trimester) often have an outcome similar to that of women who delayed surgery until postpartum. (Moosa and Mazzaferri, 1997; Yasween et al., 2005). It is convenient that women with thyroid cancer or nodules with rapid growth should receive a suppressive dosage of thyroxine during pregnancy. In differentiated thyroid cancer, the ^{131}I ablative therapy should be administered postpartum; it will be necessary to discontinue lactation and provide counselling on the circumstances of a future pregnancy.

Recommendation 5.1: FNA cytology should be performed for single or dominant thyroid nodules larger than 1 cm discovered during pregnancy. Ultrasound-guided FNA may have an advantage for minimising inadequate sampling. USPSTF recommendation level B, evidence fair, grade 1.

Recommendation 5.2: When nodules are discovered in the first or early second trimester to be malignant on cytopathological analysis or exhibit rapid growth, pregnancy should not be interrupted but surgery should be offered in the second trimester, before foetal viability. Women found to have cytology indicative of papillary cancer or follicular neoplasm without evidence of advanced disease, who prefer to wait until the postpartum period for definitive surgery, may be reassured that most well-differentiated thyroid cancers are slow growing and that surgical treatment soon after delivery is unlikely to change the prognosis. USPSTF recommendation level B, evidence fair, grade 1.

Recommendation 5.3: It is appropriate to administer thyroid hormone to achieve a suppressive but detectable TSH in pregnant women with a previously treated thyroid cancer, or an FNA positive for or suspicious of cancer, and those who choose to delay surgical treatment until postpartum. High-risk patients may benefit more from a greater degree of TSH suppression compared with low-risk patients. The free T_4 or total levels should ideally not be increased above the normal range for pregnancy. USPSTF recommendation level I, evidence poor.

Recommendation 5.4: RAI with ^{131}I should not be given to women who are breast-feeding. USPSTF recommendation level B, evidence fair. Furthermore, pregnancy should be avoided for 6 months to 1 year in women with thyroid cancer receiving therapeutic RAI doses to ensure stability of thyroid function and confirm remission of thyroid cancer. USPSTF recommendation level B, evidence fair, grade 1.

18.3.6 Iodine Nutrition during Pregnancy

18.3.6.1 Considering the Effect Low Iodine Ingestion may Cause on Mother and Foetus, what are the Recommendations to Secure an Adequate Iodine Contribution in Women of Child-Bearing Age, during Pregnancy and Breast-Feeding?

There is evidence that the iodine deficit during early pregnancy may lead to maternal hypothyroxinaemia and impaired psychoneurointellectual development of the offspring (Glinoer, 2003). That is the reason why it would be ideal to secure an adequate ingestion of iodine in the child-bearing age woman, this intake has been estimated in 150 µg/d and is usually achieved through salt iodisation. During pregnancy, the iodine intake needs to be increased up to approximately 250 µg/d, to achieve the necessary increment in thyroid hormone production (Glinoer, 2004), but without going over an upper limit of approximately 500 µg/d which may be self-defeating in women with underlying thyroid disorders (Roti and Vagenakis, 2005). Administration of exogenous iodine supplements should be taken into account, particularly in areas with a known iodine deficit and without an adequate salt iodisation programme. At the population level, the monitoring of adequate iodine intake is given by the urinary iodine concentration, but with limitations for the individual evaluation.

Recommendation 6.1: Women in child-bearing age should have an average iodine intake of 150 µg/d. During pregnancy and breast-feeding, women should increase their daily intake to 250 µg on average. USPSTF recommendation level A, evidence good, grade 1.

Recommendation 6.2: Iodine intake during pregnancy and breast-feeding should not exceed twice the daily recommended nutrient intake, i.e., 500 µg iodine/d. USPSTF recommendation level I, evidence poor.

Recommendation 6.3: To assess the adequacy of the iodine intake during pregnancy in a population, the urinary iodine concentration (UIC) should be measured in a representative cohort of the population. UIC should ideally range between 150–250 µg/L. USPSTF recommendation level A, evidence good, grade 1.

Recommendation 6.4: To reach the daily RNI for iodine, multiple means must be considered, tailored to the iodine intake level in a given population. Therefore, different situations should be distinguished: 1) countries with iodine sufficiency and/or with a well-established universal salt iodisation (USI) programme, 2) countries without a USI programme or with an established USI programme where the coverage is known to be only partial, and 3) remote areas with no accessible USI programme and difficult socio-economic conditions. USPSTF recommendation level A, evidence good, grade 1.

18.3.7 Postpartum Thyroiditis

18.3.7.1 How should Monitoring of the Thyroid Function be Performed after Delivery to Allow Diagnosis of Postpartum Thyroiditis?

The prevalence of postpartum thyroiditis (PPT) varies widely between 1.1% and 21.1%, although on the average it could be set between 5% and 9%, this being higher in patients with type 1 diabetes mellitus (DM). Almost 90% of women with PPT present positive TPOAb, so the detection of this antibody becomes the most important predicting factor for the development of PPT. Considering that, the evidence is still insufficient to justify the universal screening of all women after delivery (Amino et al., 1999; Stagnaro-Green, 2002). TSH measurement in those patients at risk (TPOAb-positive and/or with type 1 DM) seems appropriate. Regarding the possible association between either PPT or TPOAb-positivity and postpartum depression, opinions are contradictory. That is the reason why this association could not be proved in all cases (Harris et al., 1992). Regarding treatment, propranolol administration is prescribed in symptomatic women during the hyperthyroid phase; the therapeutic decision in the hypothyroid phase depends on the severity of hypothyroidism and if the patient is looking forward to a new pregnancy. PPT is usually temporary and most women return to euthyroidism, with persistent underlying chronic autoimmune thyroiditis. However, 20–64% of women later develop permanent hypothyroidism, this is the reason why a long-term follow-up should be maintained (Premawardhana et al., 2000).

Recommendation 7.1: There are insufficient data to recommend screening of all women for PPT. USPSTF recommendation level I, evidence poor.

Recommendation 7.2: Women known to be TPOAb-positive should have a TSH performed at 3 and 6 months postpartum. USPSTF recommendation level A, evidence good, grade 1.

Recommendation 7.3: The prevalence of PPT in women with type 1 DM is 3-fold greater than in the general population. Postpartum screening (TSH determination) is recommended for women with type1 DM at 3 and 6 months postpartum. USPSTF recommendation level B, evidence fair, grade 1.

Recommendation 7.4: Women with a history of PPT have a markedly increased risk of developing permanent primary hypothyroidism in the 5–10 year period following the episode of PPT. An annual TSH level measurement should be performed in these women. USPSTF recommendation level A, evidence good, grade 1.

Recommendation 7.5: Asymptomatic women, with PPT and a TSH above the reference range but below 10 mIU/L, not planning a subsequent pregnancy do not necessarily require intervention but should be remonitored after 4–8 weeks if untreated. Symptomatic women and women with a TSH level above normal, who are attempting pregnancy, should be treated with levothyroxine. USPSTF recommendation level B, evidence fair, grade 1.

Recommendation 7.6: There is insufficient evidence to conclude whether an association exists between postpartum depression and either PPT or positive thyroid antibody (in women who did not develop PPT). USPSTF recommendation level I, evidence poor. However, as hypothyroidism is a potentially reversible cause of depression, women with postpartum depression should be screened for hypothyroidism and appropriately treated. USPSTF recommendation level B, evidence fair, grade 2.

18.3.8 Screening for Thyroid Dysfunction during Pregnancy

18.3.8.1 Which Women should be Screened for TSH during Pregnancy?

So far, there is no firm evidence in favour of or against universal screening of TSH during pregnancy. Identifying patients belonging to risk groups is accepted as more reasonable. Recently, however, a prospective study in 1580 women at their first prenatal visit reported that if the criterion of only evaluating high-risk patients were adopted, 30% of overt or subclinical hypothyroid cases would be lost (CITA Vaidya).

Recommendation 8: We recommend case finding among the following groups of women at high risk for thyroid dysfunction: 1) women with a history of hyperthyroid or hypothyroid disease, PPT or thyroid lobectomy, 2) women with a family history of thyroid disease, 3) women with a goitre, 4) women with thyroid antibodies (when known), 5) women with symptoms or clinical signs suggestive of thyroid underfunction or overfunction, 6) women with type I diabetes mellitus,

7) women with other autoimmune disorders, 8) women with infertility, 9) women with prior therapeutic head or neck irradiation, 10) women with a prior history of miscarriage or preterm delivery. USPSTF recommendation level B, evidence fair, grade1.

18.4 Conclusions

The stated recommendations should constitute a useful tool allowing endocrinologists, obstetricians, etc., as a proper team work working together to achieve the adequate management of the thyroidal alterations during pregnancy and postpartum, and a optimal foetal/neonatal and maternal health.

Acknowledgments

Members of the Guidelines Task Force: N. Amino, L. Barbour, R. Cobin L. De Groot (chairman), D. Glinoer, S. Mandel, and A. Stagnaro-Green are acknowledged for their help and interest.

References

Abalovich M, Amino N, Barbour L et al. Executive Summary: Management of thyroid dysfunction during pregnancy and postpartum: an Endocrine Society clinical practice guideline. Thyroid 2007; 17: 1159–67.

Abalovich M, Amino N, Barbour L et al. Management of thyroid dysfunction during pregnancy and postpartum: an Endocrine Society clinical practice guideline. J Clin Endocrinol Metab 2007; 92: S1–S47.

Abalovich M, Gutierrez S, Alcaraz G et al. Overt and subclinical hypothyroidism complicating pregnancy. Thyroid 2002; 12: 63–8.

Alexander EK, Marqusee E, Lawrance J et al. Timing and magnitude of increases in levothyroxine requirements during pregnancy in women with hypothyroidism. N Engl J Med 2004; 351: 241–9.

Allan WC, Haddow JE, Palomaki GE et al. Maternal thyroid deficiency and pregnancy complications: implications for population screening. J Med Screen 2000; 7: 127–30.

Amino N, Tada H, Hidaka Y. Postpartum autoimmune thyroid syndrome: a model of aggravation of autoimmune disease.Thyroid 1999; 9: 705–13.

Bagis T, Gokcel A, Saygili ES. Autoimmune thyroid disease in pregnancy and the post-partum period: re-

lationship to spontaneous abortion. Thyroid 2001; 11: 1049–53

Caixas A, Albareda M, Garcia-Paterson A et al. Postpartum thyroiditis in women with hypothyroidism antedating pregnancy. J Clin Endocrinol Metab 1999; 84: 4000–5.

Casey BM, Dashe JS, Wells CE et al. Subclinical hyperthyroidism and pregnancy outcome. Obstet Gynecol 2006; 107: 337–41.

Casey BM, Dashe JS, Wells CE et al. Subclinical hypothyroidism and pregnancy outcome. Obstet Gynecol 2005; 105: 239–45.

Chan GW, Mandel S. Therapy insight: management of Graves' disease during pregnancy. Nature Clinical Practice 2007; 3: 470–8.

Cheron RG, Kaplan MM, Larsen PR et al. Neonatal thyroid function after propylthiouracil therapy for maternal Graves' disease. N Engl J Med 1981; 304: 525–8.

Dashe JS, Casey BM, Wells CE et al. Thyroid-stimulating hormone in singleton and twin pregnancy: importance of gestational age-specific reference ranges. Obstet Gynecol 2005; 106: 753–7.

Davis LE, Leveno KJ, Cunningham FG. Hypothyroidism complicating pregnancy. Obstet Gynecol 1988; 72: 108–12.

Di Gianantonio E, Schaefer C, Mastroiacovo PP. Adverse effects of prenatal methimazole exposure. Teratology 2001; 64: 262–6.

Glinoer D. Feto-maternal repercussions of iodine deficiency during pregnancy. An update. Ann Endocrinol (Paris) 2003; 64: 37–44

Glinoer D. The regulation of thyroid function during normal pregnancy: importance of the iodine nutrition status. Best Pract Res Clin Endocrinol Metab 2004; 18: 133–52.

Glinoer D, Riahi M, Grun JP et al. Risk of subclinical hypothyroidism in pregnant women with asymptomatic autoimmune thyroid disorders. J Clin Endocrinol Metab 1994; 79: 197–204.

Goodwin TM, Montoro M, Mestman JH. Transient hyperthyroidism and hyperemesis gravidarum: clinical aspects. Am J Obstet Gynecol 1992; 167: 648–52

Haddow JE, Palomaki GE, Allan WC et al. Maternal thyroid defficiency during pregnancy and subsequent neuropsychological development of the child. N Engl J Med 1999; 341: 549–55.

Harris B, Othman S, Davies JA et al. Association between postpartum thyroid dysfunction and thyroid antibodies and depression. BMJ 1992; 302: 152–6.

Kaplan MM, Monitoring thyroxine treatment during pregnancy. Thyroid 1992; 2: 147–55.

Kung AW, Chau MT, Lao TT et al. The effect of pregnancy on thyroid nodule formation. J Clin Endocrinol Metab 2002; 87: 1010–4.

Leung AS, Millar LK, Koonings PP et al. Perinatal outcome in hypothyroid pregnancies. Obstet Gynecol 1993; 81: 349–53.

Luton D, Le Gac I, Vuillard E et al. Management of Graves' disease during pregnancy: the key role of fetal thyroid gland monitoring. J Clin Endocrinol Metab 2005; 90: 6093–8.

Mandel SJ, Larsen PR, Seely EW et al. Increased need for thyroxine during pregnancy in women with primary hypothyroidism. N Engl J Med 1990; 323: 91–6.

Mandel SJ, Spencer C, Hallowell JC. Are detection and treatment of thyroid insufficiency in pregnancy feasible? Thyroid 2005; 15: 44–53.

Mandel SJ. Hypothyroidism and chronic autoimmune thyroiditis in the pregnant state: maternal aspects. Best Pract Res Clin Endocrinol Metab 2004; 18: 213–24

Momotani N, Ito K, Hamada N et al. Maternal hyperthyroidism and congenital malformations in the offspring. Clin Endocrinol (Oxf) 1984; 20: 695–700.

Montoro M, Collea JV, Frasier SD et al. Successful outcome of pregnancy in women with hypothyroidism. Ann Int Med 1981; 94: 31–4.

Moosa M, Mazzaferri EL. Outcome of differentiated thyroid cancer diagnosed in pregnant women. J Clin Endocrinol Metab 1997; 82: 2862–6.

Morreale de Escobar G, Obregon MJ, Escobar del Rey F. Maternal thyroid hormones early in pregnancy and fetal brain development. Best Pract Res Clin Endocrinol Metab 2004; 18: 225–48.

Mortimer RH, CannellGR, Addison RS. Methimazole and propylthiouracil equally cross the perfused human term placental lobule. J Clin Endocrinol Metab 1997; 82: 3099–102.

Negro R, Formoso G, Mangieri T et al. Levothyroxine treatment in euthyroid pregnant women with autoimmune thyroid disease: effects on obstetrical complications. J Clin Endocrinol Metab 2006; 91: 2587–91.

Panesar NS, Li CY, Rogers MC. Reference intervals for thyroid hormones in pregnant Chinese women. Ann Clin Biochem 2001; 38: 329–32.

Peleg D, Cada S, Peleg A et al. The relationship between maternal serum thyroid-stimulating immunoglobulin and fetal neonatal thyrotoxicosis. Obstet Gynecol 2002; 99: 1040–3.

Pop VJ, Kuijpens JL, van Baar AL et al. Low maternal free thyroxine concentrations during early pregnancy are associated with impaired psychomotor development in infancy. Clin Endocrinol (Oxf) 1999; 50: 149–55.

Premawardhana LD, Parkes AB, Ammari F et al. Postpartum thyroiditis and long term thyroid status: prognostic influence of thyroid peroxidase antibodies and ultrasound echogenicity. J Clin Endocrinol Metab 2000; 85: 71–5.

Prummel MP, Wiersinga WM. Thyroid autoimmunity and miscarriage. Eur J Endocrinol 2004; 150: 751–5.

Rotondi M, Mazziotti G,Sorvillo F et al. Effects of increased thyroxine dosage pre-conception on thyroid function during early pregnancy. Eur J Endocrinol 2004; 151: 695–700

Rotti E, Vagenakis AG. Effect of excess iodide: clinical aspects. In: The Thyroid: a fundamental and clinical text. 9th ed., Braverman LE, Utiger RD, eds. Philadelphia: Lippincott, Williams & Wilkins, 2005; 288–305.

Rovet JF. Neurodevelopment consequences of maternal hypothyroidism during pregnancy. Presented in Annual Meeting of the American Thyroid Association. Thyroid 2004; 14: 710, Abstr 88.

Stagnaro-Green A, Chen X, Bogden JD et al. The thyroid and pregnancy: a novel risk for very preterm delivery. Thyroid 2005; 15: 351–7.

Stagnaro-Green A. Postpartum thyroiditis. J Clin Endocrinol Metab 2002; 87: 4042–7.

Stoffer SS, Hamburger JI. Inadvertent ^{131}I therapy for hyperthyroidism in the first trimester of pregnancy. J Nucl Med 1976; 17: 146–9.

Van Kamp IL, Klumper FJ, Oepkes D et al. Complications of intrauterine intravascular transfusion for fetal anemia due to maternal red-cell alloimmunization. Am J Obstet Gynecol 2005; 192: 171–7.

Yasmeen S, Cress R, Romano et al. Thyroid cancer in pregnancy. Int J Gynaecol Obstet 2005; 91: 15–20.

19 Universal Screening for Thyroid Dysfunction in Pregnancy?

B. Vaidya

Department of Endocrinology, Peninsula Medical School and Royal Devon & Exeter Hospital, Exeter EX2 5DW, U.K.

Abstract

Maternal thyroid hormones play an important role in the early foetal neurological development. Recent studies have shown that even mild maternal thyroid hormone insufficiency during pregnancy is associated with impaired neuropsychological development of the children and obstetric complications. Subclinical hypothyroidism during early pregnancy is common, affecting between 2–3% of pregnant women. Furthermore, about 10% of pregnant women are positive for thyroid antibodies, with an associated increased risk of hypothyroidism, miscarriages and postpartum thyroiditis. Currently, there is no clinical trial evidence to show that thyroxine replacement in pregnant women with subclinical hypothyroidism improves the neuropsychological outcomes of the children. With increasing evidence for the association between maternal subclinical hypothyroidism and adverse pregnancy outcomes but lack of intervention trials showing beneficial effect of thyroxine to prevent the adverse outcomes, it remains controversial whether all pregnant women should be systematically screened and treated for subclinical hypothyroidism. The recent guidelines from the Endocrine Society recommend thyroxine replacement in pregnant women with subclinical hypothyroidism, justified on the basis of potential benefit-risk ratio. These guidelines do not advocate universal screening of all pregnant women, but recommend targeted case-finding in pregnant women who are at high risk for thyroid dysfunction. However, in a recent study, we found that, without universal screening, a targeted thyroid function testing of only high-risk pregnant women would miss about one-third of the women with overt or subclinical hypothyroidism.

19.1 Introduction

Thyroid hormones play an important role in the foetal neurological development (Morreale de Escobar et al., 2004). The presence of thyroid hormones in the foetal tissues is evident as early as the first trimester (Calvo et al., 2002). However, the foetal thyroid gland does not start producing thyroid hormones until about 12 weeks of gestation suggesting that the foetus depends on maternal thyroid hormones during the early phase of neurological development. Studies in hypothyroid rats have shown that maternal thyroxine passes through the placenta to reach the fetus (Morreale de Escobar et al., 1988). In humans, neonates with congenital hypothyroidism due to a total organification defect or thyroid agenesis have a detectable thyroxine level in cord blood providing evidence for the placental transfer of maternal thyroid hormones (Vulsma et al., 1989).

The importance of optimal maternal thyroid function during pregnancy for a proper neurological development of the offspring has been recognised for over a century from studies in iodine-deficient regions (McCarrison, 1908). An inadequate dietary intake of iodine leading to maternal and foetal thyroid hormone insufficiency can result in severe mental retardation and neurological deficit (cretinism) in the offspring. In the last decade, studies have shown that even mild and asymptomatic maternal thyroid hormone insufficiency during pregnancy is associated with an impaired neuropsychological development of the offspring (Haddow et al., 1999; Pop et al., 1999). These findings have raised the question as to whether all pregnant women should be systematically screened and treated for hypothyroidism. This review discusses various issues surrounding the screening of pregnant women for thyroid dysfunction.

19.2   Prevalence of Thyroid Hormone Insufficiency in Pregnancy

Hypothyroidism is common in women of reproductive age. A recent study in the general population has shown that 3.1% women in the reproductive age have overt or subclinical (mild) hypothyroidism (Aoki et al., 2007). In pregnancy, the prevalence rate of overt hypothyroidism is estimated between 0.3–0.7%, and between 2–3% for subclinical hypothyroidism (Klein et al., 1991; Glinoer, 1997; Casey et al., 2005; Vaidya et al., 2007). In addition, between 1.3–2.3% pregnant women have isolated hypothyroxinaemia [normal thyrotropin (TSH) and free T_4 < 2.5th percentile) (Cleary-Goldman et al., 2008; Casey et al., 2007). Thyroid antibodies are present in about 10% of pregnant women and associated with an increased risk of hypothyroidism, postpartum thyroiditis and spontaneous miscarriages (Glinoer, 1997; Lazarus and Koknadi, 2000).

19.3   Association between Mild Maternal Thyroid Hormone Insufficiency and Impaired Neuropsychological Development of the Offspring

About 40 years ago, Evelyn Man and colleagues first showed that offspring born to mothers with inadequately treated hypothyroidism have a low intelligence quotient (IQ) (Man et al., 1971). In 1999, Haddow and colleagues found that children born to untreated mothers with mild hypothyroidism (TSH > 98th percentile) have a significantly lower IQ score than the controls (Haddow et al., 1999), and that the offspring's IQ score correlates negatively with the severity of maternal hypothyroidism (Klein et al., 2001). The study also found that two-thirds of the women with undiagnosed hypothyroidism during the pregnancy were subsequently confirmed to have hypothyroidism at follow-up 11 years after the pregnancy (Haddow et al., 1999). Another smaller study of 20 pregnant women with known thyroid disease showed that infants of mothers with subclinical hypothyroidism during pregnancy have a decreased mental development index during the first year of life (Smit et al., 2000).

Maternal hypothyroxinaemia has also been shown to be associated with impaired neuropsychological development of the offspring. Pop and colleagues found that offspring of pregnant women with hypothyroxinaemia (free T_4 < 10th percentile) during early gestation have a delayed psychomotor development at 10 months and 2 years (Pop et al., 1999; Pop et al., 2003). The same group recently showed that the deleterious effect of maternal hypothyroxinaemia on neuropsychological development of the offspring is evident as early as 3 weeks of age (Kooistra et al., 2006).

19.4   Association between Mild Maternal Thyroid Hormone Insufficiency and Poor Obstetric Outcome

Untreated maternal overt hypothyroidism is well known to be associated with several obstetric complications, including gestational hypertension, miscarriages, and premature birth (Glinoer, 1997; Lazarus and Kokandi, 2000). Recent studies have suggested that maternal subclinical hypothyroidism is also associated with an increased risk of obstetric adverse events, such as premature birth (Casey et al., 2005; Stagnaro-Green et al., 2005; Abalovich et al., 2002), placental abruption (Casey et al., 2005), pre-eclampsia (Leung et al., 1993), admission to intensive care (Casey et al., 2005), impaired foetal growth (Blazer et al., 2003) and increased foetal mortality (Allan et al., 2000). However, the association between maternal subclinical hypothyroidism and the obstetric complications have not been consistent across the studies (Cleary-Goldman et al., 2008). A recent study did not find an association between isolated maternal hypothyroxinaemia and obstetric complications (Casey et al., 2007).

19.5   Does the Treatment of Mild Thyroid Hormone Insufficiency Improve the Pregnancy Outcome?

Currently, there is no clinical trial evidence to show that thyroxine replacement in maternal subclinical hypothyroidism improves the offspring's neuropsychological development. One randomised controlled trial in euthyroid pregnant women with positive anti-thyroid peroxidase (anti-TPO) antibodies has shown that thyroxine treatment in such women reduces miscarriage rate and premature birth (Negro et al., 2006). The TSH levels in the untreated group progressively increased during the study and were significantly higher than those in the treated group at the end of the study, providing indirect evidence that thyroxine replacement in maternal

Table 19.**1**   Which of the screening criteria does screening pregnant women for thyroid dysfunction fulfill?

Criterion	Fulfilled?
Is the condition an important public health problem?	Yes
Is the epidemiology and natural history of the condition adequately understood?	Yes
Have all the cost-effective primary preventions been implemented?	No
Is there a simple, safe, precise, validated and acceptable screening test?	Yes
Is there a suitable cut-off level of the test and a policy on the further investigation of individuals with a positive result?	Partly
Is there an effective treatment?	Yes
Is there an agreed evidence based policies to determine which patients should and should not be treated?	No
Is there evidence from high quality randomized controlled trials that screening improves health outcomes?	No
Do the benefits from the screening outweigh the harm caused by the test, investigations or treatment?	Yes
Is the screening cost effective?	Yes

subclinical hypothyroidism may reduce obstetric complications.

19.6   Would Screening Pregnant Women for Thyroid Dysfunction be Cost-Effective?

Dosiou et al. (2008) have carried out a cost-effectiveness analysis of screening pregnant women for thyroid dysfunction, by developing a state-transition Markov model simulation. The analysis showed that screening pregnant women with either TSH or anti-TPO antibodies in the first trimester is cost saving as compared to not screening. Screening pregnant women for thyroid dysfunction was found to be as cost-effective as other well established screening programmes.

19.7   What are the Potential Harms Caused by Screening Pregnant Women for Thyroid Dysfunction?

The potential harms caused by screening pregnant women for thyroid dysfunction include increased anxiety, misdiagnosis, unnecessary treatment and adverse effects from the treatment. Studies in pregnancies associated with untreated Graves' disease, thyroid hormone resistance and non-autoimmune hyperthyroidism due to activating TSH-receptor mutation have shown that an overt excess of thyroid hormone is associated

with several obstetric complications, including miscarriage, premature delivery and low foetal birth weight (Lazarus and Kokandi; 2000; Anselmo et al., 2004; Vaidya et al., 2004). However, it is reassuring that a recent study did not find an increased incidence of obstetric complications in association with subclinical hyperthyroidism in pregnancy (Casey et al., 2006). Together, these studies suggest that thyroxine replacement in pregnant women with subclinical hypothyroidism carries minimal risk, provided thyroid function is monitored carefully.

19.8   Does Screening Pregnant Women for Thyroid Dysfunction Fulfill Criteria for Systemic Screening?

Screening is a strategy to detect a disease in asymptomatic individuals with an aim to improve health outcomes by early diagnosis and treatment of the disease. A series of criteria should ideally be fulfilled before considering screening as a public health policy (Table 19.**1**) (Wilson, 1968; UK National Screening Committee, 2008).

Mild maternal thyroid hormone insufficiency during pregnancy is an important public health problem with a high prevalence rate and an association with a serious adverse effect on the offspring's neuropsychological development and several obstetric complications. It can be detected easily by measuring the serum TSH level, which is a simple, safe, precise and relatively cheap investigation. More recently, trimester-specific TSH reference ranges for different populations have become available (Soldin et al., 2007). Thyroxine is an effective treatment for maternal subclinical hypothyroidism during pregnancy, and an expert panel has justified its use in this condition on the basis of favourable potential benefit-risk ratio (Surks et al., 2004). A recent study has shown that systematic screening of pregnant women for thyroid dysfunction would be cost-effective (Dosiou et al., 2008).

However, there remain several uncertainties regarding screening pregnant women for thyroid dysfunction. For example, when is the most appropriate time for screening? Should free T_4 and anti-TPO antibodies be included in the screening? At what level of TSH should thyroxine be started? Should pregnant women with isolated hypothyroxinaemia be treated with thyroxine? How should the thyroxine treatment be monitored? In 1998, Glinoer proposed an algorithm for systematic screening of pregnant women for thyroid dysfunction addressing some of these issues (Glinoer, 1998). Another important question is that iodine deficiency, which is a major risk factor for maternal thyroid hormone insufficiency, remains endemic in many parts of the world and should

public health efforts be directed at ensuring adequate dietary iodine intake amongst pregnant women before implementing systematic screening for thyroid dysfunction in pregnancy (Utiger, 1999)? Lastly, and critically, there is no randomised controlled trial evidence to show that thyroxine replacement in maternal subclinical hypothyroidism during pregnancy improves foetal neuropsychological outcome.

19.9 What do the Guidelines Say?

In the recent years, several guidelines on screening thyroid function in pregnancy have been published (Table 19.2). However, the recommendations have been inconsistent, with some guidelines advocating universal screening of all pregnant women while the others favouring an aggressive case finding in high-risk group. The recent guidelines from The Endocrine Society have not endorsed universal screening of all pregnant women for thyroid dysfunction but have recommended targeted case finding in high-risk pregnant women by TSH measurement in early pregnancy (Table 19.3) (Abalovich et al., 2007).

Table 19.**2**   Guidelines on screening thyroid dysfunction in pregnancy.

Authorities	Year	Recommendations
American Association of Clinical Endocrinologists (2002)	2002	Universal screening
Expert panel of American Thyroid Association, American Association of Clinical Endocrinologists and The Endocrine Society (Surks et al., 2004)	2004	Case-finding in high-risk group
Second panel of American Thyroid Association, American Association of Clinical Endocrinologists and The Endocrine Society (Gharib et al., 2005)	2005	Universal screening
British Thyroid Association, Association of Clinical Biochemists, British Thyroid Foundation. UK Guidelines for the Use of Thyroid Function Tests. http://www.british-thyroid-association.org/info-for-patients/Docs/ TFT_guideline_final_version_July_2006.pdf – date accessed 1 September 2008.	2006	Case-finding in high-risk group
American College of Obstetrics and Gynecology (2007)	2007	Case-finding in high-risk group
The Endocrine Society (Abalovich et al., 2007)	2007	Case-finding in high-risk group

Table 19.**3** Selected high-risk pregnant women in whom The Endocrine Society Clinical Practice Guidelines recommend targeted case-finding (Abalovich et al. 2007).

No.	Risk Group
1	Women with a history of thyroid disease (including hyperthyroidism, hypothyroidism and postpartum thyroiditis) or thyroid surgery
2	Women with a goitre
3	Women with symptoms or signs suggestive of hypothyroidism or hyperthyroidism
4	Women with a family history of thyroid disease
5	Women with thyroid antibodies (when known)
6	Women with type 1 diabetes or other auto-immune disorders
7	Women with a history of infertility (as part of their infertility work-up), miscarriage or pre-term delivery
8	Women with a history of head or neck irradiation

19.10 Does a Targeted High-Risk Case Finding Approach Work?

In a recent study of 1560 women in early pregnancy, we have analysed whether a targeted high-risk case finding approach can identify all women with thyroid dysfunction during pregnancy (Vaidya et al., 2007). Overall, 2.6% of these women had overt or subclinical hypothyroidism. We found that high-risk women (with a personal or family history of thyroid disorders or a personal history of other autoimmune diseases) have more than a 6-fold increased risk of hypothyroidism. However, we also found that screening only the high-risk group fails to identify about one-third of the women with hypothyroidism. Furthermore, our audit on clinical practice has highlighted practical difficulties in implementing the targeted case finding approach since, despite the development of local district guidelines to screen high-risk pregnant women for thyroid dysfunction, only 18% of these women were screened (Vaidya et al., 2002).

19.11 Conclusions

With increasing evidence for the association between maternal subclinical hypothyroidism and adverse pregnancy outcomes but lack of intervention trials showing beneficial effect of thyroxine to prevent the adverse outcomes, it remains controversial whether all pregnant women should be systematically screened and treated for subclinical hypothyroidism (Spong, 2005; Brent, 2007). The current guidelines recommend case-finding in high-risk pregnant women; however, this approach fails to identify one-third of pregnant women with hypothyroidism (Abalovich et al., 2007; Vaidya et al., 2007). The controversy surrounding screening thyroid function in pregnancy can only be resolved through further studies. Currently, there are two ongoing randomised controlled trials of thyroxine replacement in mild maternal thyroid hormone insufficiency in pregnancy (Randomised Controlled Trial ..., 2008; The Effect of Thyroid Hormone ..., 2008). The outcome data from these clinical trials will be vital before introducing universal screening of pregnant women for thyroid dysfunction.

References

Abalovich M, Amino N, Barbour LA, Cobin RH, De Groot LJ, Glinoer D et al. Management of thyroid dysfunction during pregnancy and postpartum: an Endocrine Society Clinical Practice Guideline. J Clin Endocrinol Metab 2007; 92 (Suppl. 8): S1–47.

Abalovich M, Gutierrez S, Alcaraz G, Maccallini G, Garcia A, Levalle O. Overt and subclinical hypothyroidism complicating pregnancy. Thyroid 2002; 12: 63–8.

ACOG Committee Opinion No. 381: Subclinical hypothyroidism in pregnancy. Obstet Gynecol 2007; 110: 959–60.

Allan WC, Haddow JE, Palomaki GE, Williams JR, Mitchell ML, Hermos RJ et al. Maternal thyroid deficiency and pregnancy complications: implications for population screening. J Med Screen 2000; 7: 127–30.

American Association of Clinical Endocrinologists medical guidelines for clinical practice for the evaluation and treatment of hyperthyroidism and hypothyroidism. Endocr Pract 2002; 8: 457–69.

Anselmo J, Cao D, Karrison T, Weiss RE, Refetoff S. Fetal loss associated with excess thyroid hormone exposure. JAMA 2004; 292: 691–5.

Aoki Y, Belin RM, Clickner R, Jeffries R, Phillips L, Mahaffey KR. Serum TSH and total T_4 in the United

States population and their association with participant characteristics: National Health and Nutrition Examination Survey (NHANES 1999–2002). Thyroid 2007; 17: 1211–23.

Blazer S, Moreh-Waterman Y, Miller-Lotan R, Tamir A, Hochberg Z. Maternal hypothyroidism may affect fetal growth and neonatal thyroid function. Obstet Gynecol 2003; 102: 232–41.

Brent GA. Diagnosing thyroid dysfunction in pregnant women: Is case finding enough? J Clin Endocrinol Metab 2007; 92: 39–41.

British Thyroid Association, Association of Clinical Biochemists, British Thyroid Foundation. UK Guidelines for the Use of Thyroid Function Tests. http://www.british-thyroid-association.org/info-for-patients/Docs/TFT_guideline_final_version_July_2006.pdf – date accessed 1 September 2008.

Calvo RM, Jauniaux E, Gulbis B, Asuncion M, Gervy C, Contempre B et al. Fetal tissues are exposed to biologically relevant free thyroxine concentrations during early phases of development. J Clin Endocrinol Metab 2002; 87: 1768–77.

Casey BM, Dashe JS, Spong CY, McIntire DD, Leveno KJ, Cunningham GF. Perinatal significance of isolated maternal hypothyroxinemia identified in the first half of pregnancy. Obstet Gynecol 2007; 109: 1129–35.

Casey BM, Dashe JS, Wells CE, McIntire DD, Byrd W, Leveno KJ et al. Subclinical hypothyroidism and pregnancy outcomes. Obstet Gynecol 2005; 105: 239–45.

Casey BM, Dashe JS, Wells CE, McIntire DD, Leveno KJ, Cunningham FG. Subclinical hyperthyroidism and pregnancy outcomes. Obstet Gynecol 2006; 107: 337–41.

Cleary-Goldman J, Malone FD, Lambert-Messerlian G, Sullivan L, Canick J, Porter TF et al. Maternal thyroid hypofunction and pregnancy outcome. Obstet Gynecol 2008; 112: 85–92.

Dosiou C, Sanders GD, Araki SS, Crapo LM. Screening pregnant women for autoimmune thyroid disease: a cost-effectiveness analysis. Eur J Endocrinol 2008; 158: 841–51.

Gharib H, Tuttle RM, Baskin HJ, Fish LH, Singer PA, McDermott MT. Subclinical thyroid dysfunction: a joint statement on management from the American Association of Clinical Endocrinologists, the American Thyroid Association, and the Endocrine Society. J Clin Endocrinol Metab 2005; 90: 581–5.

Glinoer D. The regulation of thyroid function in pregnancy: pathways of endocrine adaptation from physiology to pathology. Endocr Rev 1997; 18: 404–33.

Glinoer D. The systematic screening and management of hypothyroidism and hyperthyroidism during pregnancy. Trends Endocrinol Metab 1998; 9: 403–11.

Haddow JE, Knight GJ, Palomaki GE, McClain MR, Pulkkinen AJ. The reference range and within-person variability of thyroid stimulating hormone during the first and second trimesters of pregnancy. J Med Screen 2004; 11: 170–4.

Haddow JE, Palomaki GE, Allan WC, Williams JR, Knight GJ, Gagnon J et al. Maternal thyroid deficiency during pregnancy and subsequent neuropsychological development of the child. N Engl J Med 1999; 341: 549–55.

Klein RZ, Haddow JE, Faix JD, Brown RS, Hermos RJ, Pulkkinen A et al. Prevalence of thyroid deficiency in pregnant women. Clin Endocrinol (Oxf) 1991; 35: 41–6.

Klein RZ, Sargent JD, Larsen PR, Waisbren SE, Haddow JE, Mitchell ML. Relation of severity of maternal hypothyroidism to cognitive development of offspring. J Med Screen 2001; 8: 18–20.

Kooistra L, Crawford S, van Baar AL, Brouwers EP, Pop VJ. Neonatal effects of maternal hypothyroxinemia during early pregnancy. Pediatrics 2006; 117: 161–7.

Lazarus JH, Kokandi A. Thyroid disease in relation to pregnancy: a decade of change. Clin Endocrinol (Oxf) 2000; 53: 265–78.

Leung AS, Millar LK, Koonings PP, Montoro M, Mestman JH. Perinatal outcome in hypothyroid pregnancies. Obstet Gynecol 1993; 81: 349–53.

Man EB, Jones WS, Holden RH, Mellits ED. Thyroid function in human pregnancy VIII: retardation of progeny aged 7 years; relationships to maternal age and maternal thyroid function. Am J Obstet Gynecol 1971; 111: 905–16.

McCarrison R. Observations on endemic cretinism in the Chitral and Gilgit Valleys. Lancet 1908; ii: 1275–80.

Morreale de Escobar G, Obregon MJ, del Rey FE. Maternal thyroid hormones early in pregnancy and fetal brain development. Best Pract Res Clin Endocrinol Metab 2004; 18: 225–48.

Morreale de Escobar G, Obregon MJ, Ruiz de Ona C, Escobar del Rey F. Transfer of thyroxine from the mother to the rat fetus near term: effects on brain 3, 5, 3′-triiodothyronine deficiency. Endocrinology 1988; 122: 1521–31.

Negro R, Formoso G, Mangieri T, Pezzarossa A, Dazzi D, Hassan H. Levothyroxine treatment in euthyroid pregnant women with autoimmune thyroid disease: effects on obstetrical complications. J Clin Endocrinol Metab 2006; 91: 2587–91.

Pop VJ, Brouwers EP, Vader HL, Vulsma T, van Baar AL, de Vijlder JJ. Maternal hypothyroxinaemia during early pregnancy and subsequent child development: a 3-year follow-up study. Clin Endocrinol (Oxf) 2003; 59: 282–8.

Pop VJ, Kuijpens JL, van Baar AL, Verkerk G, van Son MM, de Vijlder JJ et al. Low maternal free thyroxine concentrations during early pregnancy are associated with impaired psychomotor development in infancy. Clin Endocrinol (Oxf) 1999; 50: 149–55.

Randomised controlled trial of the effect of gestational thyroid hormone intervention therapy on childhood development. http://www.controlled-trials.com/mrct/trial/229189/thyroid – date accessed 1 September 2008.

Smit BJ, Kok JH, Vulsma T, Briet JM, Boer K, Wiersinga WM. Neurologic development of the newborn and young child in relation to maternal thyroid function. Acta Paediatr 2000; 89: 291–5.

Soldin OP, Soldin D, Sastoque M. Gestation-specific thyroxine and thyroid stimulating hormone levels in the United States and worldwide. Ther Drug Monit 2007; 29: 553–9.

Spong CY. Subclinical hypothyroidism: should all pregnant women be screened? Obstet Gynecol 2005; 105: 235–6.

Stagnaro-Green A, Chen X, Bogden JD, Davies TF, Scholl TO. The thyroid and pregnancy: a novel risk factor for very preterm delivery. Thyroid 2005; 15: 351–7.

Surks MI, Ortiz E, Daniels GH, Sawin CT, Col NF, Cobin RH et al. Subclinical thyroid disease: scientific review and guidelines for diagnosis and management. JAMA 2004; 291: 228–38.

The Effect of Thyroid Hormone Levels in Pregnant Women on the Intelligence Quotient (IQ) of Their Children. http://clinicaltrials.gov/ct2/show/NCT00147433?term=thyroxine+in+pregnancy&rank=3 – date accessed 1 September 2008.

UK National Screening Committee criteria for appraising the viability, effectiveness and appropriateness of a screening programme. http://www.nsc.nhs.uk/pdfs/criteria.pdf – date accessed 1 September 2008.

Utiger RD. Maternal hypothyroidism and fetal development. N Engl J Med 1999; 341: 601–2.

Vaidya B, Anthony S, Bilous M, Shields B, Drury J, Hutchison S et al. Detection of thyroid dysfunction in early pregnancy: Universal screening or targeted high-risk case finding? J Clin Endocrinol Metab 2007; 92: 203–7.

Vaidya B, Bilous M, Hutchinson RS, Connolly V, Jones S, Kelly WF et al. Screening for thyroid disease in pregnancy: an audit. Clin Med 2002; 2: 599–600.

Vaidya B, Campbell V, Tripp JH, Spyer G, Hattersley AT, Ellard S. Premature birth and low birth weight associated with nonautoimmune hyperthyroidism due to an activating thyrotropin receptor gene mutation. Clin Endocrinol (Oxf) 2004; 60: 711–8.

Vulsma T, Gons MH, de Vijlder JJ. Maternal-fetal transfer of thyroxine in congenital hypothyroidism due to a total organification defect or thyroid agenesis. N Engl J Med 1989; 321: 13–6.

Wilson JMG. Principles and Practice of Screening for Disease. Geneva: WHO; 1968.

Short Communications

Chairpersons: J. Lazarus (Cardiff), V. Pirags (Riga)

1 Biochemical Markers of Thyroid Function in Pregnant Women in the Republic of Macedonia

S. Miceva Ristevska*, S. Loparska, O. Vaskova, S. Kuzmanovska, B. Karanfilski, V. Bogdanova, Gj. Sestakov

Institute of Pathophysiology & Nuclear Medicine, Vodnjanska 17, Skopje, Republic of Macedonia

Aim: Normal thyroid function is necessary for normal physical as well mental development in humans. Pregnancy is a special status in women when special demands are required among which normal thyroid function is very important for normal evolution of the embryo. The aim of the study was to assess the biochemical thyroid markers in pregnant women which had not been done until now in our region.

Material and Methods: 202 pregnant women (pw) prospectively were included in the study – aged from 17 to 42 years (mean age: 26.6 ± 4.7 years); they were divided into 3 subgroups related to the I[st] trimester (tr) = 99 pw, IInd tr = 46 pw, IIIrd tr = 46 pw and 56 were examined 3–5 months after delivery. Biochemical thyroid markers: FT_4, TSH, hTg, Tab, urine iodine excretion (UIE) and thyroid volume (TV) by ultrasound were determined.

Results: The results showed significant differences of FT_4 between I[st] and IInd tr, as well between I[st] and IIIrd tr; it was less significant between IInd and IIIrd tr, (p < 0.001, 0.001, 0.01). There was a significant difference between the median of each tr and values of FT_4 of the control group (non-pregnant women). No significant difference was noticed between the control group and examinees after delivery. A significant difference of the median of TSH between I[st] and IInd tr (p < 0.05) was found. No significance was noticed for the value of hTg between any of the groups. Positive a-TPO Ab were detected in 12/122 pw in the I[st] tr, and in 4/54 in the IInd tr.

A slight but not significant increase in TV during IInd – IIIrd trimester was observed.

Conclusion: Taking into consideration all data from this study we have concluded that administration of iodide is recommended during pregnancy and lactation in women to prevent an increase of TV and the appearance of goitre as well to facilitate a successful ending of the pregnancy.

UIE	I[st] tr	IInd tr	IIIrd tr
< 150 µg/L	29.6%	37.8%	39.1%
150–249 µg/L	39.8%	28.9%	32.6%
250–499 µg/L	29.6%	31.1%	26.1%
> 500 µg/L	1%	2.2%	2.2%

2 Iodine Intake in Portuguese Pregnant Women: Preliminary Results

E. Limbert,[1]*, S. Prazeres[2], M. São Pedro[2],
A. Miranda[3], M. Ribeiro[3], J. Jacome de Castro[4],
F. Carrilho[5], H. Reguengo[6], F. Borges[7]

[1] Department of Endocrinology, Instituto
  Português de Oncologia, Lisboa, Portugal
[2] Laboratory of Endocrinology, Instituto
  Português de Oncologia, Lisboa, Portugal
[3] Department of Epidemiology, Instituto
  Português de Oncologia, Lisboa, Portugal
[4] Department of Endocrinology, Military
  Hospital, Lisboa, Portugal
[5] Department of Endocrinology, University
  Hospital, Coimbra, Portugal
[6] Laboratory of Clinical Pathology St António
  Hospital Porto, Portugal
[7] Department of Endocrinology St António
  Hospital Porto, Portugal

Introduction: Iodine is essential for the synthesis of thyroid hormones and its intake modulates the physiology and physiopathology of the thyroid gland. In Portugal, endemic goiter has been practically eradicated. However, some data indicate that iodine intake, as in other European areas, is not sufficient. Taking into account the potential harmful effects of moderate iodine deficiency during pregnancy, when needs are increased, and the absence of recent data on iodine intake in Portugal, a countrywide study on urinray iodine was undertaken in pregnant women and school children. Results of this ongoing study from pregnant women are presented.

Material and Methods: The target population consisted of pregnant women from maternity hospitals and school children from strategic geographical areas (coast line and inland); 3073 urine samples from 15 maternity hospitals were analysed. For urinary iodide a fast colorimetric method (Gnat et al., Clin Chem 2003) was used. Statistical analyses included central methods and proportional comparison tests.

Global Results: Median urinary iodide concentration was 85.6 µg/L, with 23.3% being below 50 µg/L while 17% had values above 150 µg/L.

Results by Hospital: Median urinary iodine varied from 68 to 124 µg/L; 13.9% to 37.4% of women had values below 50 µg/L and 6.1% to 34% had values above 150 µg/L.

Conclusions: These data point to an inadequate iodine intake in pregnant women admitted in most maternity hospitals. Taking into account these preliminary results, the ongoing study needs to be completed, namely with the school population, and more detailed analysis is warranted in order to explain the observed differences between regions. Considering the potential deleterious effects of an inadequate iodine supply during pregnancy, iodine supplementation is recommended in this period of life.

3 Clinical Case: Subclinical Hyperthyroidism in Pregnancy

U. Gailisa, I. Dzivite

Paula Stradina Clinical University Hospital;
Children University Hospital, Pilsonu street 13,
Riga, Latvia

Clinical Case: Patient with hyperthyroidism diagnosed during first pregnancy and subclinical hyperthyroidism during first trimester of second pregnancy.

First pregnancy in year 2007 at age of 25. In first 3 months of pregnancy patient has hyperemesis gravidarum. 18.6.2007. Hospitalisation due to partus imminens. Diagnosed overt hyperthyroidism. TSH 0.007 mIU/ml (N: 0.4–4.0); FT4 2.36 ng/dl (N: 0.8–1.9), FT3 4.37 ng/ml (N: 1.8–4.2), avTPO 188 IU/ml (N: < 34). Thyroid ultrasound: thyroid volume slightly increased and inhomogenous. Started therapy with methimazole 20 mg/d.

21.6.2007: Graviditas I in septima 23–24, partus I spontaneus. Diruptio velomentorium ovii praecox spontaneus. Presentatio pelvica. Child weight 710 g, height 29 cm. Apgar scale 4–6–6. Severe ventilation problems (Silverman score 6 points), mechanical ventilation 16 days. Child TSH 4.1 mU/L, FT4 10.9 pmol/l – normal (on 5th day of life). No maternal complications post partum.

19.7.2007: Child died at Childrens University hospital intensive care unit.

Diagnosis: Prematurity IV. Intraventricular haemorrhagia III. Ulcerative necrotic enterocolitis I. Bronchopulmonar dysplasia. Candydosis with purulent meningitis. Anemia. Necrosis *septum nasi*. After pregnancy patient used methimazole and Jod activ. Last 3 months methimazole stopped, 24.1.2008 Graviditas II in septima 7–8. Patient used Jod activ and multivitamins – elevit. No complaints. TSH 0.015 mU/L (N: 0.4–4.0); FT4 17.0 pmol/L (N: 10.3–24.5); FT3 5.1 ng/ml (N:

2.8 – 8.0), avTPO 2352 U/mL (N: < 35), avTg 50 U/mL (< 50).

Diagnosis: Thyroid autoimmunity. Subclinical hyperthyroidism. Graviditas II in septima 7 – 8.

Recommendations: Stop usage of Jod activ. Consult endocrinologist after 3 weeks. No evidence that treatment of subclinical hyperthyroidism improves pregnancy outcome and treatment potentially adversely affect fetal outcome, but anti TPO antibodies is a predictor of thyroid dysfunction during pregnancy.

Object of Discussion: Treatment of subclinical hyperthyreosis in first trimester of pregnancy for patient with hyperthyreosis in anamnesis and thyroid autoimmune activity.

4   Thyroid Nodules in Pregnancy

I. Lase

Department of Endocrinology, Pauls Stradiņš Clinical University Hospital, Pilsoņu iela 13, LV-1002 Riga, Latvia

Introduction: Thyroid problems are common in women who are pregnant and thyroid nodules in pregnant women have a greater chance of being malignant than nodules in non-pregnant patients.

Case Report: A 28-year-old pregnant woman (4th pregnancy; week 28/29) was investigated in the Department of Endocrinology. One month previously she had noticed a nodule on the right side of the neck. She had no other complaints.

Examination: There was 4 cm firm smooth node on the right side of the larynx that moved with swallowing. No other abnormality was found.

Test Results: Thyroid function tests showed mild hyperthyroidism (TSH 0.04 µIU/mL [normal: 0.4 – 4.0]; fT_3 4.31 pg/mL [normal: 1.8 – 4.2]; fT_4 0.8 ng/dL [normal: 0.8 – 1.9], but patient did not have any complaints or clinical symptoms of hyperthyroidism. An ultrasound examination confirmed a 4.4 × 3.3 cm multicystic node in the right thyroid lobe. The left thyroid lobe appeared normal. Fine-needle aspiration and core-needle biopsy were performed. The cytological examination did not show any malignant cells. The histological examination suggested diagnosis of trabecular adenoma.

Management: The patient was referred to the thyroid surgeon, who recommended surgery after delivery.

Discussion and Conclusions: We reported this case because we wanted to show the tactics of examination and possible treatment in patients with thyroid nodes, found during the pregnancy. Ultrasound examination of the thyroid is safe during pregnancy, but does not usually help in excluding the possibility of cancer. The best test to perform is a fine-needle aspiration biopsy to determine whether the nodule is benign or malignant, but the success of a biopsy depends on the adequacy of the specimen and skill of the cytopathologist. If examination of the biopsy suggests that a cancer is present, the necessary surgery can be performed. If a nodule is discovered later in pregnancy, investigation and treatment can probably be deferred until the postpartum period.

5   Colour Flow Doppler Sonography Enables Distinction between the Hyperthyroid Phase of Postpartum Thyroiditis and Graves' Disease

S. Gaberscek, J. Osolnik, K. Zaletel, E. Pirnat, S. Hojker

Department of Nuclear Medicine, University Medical Centre, Zaloska 7, 1525 Ljubljana, Slovenia

The aim of this study was to determine the role of colour flow Doppler sonography (CFDS) for distinction between the hyperthyroid phase of postpartum thyroiditis and Graves' disease. A reliable distinction enables a prompt decision about the treatment of hyperthyroidism in the postpartum period (wait and see in postpartum thyroiditis and antithyroid drugs in Graves' disease). For this purpose, we included 33 hyperthyroid women in the postpartum period, among them 25 women in the hyperthyroid phase of postpartum thyroiditis (group 1) and 8 women with Graves' disease (group 2), first appearing in that period. Measurements of TSH, free thyroid hormones, thyroid peroxidase antibodies (antiTPO), thyroglobulin antibodies (antiTg) and thyroid stimulating immunoglobulins (TSI) were performed. Graves' disease was confirmed by increased levels of TSI antibodies. Women with postpartum thyroiditis were negative for TSI antibodies. By using a 7.5 MHz linear transducer we estimated colour flow Doppler sonography patterns 0, I, II, III, where thyroid vascularity increased from pattern 0 to III. Additionally, we measured peak systolic velocity

(PSV) at the level of the intrathyroid arteries. PSV was expressed as the mean of five measurements. In our study, the hyperthyroid phase of postpartum thyroiditis appeared 5.2 ± 2.5 months after delivery, while Graves' disease appeared 8.1 ± 3.4 months after delivery. Estimating CFDS patterns, we did not observe CFDS pattern 0 in group 2 or CFDS pattern III in group 1. The prevalent CFDS pattern in group 2 was III (in 50% of women), whereas in group 1 the dominant pattern was I (in 50% of women). Similarly, in group 2, PSV was significantly ($p = 0.017$) higher than in group 1 (mean $\pm$ SD, 16.3 ± 6.8 cm/s and 9.7 ± 2.8 cm/s, respectively). Our results demonstrate that CFDS is a useful method for distinction between the hyperthyroid phase of postpartum thyroiditis and Graves' disease, first appearing in the postpartum period. The present findings are proposed to have a significant clinical relevance – they will allow for a prompt and correct decision about the treatment of hyperthyroidism in the postpartum period.

Poster Presentations

1 Impact of Pregnancy on Prevalence of Goitre And Nodular Thyroid Disease in Women Living in a Region of Borderline Iodine Deficiency

S. Karger*, S. Schötz, M. Stumvoll, D. Führer

Department of Internal Medicine III, University of Leipzig, Ph.-Rosenthal-Str. 27, 04103 Leipzig, Germany.

Purpose: An interplay of genetic, epigenetic and environmental factors contributes to thyroid disease. In a cross-sectional study we aimed to determine the actual influence of parity on goitre and nodular thyroid disease (NTD) in women living in a region with borderline iodine deficiency.
Methods: Thyroid ultrasonography (7.5 MHz; Merck Thyromobil) was performed by the same investigator in 731 women living in Thuringia and Saxony. Furthermore, age and BMI were documented and all women were asked about the number of previous pregnancies, family history of thyroid disease and past or present smoking.
Results: Goitre prevalence was 17.6%. Solitary thyroid nodules were detected in 21.2%, multiple nodules in 24.6% of the study population. Age was positively correlated with goitre prevalence and NTD (due to multiple but not solitary nodules). No association was found between parity and goitre prevalence. In contrast, a significant increase in both solitary (22.2%) and multinodular thyroid disease (23.7%) was observed in women with at least one pregnancy compared to nullipara (11.9% and 16.9%, respectively). The BMI in women with goitre (27.3 kg/m²) was significantly higher than in women without (24.8 kg/m²). In addition, a significant correlation was detected between BMI and the presence of multinodular disease (26.5 kg/m²). 24.5% of women with goitre reported a positive family history for thyroid disease, as opposed to 15% of women with a normal size thyroid gland. Neither goitre nor NTD were associated with a present or past history of smoking.

Conclusion: NTD and/or goitre are present in up to 50% of women in an area with borderline iodine deficiency. Besides age, BMI and family history, parity is positively correlated with the presence of NTD, whereas smoking was not associated with goitre/NTD.

2 The Clinical Report: Graves' Disease in Combination with Primary Hyperparathyroidism

N. Fokina

Endocrinology Department, Pauls Stradiņš Clinical University Hospital, Pilsoņu str 13, LV-1002 Riga, Latvia

Introduction: Graves' disease and primary hyperparathyroidism are reported usually not to have any association and occur just as a chance combination of two different diseases.
Case Report: The patient is 62-year-old woman who was admitted to the Endocrinology Department in January 2008 due to untreated ophthalmopathy. She had no other complaints except some visual discharge, periorbital oedema and excessive lacrimation.
Examination: There are some signs of mild ophthalmopathy: periorbital oedema, redness of the conjunctiva, and proptosis. No signs or symptoms of thyrotoxicosis were noted. No symptoms of hyperparathyroidism were present.
Investigation: Thyroid function tests showed a slight hyperthyroidism (TSH: 0.01 µIU/mL [normal: 0.4–4,0], fT_4 1.99 ng/dL [normal: 0.8 – 1.9], fT_3 4.82 pg/mL [normal: 1.8–4.2]), thyroid immunological tests show no high activity of the process (TSH-R Ab 3.2 IU/L [normal: < 1.8]). The calcium level checked by a routine screening method was elevated (Ca 2.76 mmol/L [normal: 2.2–2.65]). The rechecked calcium was elevated (2.73 mmol/L), phosphorus was normal (P 1.08 mmol/L [normal: 0.8– 1.6]), PTH was elevated (13.3 pmol/L [normal: 0.7–5.6]). Ultrasound

examination used for the topical diagnosis showed gl. parathyreoidea sin. inf. adenoma 2.6 × 1.0 cm and specific changes in the thyroid. Orbital muscle enlargement was detected by ultrasound to a serious degree: 4.6 – 7.2 cm.

Management: The antithyroid treatment was with Thyrosol 5 mg/dn due to slight hyperthyroidism. The patient underwent two courses of glucocorticoid infusions (SoluMedroli 1000 – 500 – 500 mg) with marked improvement. Any surgery was put off until the ophthalmopathy is in remission.

Conclusions: The aim of this case presentation is to show a rare combination of Graves' disease with ophthalmopathy and primary hyperparathyroidism. The problem is about the diagnosis, because thyrotoxicosis can diminish the symptoms of hyperparathyroidism, or the latter are not specific. Another problem is about the treatment of hyperparathyroidism – surgery in the thyroid area when the patient has active autoimmune ophthalmopathy. Routine screening measurements of serum calcium are the best method for the early diagnosis hyperparathyroidism. The surgery in the thyroid region can be put off until the ophthalmopathy is in remission.

3   Thyreotoxic Struma Ovarii – Case Report

L. Puklavec[1]*, I. Takac[2]

[1] Department for Nuclear Medicine, University Hospital Maribor, Ljubljanska 5, 2000 Maribor, Slovenia
[2] Department of Gynecology and Obstetrics, University Hospital Maribor, Ljubljanska 5, 2000 Maribor, Slovenia

Introduction: Struma ovarii was first described in 1899 and is extremely rare, with only 150 reported cases in the medical literature. Struma ovarii is defined as the presence of an ovarial tumor containing thyroid tissue. They may occur as part of a teratoma but may occasionally be encountered with serous or mucinous cystadenomas. Malignant transformation is rare and only 8% of patients present with clinical hyperthyroidism.

Case Report: A 51-year-old female patient was first presented in 1982 with typical symptoms of Graves' disease with hyperthyroidism, mild exophthalmos and elevated aTg, aTPO and TSI antibodies. Since thyrostatic therapy was ineffective, a partial thyroidectomy was done in 1983. After the operation the patient was still thyrotoxic and thyrostatic therapy was continued until 1995, when treatment with ^{131}I (10 mCi) was performed. Treatment with radioiodine resulted in hypothyroidism and the patient was substituted with L-thyroxine until 2006 when hyperthyroidism with tachycardia and palpitations appeared. Ultrasound revealed a small thyroid gland with no isotope uptake on a technetium scan. ^{131}I scintigraphy showed an increased uptake in right pelvic region and struma ovarii was suspected. Adnexectomy was performed and histology revealed a lutein cyst with no thyroid cells. After the operation the patient was hypothyrotic again and substituted with L-thyroxine. Repeated ^{131}I scintigraphy showed no further uptake in the pelvic region. Two years after the operation the patient is well, performing her job as a nurse.

Discussion: Despite negative histological findings, we believe that thyroid tissue was present in the ovarial cyst. No other tissue than thyroid can accumulate ^{131}I. Also hyperthyroidism was absent after ovariectomy. For exact histology, specific immunochemistry or electronic microscopy may sometimes be necessary. When no obvious cause of hyperthyroidism is evident, struma ovarii should be suspected and iodine scintigraphy should be performed.

Keyword Index